# I FEEL LOVE

*Poached: Inside the Dark World of Wildlife Trafficking*

# I FEEL LOVE

## MDMA AND THE QUEST FOR CONNECTION IN A FRACTURED WORLD

### RACHEL NUWER

BLOOMSBURY PUBLISHING

NEW YORK · LONDON · OXFORD · NEW DELHI · SYDNEY

BLOOMSBURY PUBLISHING
Bloomsbury Publishing Inc.
1385 Broadway, New York, NY 10018, USA

BLOOMSBURY, BLOOMSBURY PUBLISHING, and the Diana logo are trademarks
of Bloomsbury Publishing Plc

First published in the United States 2023

LIBRARY OF CONGRESS CATALOGING-IN-PUBLICATION DATA IS AVAILABLE

ISBN: HB: 978-1-63557-957-4; EBOOK: 978-1-63557-958-1

2 4 6 8 10 9 7 5 3 1

Typeset by Westchester Publishing Services
Printed and bound in the U.S.A.

To find out more about our authors and books visit www.bloomsbury.com and sign up
for our newsletters.

Bloomsbury books may be purchased for business or promotional use. For information
on bulk purchases please contact Macmillan Corporate and Premium Sales Department at
specialmarkets@macmillan.com.

*To Paul, with whom I feel the love*

# CONTENTS

# AUTHOR'S NOTE

MDMA, ALSO KNOWN as Ecstasy or Molly, is currently an illegal drug. Yet evidence is building that MDMA-assisted therapy can help some individuals who are haunted by post-traumatic stress disorder and, potentially, a host of other mental health conditions. Although there is ongoing scientific investigation into therapeutic uses of MDMA, and a public conversation about decriminalizing or even legalizing the drug, it still appears on Schedule I of the U.S. Controlled Substances Act—the same list of strictly prohibited drugs that includes marijuana, heroin, and LSD. MDMA is also criminalized in most other countries around the world, including the United Kingdom. For that reason, readers are strongly cautioned to consult appropriate experts in medicine and criminal law about the risks of using MDMA before making any decision to do so.

# INTRODUCTION

CALEDONIA CURRY GREW up under the weight of what she called an unbearable truth: "I feared and hated someone I also adored and loved, who was my mother," Callie said.

Callie was born in Florida to parents heavily addicted to heroin. Her dad almost fatally overdosed when she was three years old. He managed to stay sober after that, but Callie's mother kept using. On good days, she radiated kindness, fun, and love, but on bad days, she seemed to Callie like a demon careening from hyperactivity to suicidal ideation and psychosis.

Callie left home at seventeen and embarked on a successful career as an artist under the name Swoon. Within a decade, her work had been featured in the Museum of Modern Art in New York City and the Museum of Contemporary Art in Los Angeles. At times she felt she'd broken free from her past. But her childhood, as she came to see it, was like a rubber band encircling her life: the farther she ran from her point of origin, the tighter it became, threatening to jerk her back to where she started.

To the outside world, Callie projected success. But privately she was experiencing an array of distressing symptoms. She stopped cleaning her house and kept her possessions in "huge, unorganized piles on the floor which I would just sort of walk over to get anywhere." She developed chronic pain in her lower back and neck, and carpal tunnel in her wrists. Her temper with those closest to her became explosive and sometimes erupted into violence. "I had a moment where I started punching my boyfriend in the face," she said. "It felt like a trapdoor would open under me, and I'd go from being a nice person to someone screaming and breaking shit in one second."

Callie's mother had always denied that there had been any bogeyman at the root of her own mental turmoil and problems with drugs. But as she lay dying from lung cancer, she admitted to Callie that in fact there had been an abuser: a sexual predator in the family. No one protected the children from this man, and drugs were the only relief Callie's mother ever found for the anguish she experienced as a result of her abuse. Callie had long thought of her mother as a "crazy junkie," as society labels people like her. But in finally hearing what she'd been through, Callie said, "I was able to let go of childhood ideas that my mother was just this irresponsible hedonist who chose to love drugs more than she loved her children."

It took Callie's father committing suicide a year and a half later, however, for Callie to finally realize that no amount of achievement would free her from the legacy of suffering passed down from her parents. She needed help. "I was just in so much pain," she said. "The current suffering was dredging up the old trauma so intensely."

Callie started with talk therapy, but she wanted to go deeper. So in 2016 she sought out an underground therapist willing to give her MDMA, the illegal drug also known as Ecstasy or Molly. On the morning of her appointment she swallowed a capsule and lay back on a futon in a sunlit library-like room, her therapist stationed nearby. She quietly closed her eyes for the first thirty minutes or so, but soon she was up on her feet, pacing, speaking, and asking her therapist to hold her hand.

Under MDMA's influence and her therapist's guidance, Callie regressed into a childlike state that ultimately allowed her to uncover a long-buried memory from when she was around seven years old. Her mother was having another psychotic episode and had become convinced that aliens were on their way to Earth, and as soon as they arrived, they were going to eat everyone—including Callie and her sister. The only recourse they had, her mother told them, was to commit suicide by alcohol to poison the aliens. Callie's mom began forcing the girls to drink, but Callie was crying and gagging too much to finish what she had been given. Distraught, her mother dragged the girls out onto the street to prepare for the aliens' arrival. "This was sheer desperation—an animal instinct gone awry," Callie said. "I thought she was taking us somewhere to kill us."

Fortunately, Callie's father dropped by unexpectedly, and he quickly put a stop to the situation. But while Callie wasn't physically harmed, in recovering the memory of that horrific day she realized she'd been living "with this fear that my mom would kill me, and the fear had been so terrifying and unacceptable that I hadn't allowed myself to know about it."

This epiphany marked a turning point in Callie's life. She has not raged out or broken anything for years, and her chronic pain went away and has not returned. She still does MDMA-assisted therapy two to four times per year, and is working her way through her childhood memories. The lessons she's learned through those sessions have also changed her outlook on the creative process. Whereas buried pain had previously driven her work, now she knows that art can also be done in the service of healing. As she told attendees at Horizons, a psychedelics conference, "I've found that the muses love us just as much, and maybe more, when we allow ourselves to unfurl toward wholeness."

While Callie does not claim to have been "cured" by MDMA-assisted therapy, it did allow her to see fundamental things about herself that had been concealed before. She was able to begin processing what had happened to her as a child and to free up the energy her subconscious had previously spent on keeping that material repressed. MDMA-assisted therapy, she said, ultimately permitted her to "get unstuck in places in my psyche that were frozen by trauma."

\*

THERE'S A GOOD chance that you've come across a story like Callie's in the past few years, perhaps in your news feed, on a favorite podcast, or in conversation with friends. Seemingly overnight, MDMA-assisted therapy has emerged in the popular imagination as a miracle cure for otherwise intractable cases of post-traumatic stress disorder (PTSD) in combat veterans, survivors of sexual violence and childhood abuse, and others haunted by past pain. But while clinical trial results do indicate that MDMA-assisted therapy significantly outperforms all existing treatments for PTSD, too often the stories shared about its healing potential overpromise and exaggerate what the drug, when paired with therapy, can actually deliver. As Callie told me, "People think it's a panacea, but it only gives back what you put into it."

In fact, the new narrative of MDMA-as-definitive-cure-for-trauma is only the latest installment in a long history of hype that's surrounded this unique molecule. Over the past forty-five years, MDMA has ricocheted from celebrated therapeutic catalyst to vilified illicit substance, from the world's favorite party drug to federally designated breakthrough therapy. Through each of these roller-coaster twists and turns in MDMA's history—and even earlier, dating back to its original creation—misunderstandings, false promises, and skewed facts have abounded, amplifying harm caused by the molecule and curtailing its potential benefits. As we move into a vital new chapter in our relationship with MDMA, detailed, knowledgeable information about this drug is needed more than ever.

First synthesized in 1912 by the German pharmaceutical company Merck, MDMA was mostly forgotten for decades after that—save for a brief appearance in the 1950s in the U.S. Army's murky search for a chemical truth serum. In 1975 it was resynthesized by the pioneering psychedelic chemist Alexander Shulgin in California. Shulgin shared MDMA with therapists who quietly popularized its use for enhancing couples counseling, addressing trauma, and helping clients come to realizations that typically take years of traditional talk therapy to uncover. In the early 1980s MDMA escaped the confines of the therapist's office and made its debut on the dance floor, displacing cocaine as the drug of choice among patrons of major clubs in Dallas and New York City. It acquired the name Ecstasy and attracted the attention of officials invested in the war on drugs.

Government crackdown came in 1985, ushering in a quarter century of hysterical public messaging and politically motivated suppression. MDMA was said to eat holes in users' brains and, in the United States, was made more heavily punished, dose by dose, than heroin. By this time MDMA had jumped across the pond to the United Kingdom, where young revelers turned the drug into a truly global phenomenon. British youth invented raves to keep Ecstasy-fueled parties going until dawn and spread MDMA to the rest of Europe and beyond, ultimately laying the foundations for the multibillion-dollar dance music industry. Molly, as MDMA is now popularly called, remains a key ingredient propelling music festivals around the world, some of which attract hundreds of thousands of attendees.

Now, after years of persecution by the mainstream, the pendulum is swinging back to where MDMA first began: as a tool for insight and healing. A slew of recent scientific studies point to MDMA's ability to address severe PTSD, alcoholism, and social anxiety in autistic adults. Upcoming research is examining MDMA-assisted therapy's potential in cases of eating disorders, obesity, traumatic brain injury, and other difficult-to-treat conditions. Still other labs have begun investigating MDMA's use for elucidating the components of meaningful connection; for potentially helping to steer extremists away from harmful ideologies; and for shining a light on the evolutionary origins of sociality.

Developments in the scientific realm are triggering major political and social changes. In May 2022 the Biden administration issued a memo anticipating regulatory approval for MDMA-assisted therapy for PTSD within the next two years. Beating the United States to the punch, Australia became the first country to officially recognize MDMA as a medicine in February 2023. Around the world, nonprofit and for-profit groups alike are scrambling to determine how best to meet the wave of demand that will come with the new treatment's legalization, and how to ensure that MDMA-assisted medicine is equitable, affordable, and available to all who need it. Some experts also think it will only be a matter of time before MDMA follows the path blazed by marijuana, with medical approval of a once-maligned drug paving the way for legalized, socially acceptable recreational use as well.

MDMA is already one of the most popular illegal drugs on the planet, and as we head toward FDA approval for therapeutic use, interest in it is only increasing. Yet it can still be difficult to find reliable information about it. While Michael Pollan's *How to Change Your Mind* extensively explored the history, culture, and science of LSD and psilocybin—and, arguably, solidified the rise of the psychedelic renaissance—no such modern telling exists for MDMA. This isn't due to a lack of storytelling substance. MDMA has its own distinct history and compelling cast of characters, its own unique neurological mechanisms and potential for both ill and good. The tale of MDMA warrants its own telling, but more than that, a solid foundation of knowledge is needed to help us avoid the mistakes of the past and maximize gains for the future.

I wrote *I Feel Love*, first and foremost, to fill this need. On a more personal level, I pursued this project to satisfy my own curiosity about MDMA. I wanted answers to some long-standing questions I've had about the drug, and I also sought to better understand my own changing relationship with it.

\*

THE FIRST TIME I can recall hearing about Ecstasy was on Channel One, a teen news program that my junior high school played each morning. It was probably about 1999. The young news anchors issued warnings about Ecstasy's ability to cook ravers' organs "from the inside out." I didn't really need to hear those dire admonitions about the dangers of drugs, though. I was a straight-edge DARE kid whose only foray into mind-altering substances was the occasional Starbucks Frappuccino. Drugs and booze were crutches for insecure people trying to appear cool, I thought, or for burnouts with no ambitions.

I didn't hear anything else about Ecstasy until a few years later, during my first summer of college, when a friend's brother committed suicide. His older sister, my friend Courtney, had died from leukemia two years earlier, and Chris had been struggling to cope ever since. Rumor had it that he had been doing a lot of Ecstasy, and in my conservative Mississippi town, the blame for his death fell squarely on the drug. I recall being told that Ecstasy causes users to fall into a crippling depression in the days after consuming it, driving some people to take their own lives. I internalized this message and, for years after, viewed the drug as a killer. (I recently spoke with Courtney and Chris's mother to ask her permission to mention Chris's story in my book. She told me she educated herself about MDMA after Chris's death, and had come to realize that he was "100 percent looking for a way to escape the pain of living life without his sister.")

There wasn't a specific moment when I let go of the negative connotations I'd attached to MDMA. It was more of a gradual reevaluation. The mushrooms I tried in college flung open the door to the incredible experience of altered consciousness, and friends I made as I got older—a number of whom had participated in the 1990s rave scene, including my husband, Paul—gave me a more realistic idea of what it was like to take Ecstasy.

As I approached the end of my twenties, I began feeling antsy with life as usual, and yearned for something new. I can't remember exactly why, but I decided to try Ecstasy. I put out some feelers and, with some embarrassment, learned from a cooler friend that the drug had for years been called not Ecstasy but Molly. I finally got hold of the elusive Molly and tried it at a warehouse party in Brooklyn. Forty-five minutes after swallowing the awful-tasting crystals, I understood what all the fuss was about.

I had initially been nervous that MDMA would cause me to spontaneously start making out with everyone around me—it was called the love drug, after all—but I was pleased to find that even in this altered state, I had full control. I just felt really, really good. It made me think of floating on my back in a warm ocean, bobbing to the gentle rhythm of the waves under a perfectly blue sky—safe, content, and, for a brief moment, at one with a force larger than the individual me. A friend of mine once aptly described it as what the rush of joy, elation, and love would feel like if you were suddenly reunited with a good friend that you hadn't seen in years, and you stayed up all night talking because you were so happy to see each other.

The rave atmosphere enhanced the effects, too. The music felt like it was moving through me, with my heart in sync to the beat, and the lasers and aerialist performances were visually mesmerizing, like the flickering flames of a campfire. I had the energy to move to the music all night—a rarity for me—and was able to let go of any feelings of self-consciousness about my lame dance moves. Everyone else around me, friends and strangers alike, seemed to be on the same positive wavelength. I'd catch the eye of someone next to me, and rather than quickly look away, we'd exchange beaming smiles. Brushing up against other gyrating bodies in the crowd rivaled the soothing pleasure of even the best professional massage, and the group hugs with Paul and our friend Ty were simply phenomenal.

Molly became a special treat, something to indulge in every three or four months for a big night out on the town. But then came the pandemic. Paul and I spent the cold, gray months of lockdown holed up in our New York City apartment. For weeks, ambulance sirens were the only sound that broke the eerie silence outside, while the latest news about Covid-19 punctuated the anxious monotony inside. Work felt impossible and pointless, and insomnia kicked in with a vengeance. Sleep, when it did come, was a sweaty, restless affair, full of Technicolor nightmares. As the days dragged into weeks, I had the sense that we were trapped on an endless, miserable budget flight, circling an airport with no idea of if or when we'd ever be able to land, or if the plane would simply run out of gas and fall out of the sky, killing us all.

Something had to give. We concocted a plan to host a Molly night for three with Ty, with whom we'd formed a quarantine pod. He put together a killer disco playlist, and we all donned our sequin club gear, meeting in Paul's and my living room early on a Friday evening. (There's no point waiting until after dark to party when there's literally nothing to do!)

I'd never done Molly in any setting other than a club, concert, or large party, and I wasn't sure what to expect. I knew the drug was taking effect as usual, though, when I noticed that I was smiling—an anomaly in those early pandemic days. MDMA done at home, it turned out, felt just as good as MDMA taken at a club. Against the pandemic's backdrop, however, the experience seemed to hold much more significance than usual. For a few blessed hours the heavy shroud of anxiety lifted and, seemingly for the first time in weeks, I could just breathe and be. Later that night we tuned into a Zoom livestream party hosted by our favorite club, House of Yes. As a DJ broadcast from somewhere out in lockdown, the video feed cycled through attendees, all of whom were stuck, just like us, in basements, kitchens, and, for some, what looked like childhood bedrooms—dancing alone or with one or two other people. We were separate yet utterly together, and I suddenly had the conviction that we would get through this.

That night, while taking a break on the couch from dancing, I had the idea for this book. I wanted to better understand what it was that created the subjective feeling of being on MDMA, and how it came to be that this drug, despite its immense and lasting popularity—and its clear perks, as I was experiencing directly in that moment—is so heavily criminalized around the world. I realized, too, that I felt burned out after spending a decade-plus reporting on the sometimes crushingly disheartening subjects of conservation and the illegal wildlife trade. I had been craving a new challenge, even if I hadn't realized it until that moment.

The next day, for the first time since the pandemic began, I felt invigorated and excited to see what the future would bring. My conviction that I was on the right path was strengthened when I reached out to two key sources, activist Rick Doblin at the Multidisciplinary Association for Psychedelic Studies (MAPS) and neuroscientist Gül Dölen at Johns Hopkins University.

Both agreed that the time was right for a book about MDMA. Doblin told me about Phase 3 clinical trials that were wrapping up soon for MDMA-assisted therapy for PTSD (and that I would wind up writing about for the *New York Times*), and Dölen shared with me some of her groundbreaking results pointing to the neurological underpinnings behind MDMA's ability to provide lasting psychological relief.

Although I had not undergone formal therapy with MDMA, the findings both Doblin and Dölen described about the drug's clinical use made me think of my living room epiphanies. I followed my curiosity, and after a whirl-wind year of researching, reporting, and writing—including two bookshelves' worth of reading on topics ranging from the war on drugs to electronic dance music; nearly 150 interviews with scientists, ravers, parents, historians, therapists, activists, illicit chemists, attorneys, monks, journalists, traffickers, and more; and travels around the United States and United Kingdom, to destinations as varied as Baltimore, Bristol, and Berkeley, and London, Los Angeles, and Lafayette, Indiana—this book is the result.

*

I WROTE *I Feel Love* with all types of readers in mind, including those who have experienced MDMA recreationally or therapeutically, or both—or neither. Whether you've done MDMA a hundred times or zero times, though, the subjects covered in this book pertain to us all. In my reporting, I found that MDMA's ever-evolving story offers a fascinating and sometimes infuri-ating lens through which to examine the forces that shape all facets of life, including culture, politics, science, and even who we are as a species.

I also encountered ample misinformation, including erroneous "facts" frequently repeated about MDMA in major news outlets, documentaries, and books. I've tried here to set the record straight on what we know about MDMA's history, including by sharing the voices of some key players who are frequently left out—and some of whom have never been publicly quoted before. I've strived for honesty about the drug's benefits and risks by sharing the stories of dozens of people whose lives have been impacted by MDMA, for better or worse, and I have attempted to set realistic expectations for MDMA-assisted therapy by describing the experiences of some of those who have gone through it.

I also dig into the latest scientific findings, including Dölen's potentially paradigm-shifting neuroscience research that may answer, once and for all, how it is that MDMA and other psychedelics produce their therapeutic effects: by returning the brain to a state of childlike malleability, permitting new connections to be formed and harmful habits to be undone. If Dölen and her colleagues' findings withstand the test of replication and further study, then the implications may extend to a whole suite of brain-based interventions for conditions well beyond PTSD and other mental health maladies—from restoring speech or movement in stroke patients to returning sight, smell, or hearing to people who have lost those senses. Dölen's findings also indicate that, at their heart, substances as seemingly different as MDMA, ketamine, LSD, and ibogaine all work through common pathways on the molecular level, settling the long-standing question of whether MDMA is actually a psychedelic or not.

Whether discussing all-night raves, mental health interventions, or cutting-edge neuroscience, across all of my reporting about MDMA, one major theme emerged: connection. Research now points to human beings' ability to connect with each other as foundational to all we've accomplished as a species, and as the Covid-19 pandemic laid bare, this evolutionarily ordained imperative is also key to our individual happiness and mental health. We need each other not only to survive but also to thrive. MDMA's greatest asset, then, is that it enhances this feature of our biology, greasing the wheels of connection with the self, with others, and with all life on the planet.

All that said, MDMA is not going to save the world. Only we can do that. What MDMA may be able to do, instead, is improve lives by addressing trauma, bringing happiness (whether achieved on the dance floor, in the arms of a lover, or in a therapist's office), and forging stronger genuine, loving bonds. Perhaps then we would have greater bandwidth as a species to tackle the major societal and environmental problems that are behind so much suffering and loss today. That hope may be the only constant in the decades-long journey toward realizing MDMA's potential—a journey that is still ongoing, and whose end result is by no means obvious or assured. From the first confirmed use of MDMA by a human—in 1975, aboard a boat, on the sparkling waters of San Francisco Bay—it has never been merely a drug, but rather a signifier of a possible world.

# THE FERRY TO SAUSALITO

CARL RESNIKOFF WAS in eighth grade when he decided to learn how to make drugs. Growing up in Oakland in the 1960s, Carl spent weekends exploring Haight-Ashbury, the counterculture's unofficial headquarters and the epicenter of the nation's mounting interest in psychedelic drugs, across the San Francisco Bay. By junior high, Carl's reading list included accounts of esoteric drug experiences by Thomas De Quincey, Charles Baudelaire, and William S. Burroughs, and he idolized underground chemists featured in the media. He desperately wanted to embark on his own drug-induced internal journeys, but there was only one problem: he couldn't find anyone who would sell LSD to a twelve-year-old. No bother, he thought; he'd synthesize it himself.

By the time Carl enrolled as a biophysics major at the University of California, Berkeley, in 1971, he fully looked the part of that era's stereotypical drug chemist: John Lennon glasses, laid-back smile, and shaggy, shoulder-length dark hair. But he was still struggling to gather the knowledge needed to make his own LSD; the more he learned, the more he realized he did not know. He had, however, long since found hookups for buying mind-bending drugs, and he'd especially become a fan of MDA, the so-called love drug or "mellow drug of America." As Carl refined his psychedelic palate, his passion for learning to make the substances himself had only grown.

"It was about seeing the world in an entirely different way," Carl recently explained of the appeal of psychedelics. "We were exploring inner space. I'm not sure the word *psychonaut* had been coined then, but that describes it perfectly."

One day, while browsing the university library, Carl came across an intriguing 1969 article published in the respected journal *Nature*, titled "Structure-Activity Relationships of One-Ring Psychotomimetics." At the time, *psychotomimetics*—"drugs that mimic psychosis"—was another term for hallucinogenic drugs, a nod to scientists' original hypothesis that LSD induced a temporary state of madness. Carl noted with amazement that the article's lead author, a man named Alexander Shulgin, lived just fifteen minutes up the road in Lafayette, an idyllic town of rolling hills and postcard-perfect views of Mount Diablo. Shulgin's affiliation was listed not as an institution but as a home address on—even more intriguingly— Shulgin Road.

Carl pretty much memorized that first article, and he dug up every other scientific paper he could find with Shulgin's name on it, too. Shulgin, he learned, was a leading psychedelic chemist who studied not just known molecules but also brand-new drugs he created in his lab—and even, apparently, tried on himself. When Carl saw Shulgin listed as the instructor for a forensic toxicology class at UC Berkeley a couple of years later, he couldn't believe his luck. He rearranged his schedule to enroll.

Shulgin—whom everyone called Sasha—seemed to embody the quintessential kooky chemist. His snow-white hair and beard were styled like Santa's, and his wardrobe consisted of a rotating collection of brash Hawaiian shirts and black sandals always worn over socks. At six foot four, he towered over the class. Carl recalls Shulgin, a skilled raconteur, delivering lectures that meandered from meticulous instructions about how to use ninhydrin to visualize blood spatter at crime scenes to philosophical musings about chemistry's ability to reveal core truths about human nature. Shulgin also had an uncanny prescience: he issued a warning to the class about an obscure compound called fentanyl, which he predicted would become a major public health and law enforcement issue in years to come. Carl absorbed it all.

"Everybody else in the class but me was very conservative, had the goal of working in a police lab and didn't know Shulgin's background," Carl said. "I had read all of his journal articles and had tried a number of those compounds, so we immediately had a rapport."

At the end of the semester, Carl worked up his nerve to ask his renowned professor if he would mentor him in an independent study. Shulgin not only said yes but also suggested they work together on a project synthesizing street drugs under the auspices of "characterizing their impurities" for forensic use.

Shulgin secured a lab space in the basement of the life science building, and—after a few months teaching his student techniques for analyzing, synthesizing, and purifying alkaloids—suggested that Carl propose a project all his own.

Carl knew just the thing. He was already familiar with the psychedelic amphetamine MDA, one of his favorite drugs. He also knew from experience that methamphetamine is more euphoric than plain amphetamine, and that the only difference in these molecules' compositions comes down to methamphetamine's extra N-methyl group—an example of a side chain, a chemical structure that can be attached to the main body of a molecule. In this way, a difference of just a few atoms can drastically alter a drug's effect in the human brain.

Following this logic, Carl wondered what would happen if he added an N-methyl group to MDA to create MDMA (short for methylenedioxymethamphetamine). Would N-methylated MDA be even more euphoric than its parent molecule, in the same way methamphetamine is more euphoric than amphetamine? A quick literature search told him that this synthesis was not unprecedented, but he could find no record of humans ever having tried it.

The next time Carl met Shulgin in the lab, he suggested they make MDMA.

"That's a fine idea," Shulgin replied.

As it later turned out, Shulgin knew more about MDMA than he let on to Carl. "He kind of kept his cards close to the vest," Carl said. "There was a level of don't-ask-don't-tell."

Holing up in the university lab one summer afternoon in 1975, the professor and pupil needed just a few hours to complete the synthesis. Unlike LSD, a notoriously difficult drug to make, MDMA wasn't too hard to coax out of its chemical precursors—upper-division chemistry, for sure, but (with Shulgin's help, at least) not graduate-level. As Carl pointed out, "Sasha had been working with psychedelic amphetamines and related compounds for years, so he knew some shortcuts and tricks that a competent organic chemist in a different specialty would take longer to figure out." Carl's favorite part was the end, when he bubbled hydrogen chloride gas into the flask, causing white MDMA crystals to flutter to the bottom like snow.

Shulgin measured out two 120-milligram doses for Carl—a typical amount for recreational MDA use—and took the rest home with him. Carl never did find out if Shulgin tried their creation. "I was a twenty-one-year-old under-grad, and he was an experienced researcher," Carl explained. "I would not have been comfortable asking him that."

For Carl, though, the experiment would not be complete until he tried the drug himself. When he asked his then girlfriend, Judith Gips, a fellow student at UC Berkeley, if she'd like to join him, she said sure. "I knew he was in that world," Judith recently recalled. "He told me about a lot of things, including about Dr. Shulgin."

"We had already taken LSD together many times, MDA a few times," Carl added. "I mean, this was the seventies in Berkeley. Things were wild."

On a glorious September morning, Carl and Judith drove to San Francisco and boarded a ferry to Sausalito. Carl had put the MDMA powder into capsules, correctly guessing that the alkaloid would be very bitter to swallow on its own. As they set out on their literal and figurative journey, Carl recalled, "I was actually not nervous at all."

Basking in the early autumn sun and taking in views of the glittering bay and elegant arches of the Golden Gate Bridge, Carl and Judith began to feel a floating sense of euphoria.

"Everything was enhanced," Judith recalled. Strangely for a psychedelic drug, though, there were no visual distortions, and neither were there any tremors of anxiety or any sense that things might spin out of control. The most intense moments came when Judith began to feel overwhelmed by the world's beauty. "I told Carl, 'It's almost too much,'" she said. "'I feel like some guy could come walking up to us asking for help and his guts are spilling out, and we'd be grooving on how beautiful it was.'"

The warm waves of euphoria built and then finally plateaued, leaving the couple with a sense of deep love for each other, compassion for fellow human beings, and peace with the world. "This was remarkable in that I felt good the entire time," Carl said. "There were no scary moments at all, and that was unusual for most of my other psychedelic trips."

Carl and Judith's gentle, life-affirming experience was typical of the tens of millions of subsequent encounters that people around the world would have with the drug. What makes their story notable, though, is that they are the first individuals documented by name to have taken what is known for sure to be MDMA. Incredibly, their special place in history was only revealed to them some forty-two years later, when Emanuel Sferios, a friend of Judith's and founder of the drug education and safety organization DanceSafe, put the pieces together. When Carl heard, he couldn't believe it. "I am still in awe of this fact," he said. Judith thought it was "hilarious."

Under the clear blue sky in 1975, though, neither Carl nor Judith had any idea that the easygoing, heart-opening drug that filled their afternoon with smiles and laughter held all the potential that would be unlocked in the decades to come. "When I've told a few people about my history, and they say, 'MDMA saved my life,' that's good to hear," Carl said. "If not me, it's highly likely it would have been someone else. But I feel awed about possibly being the first."

\*

WHY DO WE seek out substances that alter the business-as-usual functioning of our minds? Some experts argue that there exists across the animal kingdom—in species as varied as goats, birds, ants, elephants, cats, and slugs—an innate drive to tinker with consciousness, akin to the desire for food or sex. *Homo sapiens* is no exception. Virtually every human society on Earth has used mind-altering fungi, plants, and animals for medicine, rituals, rites of passage, religion, enlightenment, entertainment, and more. As the writer and philosopher Aldous Huxley eloquently summarized it, "All the vegetable sedatives and narcotics, all the euphorics that grow on trees, the hallucinogens that ripen in berries or can be squeezed from roots—all, without exception, have been known and systematically used by human beings from time immemorial."

Mammoths still roamed, for example, when people in North America began using tobacco at least 12,300 years ago. Cannabis might have been domesticated more than 10,000 years ago in East Asia, potentially making it the first ever plant to be cultivated by humans. Alcohol brewing was taking place at least 8,000 years ago in China and in the Caucasus Mountains in Georgia, and people in modern-day Armenia started making wine 6,000 years ago. Ritual use of peyote by Indigenous peoples of the Americas also dates back at least 6,000 years, and Sumerians began cultivating opium poppies— which they called the "joy plant"—5,000 years ago. Ancient Taoist texts dating to around the same time in China indicate that shamans there sought out hallucinogenic plants and mushrooms to communicate with gods and spirits, and attain transcendence and immortality.

Psychedelics may have played a particularly important role in the founding of Western civilization. From 1200 B.C. to 395 A.D., ancient Greeks and Romans—including Socrates and Plato—took part in the Eleusinian Mysteries, a secretive rite at which initiates consumed a beer-based *kykeon* ("mixed drink" or "potion"). Women were the keepers of the fiercely protected formula for making the *kykeon*, which was likely brewed with ergot, a rye fungus that contains lysergic acid, a chemical precursor for LSD. Initiates to the rite describe the experience as practice for the awe, rapture, and transcendence of dying. "At the moment of quitting it come terrors, shuddering fear, amazement," the first-century philosopher Plutarch wrote of the experience. "Then a light moves to meet you, pure meadows receive you, songs and dances and holy apparitions." Similar rituals were also held in honor of Dionysus, the god of wine and ecstasy, using spiked wine rather than beer.

Because our tendency to seek out consciousness-altering experiences has withstood the selective pressures of evolution, scientists surmise that there must be benefits. Some of these benefits probably relate to survival: caffeine to keep us alert and enhance our abilities, opium to relieve pain, alcohol to bring us together. But evidence also indicates that our use of psychoactive substances has shaped us in subtler but perhaps equally powerful ways, by helping to mold the customs, beliefs, and traditions that have made our species what it is today.

"I do think psychoactive drugs have played a profound role in cultural evolution," said Michael Pollan, author of *How to Change Your Mind*. "We have the accounts of artists who have created breakthroughs on psychoactive drugs, we have scientists who made discoveries while on psychoactive drugs. The more we look for examples like that, the more we find them."

Scholarship investigating the role that mind-altering materials have played in the story of humanity is only in its infancy, though, because until recently, if drug research got done at all, it got done mostly by chemists, psychiatrists, and neuroscientists—not archaeologists, anthropologists, historians, archaeochemists, and ethnobotanists. But as the field expands, fascinating findings are beginning to come to light. Based on twelve years of meticulous research outlined in *The Immortality Key*, classicist Brian Muraresku pieced together compelling evidence of a pivotal psychedelic through line between prehistoric spiritual rituals, the Eleusinian and Dionysian Mysteries, and early Christianity. Muraresku provides evidence that these millennia-old, women-led ceremonies continued for several hundred years after the founding of Christianity, when the new religion was still an illegal cult and retained strong ties to worship of Dionysus. For Christianity to have had any chance of gaining popularity, "the Eucharist simply *had* to involve the kind of genuine mystical experiences so well documented in the Dionysian tradition," Muraresku writes. "Unlike the cardboard wafer and cheap boxed wine of today's Mass, it had to actually deliver."

Psychedelics likely provided the mystical core at the heart of countless religions. According to Osiris Sinuhé González Romero, a postdoctoral fellow in cognitive freedom and psychedelic humanities at the University of Saskatchewan, historical and archaeological records indicate that cultures around the world have traditionally valued psychedelic substances primarily as ritual, spiritual, and therapeutic tools. Many Indigenous societies also paired consumption of these powerful materials with complex ceremonies to prevent abuse. The substances themselves were frequently considered sacred, respected entities whose spirits infused those who consumed them.

The sacraments of both Dionysus and Jesus were also literally taken to be holy flesh and blood—and the psychedelic experiences they induced reinforced that divine guarantee. Christianity's relationship with mind-altering substances likely soured, however, when Roman Catholicism's thought leaders—"God's bouncers," as Muraresku put it—began pushing for male human intermediaries to manage the relationship between worshippers and God, a clear power play. "If anyone with the right ingredients could mix up their own Eucharist at home, and meet Jesus on their own terms, Christianity never would have consolidated the wealth and power to replace the Roman Empire as Europe's central governing authority," Muraresku writes.

The new patriarchy did not manage to stamp out psychedelics overnight. For centuries in Europe, knowledge of psychoactive substances was kept alive by pagans and heretics. In the Middle Ages, however, religious authorities began aggressively persecuting anyone who turned to nature rather than the moral authority of the church in their study of medicine or pursuit of spirituality. Over the span of three hundred years, several million healers, primarily women, were accused of practicing witchcraft and condemned to death.

In 1620 the Spanish Inquisition officially banned mandrake root, belladonna, stinking nightshade, and other psychotropic plants and recast them as "tools of Satan." The Inquisition likewise sought to control people living in the Americas who practiced ritual use of sacred mushrooms, morning glory, and peyote. According to a proclamation issued that same year by the Holy Inquisition of Mexico, anyone caught under the influence of "herbs and roots with which they lose and confound their senses" would be subject to punishments ranging from public flogging to being burned alive at the stake. Christian missionaries continued to push this form of Indigenous religious prohibition and suppression throughout the early twentieth century. In quashing Indigenous use of these materials, "the Church sought to eliminate a perceived threat to its oligarchic powers and reassert its monopoly on legitimate access to the supernatural," writes psychiatrist Charles Grob.

While extremely damaging, the church's attempt to eradicate traditional ecological knowledge and overturn Indigenous communities' human rights was not entirely successful. Some Indigenous groups quietly continued underground use of these materials for centuries, allowing their knowledge and traditions to survive unknown to Western authorities or scholars. That began to change in the 1880s, when the German pharmacologist Louis Lewin received peyote samples at his lab. Lewin isolated several alkaloids from the cactuses, but failed to identify what they were. Arthur Carl Wilhelm Heffter, a renowned pharmacologist and chemist, picked the research up from there and was able to identify mescaline, the psychoactive component of the peyote cactus—and the first ever psychedelic substance to be chemically identified—by ingesting the material himself. Mescaline was synthesized for the first time in 1919, and throughout the 1920s, German scholars published manuscripts attempting to scientifically categorize "inebriation" following consumption of the molecule.

Western interest in nonordinary states of consciousness continued to grow with the "discovery" of sacred mushrooms by a team of American anthropologists on a trip to Oaxaca, Mexico. A few years later, in 1938, the Swiss chemist Albert Hofmann synthesized LSD. Hofmann stumbled upon the incredibly mind-altering properties of his creation on April 19, 1943, when he consumed 250 micrograms of LSD and famously pedaled home on his bicycle while tripping. Now known as Bicycle Day, the anniversary of Hofmann's eye-opening journey is celebrated by psychedelic aficionados around the world.

MDMA likewise originated in a lab in recent history, and also like LSD, it took a few years for its mind-altering effects to be discovered. Probably an order of magnitude more people have taken MDMA than LSD, so the story of the first person to have consumed it would also be of great interest to potentially millions of individuals around the world. Yet there is no equivalent to Bicycle Day for MDMA. That's because we really have no idea who, exactly, was first to take it. While Carl and Judith are the earliest definitively identified users, there were probably others before them. We may never know for sure.

Still, the question of who really was the first to sample MDMA has vexed psychedelics and history buffs for years. And some speculate that this distinction could in fact belong to someone who took the drug under much darker circumstances. As MDMA gains notoriety as an agent of connection and healing, it becomes all the more important to acknowledge its murky origins and the possibility that the first person who ever experienced it might have done so under duress.

*

MDMA'S OFFICIAL STORY begins on Christmas Eve 1912, when Merck, the German pharmaceutical company, filed a patent application for "methylsafrylamin"—now known as MDMA. Anton Köllisch, a young chemist who was killed four years later in World War I, had identified MDMA as one of a handful of chemical intermediates—also among them MDA—for "manufacturing of therapeutically effective compounds." Specifically, Köllisch and his colleagues at Merck were trying to develop a drug to promote blood clotting, to compete with a rival product recently licensed by Bayer. (Much later an urban myth emerged—untrue, but oft-repeated—that Merck originally developed MDMA to suppress the appetites of soldiers in World War I.)

Merck revived its interest in MDMA in 1927, when a chemist named Max Oberlin hypothesized that the molecule might mimic adrenaline. Oberlin described the tests he was carrying out in the lab as producing "partly remarkable results"—yet oddly, he did not indicate if those tests had been carried out in animals, humans, or Petri dishes. His research was halted due to what Merck has reported to be steep price increases, but not before Oberlin noted that this avenue of investigation was something "to keep an eye on."

In 1959, yet another Merck chemist, Wolfgang Fruhstorfer, resumed investigations of MDMA as a possible new stimulant. According to a paper published in 2006 by researchers from Merck and the University of Ulm, at this time there were also "some insinuations of a cooperation with an institute for aviation medicine." There was precedent for this in Germany: a few years earlier, the Nazis had discovered that they could keep their pilots going with methamphetamine.

"In the Merck archives is a file card that explicitly refers to military research, but what happened to the MDMA is not known," said Torsten Passie, a professor of psychiatry at Hannover Medical School who has published extensively about MDMA's history. If MDMA was tested in German fighter pilots, Passie guesses that it was probably quickly abandoned. As he said, "If they feel full of love for their victims on the ground, they might not throw down the bombs!"

Merck has emphasized that MDMA "was not tested in humans" under the company's watch. But this assertion is something "they can't say for sure, because their records are incomplete," said David Carlson, an independent organic chemist in Northern California who has been researching the Merck story for years. Carlson and others have questioned Merck's official version of events, particularly the company's insistence that it did not know about MDMA's psychochemical properties or engage in any human tests of the drug.

Sabine Bernschneider-Reif, the head of corporate history at Merck, and her colleagues stated in their 2006 paper that all relevant materials related to MDMA are "available at request at Merck's historical archive for further studies." But Carlson said he has run into issues trying to source key documents from Merck. Bernschneider-Reif also declined my request for a phone interview, through a press officer who then stopped responding to my emails.

"We have all these bits and pieces of circumstantial stuff," Carlson said of the lingering mysteries. "We haven't been able to tie it all together and might never be able to."

By the 1950s, MDMA had found its way across the Atlantic. Its first known synthesis in the United States was in connection to an exceptionally shameful and infamous chapter of American history. Under the dark cloud of the Cold War, U.S. officials feared that the Soviets, Chinese, and North Koreans could be developing drugs to brainwash, control, or otherwise sabotage Americans. To get ahead of this threat, the CIA and the U.S. Army set out to secretly develop their own psychochemical weapons. While these two governmental efforts overlapped, they differed in scope: the CIA focused on control of individuals, while the Army was concerned with mass distribution of drugs to take out entire military units or even populations.

"The CIA wanted to be able to put something into a Soviet diplomat's drink at a cocktail party that would make him their agent," said John Marks, author of *The Search for the "Manchurian Candidate,"* which the *New York Times* called "the definitive book on the experiments." The military, on the other hand, was interested in "whether you could drop a cloud over the enemy that would make them drop their weapons."

From 1953 to 1973, at least eighty-six universities and institutions were involved in top-secret psychochemical and behavioral warfare programs. Hundreds of drugs were tested on some seven thousand soldiers and one thousand citizens—at times without their knowledge, an apparent violation of the Nuremberg Code, the 1947 war-crimes tribunal judgment mandating informed consent in medical testing, among other human-rights protections. At least two participants died, and countless others suffered long-term psychological damage. Little, if anything, was gained. Before he retired, Sidney Gottlieb, the CIA scientist who oversaw the notorious umbrella project, MK-ULTRA, concluded that the experiments had been useless.

Mind control had been a special interest of the Nazis, who interrogated prisoners forced to take mescaline at the Dachau and Auschwitz concentration camps. The goal, according to a Nazi nurse involved, was "to eliminate the will of the person examined." After learning of the Nazis' work, the U.S. Army was inspired to conduct its own experiments using mescaline-like compounds as possible truth serums. MDMA, code-named EA-1475, was on the Army's list of drugs of interest. Whether the U.S. military carried out tests of MDMA in people has never been clarified.

Some experts hypothesize that MDMA did not make it into humans because of a fatal error caused by closely related MDA. In November 1952 the Army Chemical Corps sent five or six newly synthesized mescaline derivatives to Paul Hoch, the head of the experimental psychiatry division of the New York State Psychiatric Institute, a well-respected mental health hospital in Manhattan. Hoch's hospital had contracted with the Army to study the effects of various mind-altering drugs in patients, "both for offensive use as sabotage weapons and for protection against them," according to court documents. None of the drugs Hoch received that fall had been previously tested in humans, Passie said, and "animal testing was grossly deficient."

Less than a month after Hoch received the latest shipment of drugs, a forty-two-year-old professional tennis player named Harold Blauer checked himself into the institute for severe depression brought about by a recent divorce. In addition to the usual talk therapy, Blauer received mystery injections. From the beginning, Blauer was "very apprehensive" about the injections, and it took "considerable persuasion" to get him to agree, according to notes made by James Cattell, the senior research scientist at the hospital. Blauer was not informed that the injections had nothing to do with treating his depression, or that he was "a guinea pig in an experiment" being run by the government, according to a federal district court judge who oversaw a wrongful death lawsuit brought by Blauer's daughter in 1987.

As a result of the injections, Blauer experienced pressure in his head, uncontrolled tremors, hallucinations, and chills. By the time he was due to receive a fifth shot, Blauer had clearly stated to his doctors that he no longer wanted to participate. Nevertheless, just before ten A.M. on January 8, 1953, Blauer received an injection of 450 milligrams of MDA—a monstrously high dose. Moments later he began sweating profusely, wildly flailing his arms, and clenching his teeth. His body stiffened and he frothed at the mouth. After an hour, he fell into a coma. At twelve fifteen, he was pronounced dead.

By way of explanation, Blauer's death certificate indicated that "a chemical compound had activated a previously unknown heart condition, causing a fatal coronary attack." The actual circumstances probably would have remained hidden were it not for an unrelated congressional inquiry in 1975 that uncovered documents stamped "secret" detailing the incident. In the immediate aftermath, though, the Army tried to cover its tracks by conducting toxicology studies in animals—something that should have been done before any drugs were ever given to humans.

"If you look at the timing of when that research seems to be done, they were like, 'Oh crap, we just killed someone. We need to quickly do some animal toxicology studies,'" said Matthew Baggott, a neuroscientist, history enthusiast, and cofounder and CEO of Tactogen, a company trying to develop new MDMA-like molecules. "If they hadn't killed Harold Blauer, they probably would have gotten around to doing MDMA, too. But his death probably stopped all that work."

From 1953 to 1954, MDMA was one of the eight chemicals tested in mice, rats, guinea pigs, dogs, and monkeys by scientists at the University of Michigan, who quietly conducted experiments on the Army's behalf. The animal studies, which were declassified in 1969, revealed that none of the compounds, including MDMA, were particularly dangerous or unusually toxic in smaller doses. In a scientific paper published about the experiments, the researchers state that the effects of MDMA in dogs were similar to those of mescaline— that is, causing the animals to first assume "bizarre body attitudes," then become "weak and sleepy," and finally run "wildly about the room bumping into walls and furniture." According to a formerly classified 1955 report, in monkeys MDMA produced "difficulty in vision," which researchers "inferred from the animal bumping into obstacles as he moves from place to place."

As with Merck, though, the lack of definitive evidence about MDMA's use in humans hasn't stopped some people from wondering whether the first Americans to take the drug might have been given it as part of a covert government experiment. Nicholas Denomme, a doctoral candidate in pharmacology at the University of Michigan Medical School, has been obsessed with finding a definitive answer to this question ever since he learned of his department's involvement in the 1950s animal trials. Given that MDMA is just another mescaline analogue, Denomme said, it's logical that the Army would have included it on its list of drugs to test. Human testing of MDMA-like drugs also continued for years after the Blauer incident, Denomme pointed out, and MDA was even rumored to have hit the recreational scene after escaping from a Bay Area military facility in the 1960s. It simply would not make sense that MDMA never made it into humans. "MDMA matched the psychological profile of what they were looking for," Denomme said. "It produces little to no hallucinations and enhances empathy in a manner that could be of interest to someone in search of a pharmacological interrogation aid."

My Freedom of Information Act (FOIA) request to the Army has so far gone unanswered, which isn't surprising. According to James Romano, a retired Colonel who formerly commanded the U.S. Army Medical Research Institute of Chemical Defense, information about the work of government scientists from earlier eras "is protected, intentionally or unintentionally, by a web of disuse, movement of files and the pernicious delays and obfuscation of the FOIA."

But persistence pays off, and Denomme has made headway on his FOIA requests—which he's been chipping away at since 2016. "It's just something that personally bothers me and I can't let it go," he said.

At the end of 2021 Denomme received a formerly redacted 1955 status report from the Chemical Warfare Laboratories's Psychochemical Program outlining toxicity data for thirty-six compounds, including MDMA. Cited in reference to EA-1475 (MDMA) was a clinical report that led Denomme to a study performed from 1955 to 1959 by Army-contracted scientists in Tulane University's Department of Psychiatry and Neurology for "research in abnormal brain functioning as related to mental illness." The Tulane study was acknowledged in a 1975 U.S. Inspector General report, which stated that "the few Army records available regarding the experiments conducted under the terms of the Army grant revealed that mental patients, normal volunteers and neurological patients were used by the Tulane medical investigators."

It could very well be, then, that MDMA was experimentally given to patients at Tulane in the 1950s. However, when Denomme reached out to the

U.S. Army Medical Research and Development Command office requesting a copy of the Tulane report—the document most likely to give a definitive answer about MDMA's experimental use in humans—he was told by a government information specialist that "a search was conducted and no responsive documents were located."

Denomme was floored. "As a scientist, I try to avoid being conspiratorial, but the writing seems to be on the wall here," he said. "Literally, there could not be a more detailed description of a document. It's dated to the day. Why would the Inspector General not have their own documents? It's ridiculous."

If the Army did give MDMA to human subjects, that would set the clock back on the first confirmed human consumption of the drug by twenty years. It would also add chilling context to MDMA's history in the United States. As Denomme said, "It would be mind-blowing to know that a compound that's about to be approved by the FDA for the treatment of PTSD in veterans and others was essentially being used in an unethical manner by the military seventy years ago."

*

WHISPERS OF MDMA had already begun to appear several years before Carl's 1975 synthesis with Shulgin—a development most likely tied to closely related MDA being made illegal in 1970, with the creation of the Controlled Substances Act. Up until then, MDA was easily available—it could even be ordered from chemical supply catalogues—but now that it was a banned substance, anyone synthesizing or selling it risked run-ins with law enforcement. In light of this development, savvy chemists probably followed Carl's logic of adding an N-methyl group to MDA—in this case, with the intention of creating a "designer drug" to skirt the new ban, rather than to explore new realms of consciousness. Indeed, the same year MDA was banned, a mystery substance picked up by the Chicago police turned out to be MDMA, and several more samples of MDMA were confirmed in 1972 in Chicago and Gary, Indiana. The year after that, in Cedar Hill, Tennessee, federal agents confiscated nearly nine hundred grams of what they thought was MDA (and enough precursors to make another ten kilograms), but that turned out to be pure MDMA. Nothing is known about the chemists who made these batches of MDMA, or about who their customers might have been.

MDMA was also on Shulgin's radar earlier than he sometimes liked to let on. He first synthesized the drug in 1965, as confirmed by an unpublished page in his lab notes, and by 1970, well before he met Carl, he had already shared the formula for making MDMA with someone he described as "a very competent chemist" in Los Angeles, who was interested in adding psychoactive drugs to his company's commercial catalogue. That chemist died a few years later in a sports accident—but not before sending MDMA to a psychologist in the Midwest, according to Shulgin's notes. Indeed, by the early 1970s,* "there were other indications that MDMA consumption was already widespread in some circles," he wrote.

David Obst, a retired literary agent, recalled taking what a friend told him was MDMA in the early 1970s in New York City—including right before an important pitch meeting with Richard Snyder, head of Simon & Schuster. Obst was trying to convince Snyder to publish *All the President's Men*, but at the end of the meeting, Snyder shook his head: "Sorry, David, pass."

Obst, who was feeling exceptionally emotional, "burst into tears," he recalled. "Not just tears—copious crying, weeping uncontrollably." Snyder was so nonplussed that he gave Obst a hug and told him, "Fine, I'll buy it if it means so much to you!"

"So thanks to MDMA, we have *All the President's Men*," Obst said.

Based on Shulgin's writing,† it seems likely that he didn't try MDMA himself until 1976, after a chance encounter with a chemistry graduate

---

* Shulgin might have given out samples of an early batch of MDMA to trusted associates to try and report back to him. Celebrity doctor Andrew Weil remembers receiving a sample of MDMA from Shulgin in what he is fairly sure was 1974 or 1975. "I thought it was great," Weil said in a December 2021 interview by the author. "He sent me more and I shared it with friends and turned people on to it." David Smith, director of the Haight Ashbury Free Clinics, was one of the people Weil shared it with, but in a November 2021 interview by the author, Smith put the date closer to 1973.

† Years after Carl synthesized MDMA with Shulgin, he discovered that his old mentor had written about him in *PIHKAL* under the pseudonym "Klaus." But Shulgin had either intentionally or accidentally gotten many details of their story wrong. For one, Shulgin wrote that Carl, who has a stutter, had been miraculously cured of it after taking MDMA, and that he had decided to become a speech therapist because of the experience. Neither are true. Shulgin also implied that his experience with Carl happened in 1976, a year after he and Carl had made MDMA together. Carl was bothered by

student. In *PIHKAL*—the thinly veiled autobiography slash drug manual that Shulgin and his wife, Ann, published in 1990—he stated that a mentee of his, whom he calls "Merrie Kleinman," inspired him to try MDMA after she told him about her own experience with the drug. The "dear, dear sprite," as Shulgin described her, "shared very little about the experience, but implied that it was quite emotional, and that there had been a basically good reaction."

It took me six months to discover the identity of Merrie Kleinman, and when I reached her, she asked that her real name not be disclosed for personal and professional reasons. Kleinman recalled spending many an afternoon with Shulgin and two other chemistry graduate students at Golden Gate Park, just across from the University of California, San Francisco. "We'd listen to his stories that a methyl group here would make greens and blues appear, a methylenedioxy group there would make noises different or smells more acute," she said. "At the time, we were totally enchanted. Shulgin was kind of our guru." Inspired, Kleinman started trying her hand at synthesizing and sampling certain drugs on her own—something she now views as "dangerous, reckless, and stupid."

"Looking back, you'd have to say that was not a good idea," she said. "But who has good judgment at that age?"

At some point, she doesn't remember where or how, she came across the structure of MDMA. She decided to make it—a very straightforward synthesis, she found—and tried it with a friend. "It was very warm and open and loving," she recalled. "This rush of empathy, the whole world is good and protective, and the people you're with are especially warm and protective and loving. It was very positive." It was a given, she added, that she would share the story with Shulgin. "I'd made this thing and tested it on myself, and that was what Sasha was all about."

---

these inaccuracies, and he eventually asked Shulgin about it; Shulgin apologized and said he meant no harm. "We talked about it and worked it out, so it was fine," Carl said, adding, "I think *PIHKAL* has a lot of embellishment." Emanuel Sferios suspects that Shulgin could have also been deliberately vague about his involvement with Carl to conceal the fact that he had not synthesized MDMA in his home lab, but on the campus of UC Berkeley. Alexander Shulgin and Ann Shulgin, *PIHKAL: A Chemical Love Story* (San Francisco: Transform Press, 1990), 66; Sferios, interview by the author.

Shulgin already had a sample of MDMA on his laboratory bench but still had not tried it, and the conversation with Kleinman seemed to be the nudge he needed. In September 1976 he decided to finally see for himself what this drug was all about.

Until I reached out to her, Kleinman said, she had no idea she had played this small but significant role in influencing MDMA's historical trajectory. "I was just a chemist in a little cubbyhole in Berkeley doing something on the weekend I shouldn't be doing," she said. "I heard he wrote a book but I never read it or knew he had given me another name."

Today she doesn't feel particularly connected to MDMA, and hasn't paid much attention to its medical or research development. "As a friend of mine once said, the midwife doesn't keep the baby."

But having successfully delivered that crucial nugget of an idea to Sasha Shulgin, Kleinman enabled MDMA's story to really begin.

# PENICILLIN FOR THE SOUL

IT'S EASY TO miss the turn for Shulgin Road. Curtained by the golden brush of Northern California, it appears suddenly, just after a blind corner near the top of a hill. If you do manage to make the exit, you'll follow a gravel road climbing past sunny fields of tall grass and majestic bent oaks, until you reach a modest white ranch house. The house itself is unremarkable, but that's not what you came to see.

You follow a narrow footpath past rows of cacti springing from the ground like exclamation marks to a hobbit hole of a shed out back. A rusted sign on the door reads CAUTION RADIOACTIVE MATERIALS. Turning the antique handle, you step into what could be a movie set for "mad scientist's lair." From floor to ceiling, all manner of chemical paraphernalia crowd the small space: beakers and tubes, flasks and funnels, pipettes and condensers. Amid the cobwebbed shelves of bottles with fading labels, you spot a plastic figurine of Mickey Mouse. He's dressed as his character from "The Sorcerer's Apprentice," and he seems to be casting a spell over a little silver urn.

The urn, unlike the bottles, bears no label. But should you open it, you'll find yet another chemical mixture: a powder primarily composed of phosphate and calcium, plus a few pinches of sulfate, potassium, and sodium. It's all that's left of the earthly remains of Alexander "Sasha" Shulgin, the reluctant "stepfather of MDMA," as he called himself, and the sorcerer who once presided over this fantastical domain.

*

SASHA SHULGIN WAS born in 1925 in Berkeley. His family always called him by the fondly diminutive nickname for Alexander, in keeping with the tradition of his Russian father. Both of his strict parents were public school teachers and purposefully kept no television in the house. They encouraged their children to entertain themselves instead by developing their musical talents—in Shulgin's case, piano and violin. To avoid practicing instruments, he took to exploring (or, according to his mother, hiding in) strange places, like the forgotten corners of friends' dank basements, or in the tangled tunnels of honeysuckle that grew along his family's backyard fence.

When he was just sixteen, Shulgin moved to the East Coast to study organic chemistry at Harvard University. He dropped out at age nineteen to join the Navy during World War II. While serving in Europe, he experienced his first inkling of the mind's powerful capacity to shift consciousness through a telling encounter with the placebo effect. Before surgery for a thumb infection, a nurse gave him a glass of orange juice with white crystals condensed at the bottom—what Shulgin assumed to be a crushed-up sedative. He downed the juice and passed out. Later, he learned that the crystals had been sugar.

In 1954 Shulgin earned his PhD in biochemistry from UC Berkeley and shortly after went to work as a chemist at the Dow Chemical Company—a role he later described as "academic prostitute." During his time there, a couple of friends offered to babysit him while he tripped on 400 milligrams of mescaline sulfate—"a day that will remain blazingly vivid in my memory, and one which unquestionably confirmed the entire direction of my life," he wrote. Shulgin had always dreamed in black and white and never paid much attention to color; during the trip, he was plunged into the wondrous nuances of the rainbow of hues all around him. He saw the world afresh as he had in childhood, full of beauty, magic, and "the knowingness of it and me." Most revelatory of all was the fact that a mere "fraction of a gram of a white solid," as he put it, had so emphatically revealed the miracle of existence contained within him.

Two years after that formative experience, Shulgin struck pay dirt for Dow when he developed Zectran, one of the world's first biodegradable insecticides. His bosses rewarded their star chemist by giving him carte blanche in the lab. Zectran "sounds like a motor additive, but it bought me a few years of fun research," Shulgin said. He knew exactly what he wanted to work on: psychedelic drugs—"treasures," he believed, for providing access to our interior worlds.

Using the mescaline molecule as a jumping-off point, over the next thirty years Shulgin would go on to make more than two hundred novel chemical substances. "It was not profound chemistry—lots of chemists could have done the same thing," said Solomon Snyder, a neuroscientist at the Johns Hopkins School of Medicine, who became friends with Shulgin in the 1960s. "But nobody had done it before, and he did it in great depth because he loved drugs."

In the tradition of scientists of yore, Shulgin investigated his creations' effects by first testing them on himself, starting at extremely low doses and working his way up. "It saves a lot of mice and dogs, believe me," he quipped. If a material proved interesting, he would introduce it to his wife, Ann, and to a research group composed of nine to eleven trusted friends, including scientists, psychologists, and others with ample experience in psychotropic drugs.

Compared to previous research on psychedelics in the 1940s and 1950s, this approach was unique not only in that it wasn't being done behind closed doors but also because the Shulgins and their friends were primarily interested in "taking these substances to flourish," said Erika Dyck, a historian at the University of Saskatchewan and author of *Psychedelic Psychiatry*. "It's a distinction from taking drugs to treat or address something we might think of as a deficit or something missing. They were taking them just to be more, or to be better than."

As his psychic explorations deepened, Shulgin became "completely convinced that there is a wealth of information built into us, with miles of intuitive knowledge tucked away in the genetic material of every one of our cells." Access to the interior universe is normally barred, however, for those who haven't devoted a lifetime to meditation or other practices for reaching transcendence. The gift of psychedelic drugs, Shulgin recognized, is that they give anyone a clear route of entry to the fathoms of the mind—an expressway to the profound that may lend answers to the deepest questions of existence, selfhood, and consciousness. It really is all in our heads, though: it's up to the individual to choose whether to use such drugs as mere entertainment, or as keys for unlocking cryptic realms of being and meaning.

Shulgin liked to joke that out of the hundreds of mind-altering drugs he sampled, cheap red wine was his favorite. A fast talker with a high-pitched voice and hypomanic energy, he was equally at ease discussing science and chemistry or philosophy and literature—a true Renaissance man, his friends like to say. He also loved a good wordplay. Many who knew him still groan when recalling his famously over-the-top puns, naughty limericks, and cheesy jokes. As one classic Sashaism went, "Do you know how an orchestra and a bull are the opposite of one another? With a bull, the horns are in the front and the asshole is in the back!"

For decades the Shulgins were at the center of a thriving West Coast community of like-minded intellectuals, eccentrics, healers, and artists. Their potluck Friday-night dinners (aka FNDs) and Easter and Fourth of July parties attracted the likes of Terence McKenna, Carl Sagan, Daniel Ellsberg, and Ram Dass. But Sasha and Ann were equally happy hobnobbing with novices as with luminaries. "I brought my girlfriend out to one of the parties and Sasha went into this whole lecture for her about how music and chemistry are the same," said organic chemist David Carlson. "She was blown away."

"It was like some humble, privileged family—we felt among the chosen," wrote William Leonard Pickard, an author and chemist who wound up serving twenty years in prison for synthesizing LSD. "The faces, it seemed sometimes, were those of poor children around their first Christmas tree."

"It was another world," added David Nichols, a medicinal chemist and pharmacologist who often collaborated with Shulgin, and who was based at Purdue University in Indiana for the majority of his career. "Imagine being in the middle of the corn fields and then going to the Bay Area where all these people are New Agey and hugging a lot."

By the mid-1960s the political climate was shifting, and Shulgin's bosses at Dow were no longer comfortable being associated with the prolific synthesis of mind-altering drugs. "If I was CEO of a big chemical company and I had someone popping pills, I'd be a little nervous about that, too," Snyder said. "Sasha Shulgin was doing what he does, and top management at Dow decided, 'Yeah, well, this is all interesting, but we can't do this.' "

"I worked for ten years before they finally realized the area I was really interested in, which is drugs that affect the human mind, was further and further from what they wanted to go into," Shulgin concurred. He left his job and set up a backyard lab at his twenty acres of property on Shulgin Road, fondly referred to then and now as the Farm. He enrolled in two years of medical school and postgraduate studies in psychiatry only so he could better understand how drugs affect the central nervous system, and then set off into the trepidatious world of freelancing.

Shulgin never sold any of his creations for money. Instead, he paid the bills by lecturing at UC Berkeley, Stanford, UCSF, and other universities. He also consulted, including for the government. This delicate balancing act would eventually lead him to cooperate closely with the U.S. Drug Enforcement Administration (DEA), analyzing samples picked up on the street and sometimes serving as an expert witness at trials. The government showed its appreciation by giving Shulgin a Schedule I license that allowed him to work with the most tightly regulated substances.

Shulgin's ties to the DEA were more than just professional. "One of our best friends was a top official in the DEA," Ann Shulgin told me, referring to Bob Sager, the former head of the administration's Western Laboratory. Sager was a young chemist when he met Shulgin, "gung ho [about] working with the government and doing some good," he said in a documentary interview. (Sager passed away sometime after 2010.) He was especially motivated, he said, to take down amateur drug producers who didn't know their way around a lab, and who created dangerous or even deadly substances as a result. "We really had some dummies, oh man, total idiots trying to cook drugs," Sager said, shaking his head.

Above all, though, Sager loved chemistry, and he found a kindred spirit in Shulgin. The two spent many a Sunday holed up in Shulgin's backyard lab, geeking out over the latest synthesis. Sager quickly grew to hold a special place in Sasha and Ann's life. He even had the honor of officiating their surprise wedding, held at the couple's Fourth of July party in 1981. "Bob Sager gave the most beautiful Native American marriage ceremony," recalled George Greer, the medical director of the Heffter Research Institute in Santa Fe.

"They were like brothers," Ann added. "That relationship was frowned on by the DEA."

*

SHULGIN APPROACHED MDMA as he would any other drug: starting at low doses and working his way up. At 120 milligrams, he began to experience an effect—one he most definitely enjoyed. As usual, while high, he took notes: "I feel absolutely clean inside, and there is nothing but pure euphoria. I have never felt so great, or believed this to be possible." On another trip of the same dose, he was equally impressed. "Everyone must get to experience a profound state like this," he gushed. "I feel totally peaceful. I have lived all my life to get here, and I feel I have come home. I am complete."

Reflecting on these experiences after coming down, Shulgin found the word *window* kept coming to mind. MDMA, he later wrote, "enabled me to see outside without distortion or reluctance, and to look inside myself." Echoing Carl Resnikoff's observation, Shulgin realized that MDMA was something different; it definitely was not in the same category as other conventional psychedelics like mescaline and LSD. "This substance stimulated but was not a stimulant; it disinhibited without being an intoxicant; it helped to express feelings and emotions more freely, but without impairing self-control," Shulgin puzzled. "And it smelled like 'snake oil,' i.e., those miracle drugs that used to be sold at fairs."

MDMA was so mellow, in fact, that Shulgin decided to bring it along on the Reno Fun Train one Friday night with his then wife, Nina, and another couple. In the bar car, over a tray of shellfish and avocado, Shulgin asked if anyone would mind if he drank "from a small ampoule instead of the martini bottle." Nina—who was "generally uncomfortable with drugs, but elated with alcohol," as Shulgin put it—didn't mind, and neither did their friends. The "pleasant lightness of spirit" brought on by the MDMA so closely matched the alcohol-induced intoxication of Shulgin's companions that they forgot entirely that he was using something other than vodka, Shulgin wrote. "The slight disinhibition of alcohol—it locked right into that."

Henceforth, Shulgin often compared MDMA's effects to "a low calorie martini." In 1978 he and collaborator David Nichols published a paper reflecting this sentiment—and reporting in the literature for the first time MDMA's effects in humans: "an easily controlled altered state of consciousness with emotional and sensual overtones."

But as Shulgin continued to gain more experience with MDMA, he began to sense that there might be more to this material than light, tipsy fun. In one instance, he shared MDMA with a "sensitive and realistic" couple he knew, both pharmacologists from Germany. A few weeks earlier, the husband had had "an extraordinarily complex and difficult" experience with LSD, Shulgin described, and was still struggling to process what he had been through. Remembering the "window" analogy, Shulgin suggested they take MDMA together. Over the course of just a few hours, the man resolved the trauma around his LSD experience and emerged from the MDMA high, in his words, as "newborn."

"Possibly, I thought, MDMA was perfectly suitable for use in psychotherapy," Shulgin wrote after witnessing the man's recovery. "Again, [a] touch of those miracle cures."

Following this instinct, in 1977 Shulgin decided to introduce MDMA to Leo Zeff, a psychologist in Oakland whom Shulgin described as "everyone's idea of what a grandfather should be, both in looks and demeanor." A former Army Lieutenant Colonel, Zeff stood at just five foot six and was hardly ever seen without a beaming smile. He primarily practiced run-of-the-mill Jungian talk therapy, but on the side he also quietly held underground psychedelic-assisted sessions. He'd overseen such trips for thousands of people, individually and in groups.

Now in his seventies, Zeff was planning on retiring and was clearing out his office. He asked Shulgin to drop by to see if he'd like any of the unusual knickknacks he had gathered on his travels around the world. Shulgin, however, had brought along an unusual curio of his own.

"Leo, I think this is something that might interest you," he said, handing his old friend a small bottle. The drug inside, he explained, was like MDA, but with "a special magic, which just might catch [your] attention. Give it a try."

Zeff sighed. "I'm getting too old for this."

"Just give it a try."

Zeff wouldn't commit. If he did get around to trying it, he said, he'd let Shulgin know.

A few days later, Shulgin's phone rang. It was Zeff. He'd tried the drug, and he was abandoning his plans for a quiet retirement. He had work to do.

*

MDMA WAS NOT the first mind-altering drug to catch the attention of the medical establishment. Immediately following Albert Hofmann's discovery of LSD, psychiatrists were intrigued. "People are intrinsically interested in drugs that alter in so dramatic a fashion how one perceives the world," Shulgin's friend Solomon Snyder said. "You've gotta be pretty boring not to be curious."

Some mainstream doctors originally viewed LSD as a tool for inducing temporary psychosis and for studying the biochemical basis of disorders like schizophrenia. "Psychedelics were awfully important to the creation of the field of psychopharmacology in the 1950s," said David Healy, a psychiatrist and psychopharmacologist at McMaster University. "Back then, we thought we had the key to working out what happens when people get mentally ill. But things didn't work out like that."

Soon psychiatrists began to see LSD, as well as mescaline and MDA, as potential tools—albeit imperfect ones—for enhancing psychotherapy, investigating the psyche, and (for some open-minded researchers) taking breaks from everyday existence. Inspired by this movement, in 1954 Aldous Huxley wrote about the need for "a new drug which will relieve and console our suffering species." Such a substance, he believed, should be potent in small doses, less toxic and socially harmful than things like alcohol and cocaine, and not addictive. And importantly, "it should produce changes in consciousness more interesting, more intrinsically valuable than mere sedation or dreaminess, delusions of omnipotence or release from inhibition."

Huxley seemed to be conjuring MDMA into being, but he died a few years too early to get to sample that molecule himself. Yet in the intervening two decades between Huxley penning his wish list for the perfect drug and Shulgin introducing MDMA to Zeff, a vibrant community of researchers began investigating LSD and, to a lesser extent, MDA as therapeutic tools.

The world's first public LSD clinic opened in 1953 in England, quickly followed by others in Europe and North America. Between 1950 and 1965, some *forty thousand* patients received LSD treatment for everything from obsessive-compulsive disorder and depression to relief from chronic pain or social anxiety in autistic people. More than a thousand scientific papers were published about LSD, and much of that research was federally funded. As observed by Stanislav Grof, a Czech psychiatrist who was at the helm of LSD research at the time, the potential significance of psychedelic materials for psychiatry was beginning to seem "comparable to the value the microscope has for biology and medicine, or the telescope has for astronomy."

LSD seemed well on its way to becoming a mainstream pharmaceutical, but in the early 1960s the drug began running into regulatory hitches. In 1962 Congress enacted new rules making it mandatory to prove the safety and efficacy of any new commercial drug. The rules also required that a drug be approved only to treat a specific diagnosis.

LSD, however, was not a typical pharmaceutical, and did not neatly fit these narrow requirements. In pharmacological talk, it was "nonspecific": it could not be taken to dependably relieve a certain symptom, and the experience itself could be wildly varied. As the Food and Drug Administration saw it, pharmaceuticals "are like a Big Mac hamburger—you want the same hamburger every time," Healy said. "But psychedelics don't produce the same outcome even in the same person every time." Most doctors were also highly resistant to the idea promoted by Grof and others that LSD could be used for the betterment of well people who had no specific ailment to treat. Given these complications, the FDA deemed LSD an "experimental drug," restricting its use solely to research.

Heaped atop this shift in regulatory practices was LSD's increasingly central role in the counterculture of the 1960s. Liberation of consciousness went hand in hand with political activism and rejection of mainstream culture, which hippies (and later yippies) associated with racism, repression, materialism, and the Vietnam War. Young people wanted a new way of seeing and being in the world, and LSD offered a means of turbocharging their departure from the norm.

Because drug taking and antiwar activism were so thoroughly blended, however, politicians and others invested in maintaining the status quo—and the war in Vietnam—found a convenient target they could use to attack the counterculture: LSD. Lyndon Johnson and others in power began branding LSD a dangerous drug that causes users to lose their minds, effectively undermining the credibility of groups opposed to the war. The government also aggressively promoted claims, later proved false, that LSD damages chromosomes. As one 1967 scientific editorial direly warned, "a decision today [to use LSD] may very well be reflected by the biologic fitness of the next generation." In other words, LSD users were portrayed as literally risking the future of humanity.

Additionally, according to Grof, the "Dionysian elements" of the psychedelic experience made it all too easy to present these drugs as threats to "the Puritanical values" of American society. The fact that a drug could bestow users with excessive amounts of pleasure apparently rubbed many Americans the wrong way, tapping into "the haunting fear that someone, somewhere, may be happy," as the journalist H. L. Mencken once wrote of Puritanism. Describing psychedelic drugs, one politically influential scientist of the time captured this hand-wringing sentiment: "We should not forget to assess the cost of sustained euphoria or pleasure states. We can seriously wonder if man is built to endure more than a brief chemically induced glimpse of paradise."

In 1965 Congress passed the Drug Abuse Control Amendment, banning the use and sale of LSD, peyote, mescaline, and several other substances. "Let us never forget that this is just one part of our effort to protect society from this threat," Johnson declared of the new restrictions. "The real answer—the final answer—lies in the education of our children." As Johnson's presidency came to an end, Richard Nixon readily took up the antidrug political baton and successfully campaigned on a promise of bringing "law and order" back to America. Famously declaring drug abuse to be "public enemy number one in the United States," Nixon rallied the country for a national and international "all-out offensive" against drugs.

This wasn't the first time that the United States had pledged "relentless warfare" on drugs. "Draconian drug laws had existed for decades," pointed out Matthew Oram, a historian of medicine and author of *The Trials of Psychedelic Therapy*. One of the country's most significant turning points for the politicization of drug regulation had come decades earlier, in the 1930s, when Harry Anslinger, head of the newly created Federal Bureau of Narcotics, set his sights on outlawing marijuana. As with Johnson's targeting of LSD, marijuana itself wasn't really driving Anslinger's crusade. Instead, it was his prejudice against "the two most-feared groups in the United States—Mexican immigrants and African Americans," reported journalist Johann Hari in *Chasing the Scream*. Anslinger chose to attack marijuana in particular, Hari wrote, because he perceived people of color to be "taking the drug much more than white people." Ignoring the protests of doctors and scientists, Anslinger claimed in the press that marijuana caused people to go insane and to kill, and that it drove Black men to lust after white women. Cocaine, heroin, and opiates soon joined the list of pharmaceutical excuses used to target minority populations, including Chinese immigrants.

The nation's history of racist drug campaigns cannot be solely pinned on Anslinger, though. It was the fears and prejudices of the American public, Hari pointed out, that enabled and supported Anslinger in these efforts. A devout Christian, Anslinger further won over the American public by presenting the drug issue as tantamount to a holy war—a legacy that would endure for decades. "A lot of law enforcement people think this is literally a war between good and evil, and they're supporting Christian ideology," said Keeper Trout, an independent scholar and author in Northern California. "This is something that's run through the thread of prohibition since the beginning. It was always about salvation of the human soul by removing this impediment of drugs."

From its outset, then, the war on drugs has been a war on minority communities and others whose interests do not align with those in power, propped up by the American public's prejudice and gullibility. Nixon only continued this tradition. Years after his presidency ended, John Ehrlichman, Nixon's former domestic policy advisor and a key architect of the war on drugs, spelled out this connection for the journalist Dan Baum. The Nixon administration "had two enemies: the antiwar left and black people," Ehrlichman said. Linking hippies with marijuana and Black people with heroin allowed the administration to heavily criminalize and disrupt those communities. "Did we know we were lying about the drugs? Of course we did."

In 1970 Congress passed the Controlled Substances Act to bring all "drugs of abuse" under one regulatory framework. In doing so, the federal government created "a far more powerful administrative regulatory apparatus than would have been imaginable twenty, perhaps even ten years earlier," wrote historian Joseph Spillane. The Controlled Substances Act categorized drugs into five "schedules" depending on their abuse potential, safety, and medical value. Federal authorities placed LSD and MDA into Schedule I, the most strictly controlled category, reserved for substances with the greatest abuse potential and no accepted medical use.

The Nixon administration gave the Justice Department almost complete authority to determine whether a drug should be controlled and into which schedule it should be placed. Scientists feared—correctly, it turned out—that this new system would stifle research. Stanley Yolles, director of the National Institute of Mental Health, went so far as to resign in protest against the Justice Department's encroachment into research. The voices of disgruntled scientists—as well as those of other experts who warned that bans would only spur the growth of illicit markets and harm public health—were drowned out by mainstream media hysteria and politicization of the drug issue.

By the time the Controlled Substances Act formally passed, though, the political winds had already shifted years before to the intensely antidrug, and the once-thriving field of LSD research had virtually ceased to exist. The end result was "a tragic loss for psychiatry, psychology and psychotherapy," Grof lamented—a waste of "what was probably the single most important opportunity in the history of these disciplines."

*

AFTER THE CRACKDOWN, most psychedelic-assisted therapists gave up on their practices and returned to the mainstream. Some, however, like Zeff, continued to work underground with forbidden "medicines," as Zeff preferred to call psychedelic drugs. Depending on the client, Zeff used LSD, MDA, or a number of other substances. In extreme cases he turned to the tremendously powerful plant-derived material ibogaine. In 1988, at Zeff's funeral, Terence McKenna declared that Zeff had been "the chief of a secret tribe." Henceforth Zeff was referred to as the "secret chief" among the group of 150 or so underground therapists he had mentored. Risking their reputations, their practices, and even their freedom, Zeff and those who followed his lead "decided not to sacrifice the well-being of [their clients] to scientifically unsubstantiated legislation," Grof wrote.

Zeff counted on a series of referrals and rules to keep himself and his clients safe from the law. But in *The Secret Chief Revealed*—an extended interview with Zeff, whose real name was printed posthumously—he admits to many sleepless nights spent thinking "What are you exposing yourself to all this shit for?" Invariably, though, by the morning, he'd recall all the fantastic results he'd seen in so many clients, and resolve once again that it was worth the risk.

MDMA was unlike any of the other medicines Zeff had ever worked with. He was "completely enraptured" by the effects, according to Ann Shulgin, and became "a proselytizer of MDMA in psychotherapy," as Torsten Passie put it.

"I kept him supplied with the drug and he went out and supplied the Western world with the experience itself," Shulgin said. "That was the blossoming of its use in psychotherapy."

Over the span of a few years Zeff spread the gospel of MDMA to hundreds of fellow therapists in North America and Europe—almost certainly changing the course of the drug's history. As neuroscientist Matthew Baggott noted, "I think it was inevitable that MDMA was going to become a popular drug. I don't think it was inevitable that it would be used in therapy. That was really Shulgin saying, 'Hey Leo, why don't you try this?' "

MDMA puzzled many of those who encountered it who, like Shulgin, couldn't quite decide if it was a psychedelic or not. Later Ralph Metzner, an early scholar of psychedelics, proposed calling it an "empathogen," the Greek word for "generating a feeling within" (and related to the word *empathy*). Nichols thought *empathogen* sounded too close to *pathogen*, however, and suggested instead *entactogen*—a mishmash of Greek and Latin meaning "producing touching from within." Debates over MDMA's nomenclature and proper classification continue today. But through the late 1970s and early

1980s, Zeff just called the drug Adam, a near-anagram he coined to refer to the more innocent and primordial state that MDMA seems to return the mind to, free from feelings of guilt, shame, and unworthiness.

"The profound simplicity of the Adam state is striking," Metzner and Sophia Adamson write in *Ecstasy: The Complete Guide*. "People often express this in the form of apparently banal statements—such as that one only needs love and all else falls into place."

Adam quickly became the most popular medicine at Zeff's group retreats of twelve to fifteen people, which he hosted one weekend or so a month. Zeff had certain rules that everyone who took part in the group experiences had to agree to: No physical harm to yourself or others. No sexual contact with other participants. No leaving the premises while high. If Zeff tells you to stop doing something, stop doing it. And finally, what happens in group experiences stays in group experiences—unless everyone who was present gives their permission to speak to an outsider about it.

People would arrive on Friday evening at a big house in the Bay Area, checking in first with Zeff for a private interview. Based on his determination of where they were at mentally, he would select from a menu of substances he had on hand. MDA was an option, but it became less favored as soon as MDMA entered the scene. People would take their assigned medicine late Friday night, and Zeff and his colleagues would be on hand all evening to assist with bathroom breaks, if needed, or difficult moments. Crucially, someone was assigned at all times to keep the records playing.

"The MDMA people liked to get up and do some hugging," Zeff recalled. "They'll call us over just for a big hug. They're so full of love, it's really fantastically beautiful."

By Saturday evening, everyone would be sobered up and the end of the experience would be officially marked with champagne. People would share with the group what they learned before parting ways.

Zeff eventually tapered the group sessions off in the interest of spending more time training therapists to use MDMA. One of the first people he taught was a young psychiatrist named George Greer. Zeff and Greer had met several years earlier when they happened to room together at a six-week workshop Grof led at the Esalen Institute in Big Sur. It was an auspicious place for them to meet. Founded in 1962 by two Stanford graduates, Esalen had become a hub for those interested in exploring consciousness and individual fulfill-ment. The sweeping 120-acre campus had been a nexus for the countercul-ture movement of the 1960s and later a center for scientific and spiritual seminars, research, and workshops aimed at fostering social change and helping both individuals and humanity realize their potential. In a testament to the center's cultural importance, the final episode of *Mad Men* features Don Draper at a fictional Esalen—albeit fulfilling his calling as ad man rather than enlightened student of the universe.

Requa Greer, a psychiatric nurse who was dating George Greer at the time and is now married to him, also learned MDMA-assisted therapy directly from Zeff. As Requa recalled, Zeff "told us he'd come across a new material that was quote-unquote 'really good for therapy.' "

After being briefed by Zeff, the Greers decided to test the new medicine on themselves. They found it to be unparalleled in its ability to open up inti-mate communication and for genuinely seeking and giving forgiveness. "We had our own experience of 'Oh, hey, were you angry with me when that happened?' 'Oh, yes I was.' 'Do you forgive me for it?' 'Yes, I do,' " Requa said. Once forgiveness for an incident in question was issued, she added, that was it—it was truly forgiven.

Communication around normally difficult subjects wasn't the drug's only strength. There was also sheer euphoria. As Requa put it, "You just feel good, you feel so good!" Love, she emphasized, was at the center of that feeling. "At first, we kept saying, 'Oh, this makes us feel love,' " Requa recalled. "But in the middle, I said, 'No, this is love! We are love!' What a relief, to suddenly know not just that God is love, but to know that love is what we're made of, love is our basic stuff."

"There really was no psychoactive drug known at that time even remotely like this," George added. "It was just a completely unique compound."

Zeff suggested that the couple connect with the Shulgins, and Sasha and Ann were more than receptive: they invited Requa and George to come over to meet them and take MDMA together. Not surprisingly, they all hit it off, and soon after, George made a batch of MDMA with Shulgin.

He and Requa began administering MDMA to "healthy normals," as they called them—people without diabetes, high blood pressure, or a history of serious mental health issues. Sessions were held either at the Greer's house—which Requa always made sure had fresh-cut flowers—or at the subject's home. Following Zeff's lead, the Greers did not try to direct the conversation or journey. Mostly they just sat quietly with subjects and watched over them as they reclined on a bed or sofa, listening to music with eyeshades on and doing their own internal work. Afterward they would talk through the experience to help the subjects integrate what they had learned.

In total, the Greers treated around eighty people over the course of a few years. Their subjects—who had been asked to fast for six hours ahead of time—took doses of MDMA ranging from 50 to 200 milligrams, but mostly in the 125 milligrams range. Often they also took a second 50 milligrams "booster" around the two-hour mark. Each session would last about six hours, and some people would come back for multiple sessions spaced weeks or months apart. In some early trials the Greers occasionally took a little MDMA with their subjects as a way to build trust, but they soon decided that this got in the way of being alert to the needs of the person they were watching over.

People came to them for all sorts of reasons. A forty-year-old woman experiencing "sadness at being alone," according to their notes, initially told them she believed she might never love anyone as deeply as she had loved her former boyfriend. During her session, she allowed herself "to cry my heart out," as she put it, and was surprised by "how healthy it felt to know that I'd really been there for those feelings, rather than the facade [of] trying to be strong and get on with my life and unconsciously avoid the pain." After three sessions, she told the Greers that she felt open to the possibility of a new relationship, but more than that, she now believed "that I can make myself happy."

A couple in their twenties, on the other hand, wanted to try MDMA "just to talk and think [and] have fun together," the wife said. During the session, the wife noted that "free thoughts escape under a euphoric cloud that makes it ok to say anything and everything." She and her husband left with a renewed commitment to communication, something "so, so valuable to a relationship," she said. Still other subjects were able to let go of the fear of their parents dying; to reconnect with their belief in God; to work through their sexual inhibitions; and to be more purposeful about how and with whom they chose to spend their time ("I don't put up with superficial cocktail parties [anymore]," one woman reported several months after her session).

"The molecule is so generous, it comes in and goes, 'What do you need? Oh, you need this? Let's go in that direction,' " Requa said. "It's a gift."

"Anything that psychotherapy is useful for, I think MDMA would be useful for, too," George added.

Intriguingly, people also sometimes reported physical improvements that accompanied their mental epiphanies. One person's chronic back pain cleared up, while another experienced some relief for the arthritis in her hands. No serious side effects occurred, but people did frequently report mild symptoms like teeth grinding, jaw tension, nausea, lack of appetite, feeling cold or shaky, and experiencing fatigue the next day.

MDMA was not a miracle cure. In a peer-reviewed study that George and Requa later published, they were careful to point out that the drug should not be promoted "as a social or psychological panacea." While all of their subjects experienced some benefits, the treatment had limitations that varied on an individual basis. As one woman told the Greers in a follow-up interview, "It was a pleasant experience, but it hasn't changed my life. I'm still a perfectionist."

*

MOST PEOPLE DOING MDMA-assisted therapy in the late 1970s and early 1980s seemed to be seeking various forms of self-improvement. For some, though, the treatment provided a more serious service: helping to resolve decades-old traumas. Bob Sager, the DEA agent who Shulgin was friends with, for example, was given MDMA by a psychiatrist he had started seeing for depression. Under the influence of the drug, he retrieved a repressed memory of the ceiling of his elementary school collapsing on him when he was in first grade. The plaster hit the child in front of Sager on the head, killing the boy and trapping Sager at his desk. As all the other children ran out of the room, screaming, Sager remained behind, unable to move and covered in his classmate's blood. "Oh, what a feeling," he recalled. After two sessions of MDMA-assisted therapy, he was able to get rid of "that trapped feeling" he had carried around since the incident. "Man, it totally changed my life."

Naomi Fiske, an ordained minister and psychotherapist in Santa Fe, goes so far to credit MDMA-assisted therapy with saving her life.

Naomi was born in a displaced persons camp in Germany, where her Romanian mother and Hungarian father, both Jewish Holocaust survivors, met. When she was three months old, her family left Europe to start a new life, eventually landing in Hollywood, Florida. Her parents' trauma did not respect geographic boundaries, however. They never spoke of the war, but it cast a constant shadow—one that Naomi at first did not understand, but could not avoid.

Her mother cried easily, often for no apparent reason. She always kept the blinds down and had marks on her hands from her nails constantly digging into her clenched fists. To manage her anxiety, she spent hours picking up tiny pieces of lint off the carpet. "My mother was so disassociated and fragmented that she couldn't really display affection," Naomi said. As for her father, he had an explosive, at times violent temper. He was more affectionate, Naomi said, "but his rage scared me."

Naomi spent as much time as she could at friends' houses, and as soon as she turned eighteen she left home to study in New York City. She felt drawn to work with dying people and started training in hospice. Up until that point in her life, Naomi had considered herself "a normal kid." But one evening at a retreat on death and dying, she was shown a video of concentration camps being liberated, and she felt something within herself go off-kilter. In tears, she tried to put words to what she was feeling, telling a mentor at the time, "I don't know my history, but I know I carry some of this." She attempted to put the experience behind her, but "that was the beginning, really," she said of her gradual downward spiral.

Naomi moved to Santa Fe for work and married a young holistic practitioner named Richard. But after the honeymoon phase, she began feeling inexplicably afraid of Richard, and her desire to be intimate with him faded. She had a short affair with another man, and after that began a longer affair with her tennis instructor, a woman. "She was flirting with me on the tennis court, and I liked it," Naomi said. Being with the woman made Naomi feel invigorated, empowered, and alive, but as things intensified, she began to feel like she was spinning out of control. She didn't know if she was straight or gay, if she loved Richard or wanted out. Naomi had always been healthy, but she developed asthma and had to start carrying an inhaler. At times she would be racked with tsunamis of grief that seemed to rise up out of nowhere. "I'd just be walking into the gym, and suddenly I'd be in a fetal position and have to go back into the car and just cry," she said. "I was falling apart."

Richard, who knew about the affair with the woman, was miserable, too. In 1984, when a colleague introduced him to a therapist in Oklahoma who used MDMA in her practice and who was willing to travel to Santa Fe, Richard suggested that he and Naomi try the drug together under the therapist's supervision.

The first trip helped Naomi clearly recognize the underlying drivers behind her feelings and behavior. She realized that she had been projecting her mother—and her yearning for her mother's love—onto the woman she was having an affair with, and projecting onto Richard her fear of her father. More than that, she saw that she had been carrying her parents' bottled trauma and pain, which they had never faced themselves and passed on to their daughter as a result. "All our acting out is because we're not integrating with whatever our deepest feelings are," Naomi said. "It goes on and on, generation after generation."

The MDMA, she continued, gave her the insight to break that cycle. It allowed her to be with the pain, transforming it into a liberating rather than oppressive force. This wasn't a one-and-done experience, though. For two years Naomi did an MDMA-assisted therapy session every two months—a regimen that was definitely too frequent, she now realizes. "Some of my most powerful journeys were going into the trauma of what my parents must have witnessed or known about," she said. "On one of those journeys, I actually smelled the gas, and I thought I was going to die. In another, I went down this vortex and I could hear people's screams and cries."

In what was perhaps her most powerful therapeutic session with MDMA, Naomi realized that her asthma—this new inability to breathe—was connected to a deep-seated conviction that she did not have the right to be alive when so many others had died in the Holocaust. Yet dying now, she realized, would dishonor those who did not make it and whose legacies she now kept alive. She opened her heart to her relatives and all the others who were murdered in the camps, and felt their light coming through her. "That was really the epitome of liberating myself from my past," she said. Her asthma never came back.

"This medicine gives us the capacity, the strength, the courage, to be willing to feel our pain and know that love holds us through it," Naomi said. "To me, that is the greatest gift of this substance."

*

ZEFF AND HIS fellow therapist converts to MDMA had no idea how this new medicine produced such stunning results. All they knew was that it seemed to catalyze mental breakthroughs that normally would take months, years, or even a lifetime of traditional therapy to achieve. Some mental health practitioners even ventured that MDMA could be the ideal substance long sought by Huxley and others—the medicine to "relieve and console our suffering species."

As stories like Naomi's poured in, though, enthusiasm was tainted by worry. Ronald Reagan had just taken office and had vowed to reignite Nixon's war on drugs. In the current feverishly antidrug climate, Zeff and others feared that should word about MDMA get out, the molecule would succumb to the same fate as LSD and MDA before it: federally blacklisted, banned from legal therapeutic practice, and all but impossible for scientists to work with. So they vowed to keep their practice a secret, avoiding media attention and doing what they could to ensure MDMA stayed safely confined within the walls of the therapist's office. As Ann Shulgin said, "MDMA is penicillin for the soul, and you don't give up penicillin, once you've seen what it can do."

Their concern, it turned out, was very much warranted.

# "Y'ALL DO X?"

MONICA GREENE ARRIVED at the Starck Club to find a line stretching around the block. Am I in Dallas, she thought, or at Studio 54? The hulking former warehouse had been difficult to find, concealed beneath a freeway overpass in a desolate part of the city that, until the club's arrival, hardly anyone came to. Now it seemed like everyone from Big D was here, vying to get through the door.

When Monica finally got to the front of the line, the stern French door-woman, Edwige Belmore—a figurehead of punk culture in Paris and New York City—looked her up and down. Monica felt incredibly nervous, not because she was afraid of getting turned away but because this was the first time she had ever been out in public as Monica. This was 1984, and it was against the law in Dallas to cross-dress. Monica—who was born Eduardo—also had a lot to lose personally. Eduardo had a family and had built a successful business in Dallas after moving there from Mexico City. Being seen as Monica "would have just ruined me at that time," she said. Yet living life as Eduardo was becoming increasingly intolerable, and Monica felt that it was now a matter of survival to explore who she really was. And the Starck Club, she'd heard, was the perfect venue for doing so.

Monica's Donna Karan miniskirt, shoulder-padded blouse, and strappy heels apparently met with Belmore's approval. Stepping through the vault-like entrance, she found a scene that seemed to channel Sodom and Gomorrah, before divine wrath. Two palatial staircases led down from a columned entryway to a sunken dance floor where writhing bodies moved like a single organism to pumping, infectiously catchy New Wave beats. Sheer curtains half concealed white couches holding couples "acting out their desires, with no regrets, no apologies," Monica recalled. The bathrooms, which were unisex—the first Monica or the city of Dallas had ever seen—were the site of equally jaw-dropping shenanigans.

The lack of inhibitions wasn't the only notable feature of the Starck crowd. There was also a level of diversity seen nowhere else in the Bible Belt. "No one cared if you were Mexican, Black, Jewish, gay, transgender, whatever," Monica said. "The Starck club provided an incredible opportunity for people like myself to express themselves, and that's so important if you've never been accepted."

The social lubricant that fueled this radical temple of acceptance was not alcohol or cocaine but Ecstasy—lots and lots of Ecstasy. "You have to remember, it was legal at the time," Monica said. "You could go to your favorite bartender and order a beer and an Ecstasy." She estimates that on any given night, 70 to 90 percent of Starck patrons were rolling, the colloquial term for Ecstasy's blissed-out high. "The kaleidoscope of emotions that brought on was incredible," Monica said. "It elevated people mentally, they were always happy. And the dancing was never ending."

The Starck Club's creators had set out to make the best club in the world, and for the five years the venue was open, it just might have been. Grace Jones and Stevie Nicks performed on opening night, immediately turning the club into a destination for people flying in from out of state or even out of country. Tom Cruise, Owen Wilson, Timothy Leary, Jack Nicholson, Allen Ginsberg, Andy Warhol, and Jean-Michel Basquiat—not to mention George W. Bush—all partied there, along with some thousand to fifteen hundred people every Friday and Saturday night.

"They didn't close," said Michael Cain, director of *The Starck Club*, a documentary film about the venue. "They'd quit serving alcohol at two A.M., but by that point you didn't need the alcohol. You might need another hit of E."

Ecstasy found its way to the Starck Club within a week of opening night, when the DJ Kerry Jaggers, a native Texan, brought a fist-sized sandwich bag of pills down with him from New York City. "Just give them out," he told one of the owners, handing her the bag. "Let people try them!"

Within a few months, "Y'all do X?" became a common refrain on the dance floor. Someone called the owners, offering to supply them with wholesale tablets at seven dollars a pop, which they could resell for twenty dollars. They passed on getting officially involved, but they turned a blind eye to bartenders who would slide tablets under napkins, or cigarette girls who would tuck pills into matchbooks.

"It set the club off," Cain said. "To have everybody in a room loving each other, it just began the fame of the club."

Whether it was the Starck Club itself or the Ecstasy consumed there that created this special moment in Dallas's history was a chicken-or-the-egg question, Monica said. But the club—and, by extension, the drug—"certainly helped Dallas become the city it is today," she said. The nights Monica spent there also helped her personally come into her own, giving her the first burst of confidence she needed to fully transition a few years later. She now owns the popular restaurant Monica's Mex-Tex Cantina, and in 2021 she was featured by *D Magazine* as one of the region's most influential business leaders, and after a long career as a restauranteur, she recently retired and now lives "blissfully" in a beachside town in Mexico, she said.

"The Starck Club showed us that Dallas was more generous than we thought it was, that it was not as segregated as we thought it was, and that it was full of opportunity," Monica said. "The perception of what a southern city was came tumbling down."

*

IN 1981 ANALYSIS Anonymous, a confidential mail-in drug testing service that provided results by answering machine, received the first sample ever submitted under the name Ecstasy. Until the early 1980s, MDMA had remained primarily in the realm of therapy and personal exploration by spiritually minded New Age types. These users tended to think of MDMA as a cherished and respected medicine, something to assist with transcendence, growth, and healing.

But as word spread, so did interest in more varied contexts—namely, partying. In 1987 Jerome Beck, now an independent drug researcher in

Portland, Oregon, and Marsha Rosenbaum, the director emerita of the Drug Policy Alliance's San Francisco office, secured a grant from the National Institute on Drug Abuse (NIDA) to put together the first ethnographic survey of MDMA users, which they later published in a book, *Pursuit of Ecstasy: The MDMA Experience.* Academic researchers normally struggle to recruit people willing to be interviewed about their drug use, but Beck and Rosenbaum easily found a hundred MDMA users eager to share their stories. As they wrote, "A surprisingly difficult part of this phase of research was having to turn people away. Users were often not only willing but anxious to express their opinions and feelings about MDMA."

In the late 1970s and early 1980s, MDMA, Beck and Rosenbaum learned, was popular among a number of diverse social groups and a wide array of professionals. Their sample included interviews with postal workers, jewelry designers, wine salespersons, physicians, carpenters, businesspersons, secretaries, teachers, and more. MDMA spread across college campuses, at first at schools typically associated with liberal values and then to more mainstream universities, where it became a staple of fraternities and sororities. The new drug also appealed to educated professionals in their thirties and forties looking for a taste of danger without the commitment or "fearsome existential challenges" of LSD, Beck and Rosenbaum wrote, as well as to those simply seeking for a break from the norm. As Gail, a busy thirty-seven-year-old lawyer, told the two researchers, "It's like taking a vacation to Mexico for a week, only I'm going to do it in a day because that's all I've got." MDMA's popularity among middle-aged, upper-middle-class people like Gail soon earned the drug the nickname "the yuppie psychedelic."

Gay clubgoers at places like the Saint in New York City had also readily adopted MDMA, frequently using it as a substitute for MDA. Somewhat counterintuitively, Deadheads constituted another early user group. Grateful Dead concerts had traditionally been associated with LSD, magic mushrooms, and marijuana, but MDMA—while not essential to the scene—became "a welcome latecomer to a time-tested menu of psychedelic options," Beck and Rosenbaum wrote. "L&M's"—a combination of LSD and MDMA, now known as candy flipping—became a new go-to cocktail for some Deadheads.

And then there was Dallas—a true mecca for Ecstasy in the early to mid-1980s. MDMA was popular among everyone from conservative Southern

Methodist University students to "flash and trash" socialites, as one user described her cohort—those riding the wave of the 1980s oil, airline, and real estate boom. Dancers at Dallas topless bars also turned to MDMA to help them accept some of their clients' "more gross behaviors and make more tips," as one interviewee explained, as did gay male sex workers for creating good vibes with johns.

For many otherwise square Dallas users, the fact that MDMA was legal and popular among their peers gave them permission to partake. Taking the drug became akin to drinking alcohol or smoking cigarettes—a mind-altering indulgence given a special carve-out. As one Sunday school teacher and former high school cheerleader who loved MDMA told Beck and Rosenbaum, "I never hung around with [drug-taking] people. Those were like scums. Those were like yuckies. . . . Drugs are wrong."

"It was a fascinating scene in Texas," Beck told me. "You had different user groups—cocaine-sniffing yuppies and otherwise fairly non-drug-using SMU students—who, once they tried Ecstasy, and found out it was legal, really made it take off there."

Conveniently, MDMA could often be paid for with a credit card. One record store that sold it on the side rang it up as "accessories." It was also available everywhere, from private "X parties" to spas that offered MDMA massages. Clubs and bars reigned supreme, though, as the venues of choice for taking Ecstasy. "Starck was one of a hundred clubs just in the Dallas–Forth Worth area that had Ecstasy being dealt in it," Cain said. "It could be a Western bar, a lesbian bar, a gay bar—every different kind of bar had their own unique experience with Ecstasy. Because of the legality of it, everybody was open to it."

Compared to therapeutic or spiritual users who were generally seeking something deeper from the MDMA experience, those in the Lone Star State overwhelmingly used Ecstasy for enjoyment. Rosenbaum wrote that she was particularly struck by the word choice of one Dallas interviewee: "It's fun," the woman told her. "[People] escape, they have fun, and they just, you know, it's a fun drug. It's not like cocaine where it's fun for twenty minutes and you have to do more. I mean, you get hours of fun."

Mixed in with all that fun, though, some Dallas revelers did experience "fortuitous therapy," as Beck and Rosenbaum put it. Under the influence of

MDMA, a thirty-six-year-old advertising executive, for example, realized that his marriage had fallen apart and "I had created this absolutely false life around myself." The drug caused him, for the first time, to take a close, honest look at the life he was living, and as a result he started to make changes to improve his health and well-being. Whether intentionally sought or not, this added layer of depth made MDMA more than just mindless pleasure for many people who took it. As Cain pointed out, "There's no one who's done cocaine or crystal meth who comes out of it and says 'I'm a better person for having done that!' "

\*

AS DEMAND FOR MDMA ramped up, so too did production. Chemists tended to serve specific crowds. Darrell Lemaire, for example, was a lanky cowboy type in Northern California who began producing MDMA after Sasha Shulgin told him about therapists in need. As reported by the journalist Hamilton Morris, Lamaire kept the therapeutic community supplied with wholesale-priced MDMA, which he produced by the hundreds of kilos in a secret lab that he built in the blasted-out center of a dormant volcano.

Another prominent early collective of MDMA chemists, the Boston Group, made more modestly sized batches of the drug for therapeutic, spiritual, and quiet recreational use. Producers like Lemaire and the Boston Group saw themselves as providing a vital service. As one psychiatrist cum MDMA distributor told Beck and Rosenbaum, "There are lots of places to chip at the great stone of uncaring, and this is where I chose to do my chipping."

Members of the Boston Group also sometimes brought MDMA along with them on trips to places like Thailand and Bali, helping to spread the word among a more international crowd. But they did not produce on demand, and "droughts" would regularly occur when members would take breaks for lengthy vacations abroad.

"It wasn't about making money, but about sharing a precious gift that had been bestowed on us," said Debby Harlow, a Bay Area therapist. She became involved in the MDMA-assisted therapeutic community in the early 1980s and would go on to serve as one of its key figures during a pivotal moment in the years to come. "In those days, 'one person touched two,' as one of the

Boston Group's distributors told me. But we all knew it could be taken away if someone got greedy and went into mass production, or if someone wound up in the hospital, as later happened with the rave scene. We did not want to repeat what happened with LSD, so we acted responsibly: limiting how much we distributed and to whom. The people I knew in those days made little to no money from selling MDMA, although in retrospect, many of us gained profound social capital."

Inevitably, though, there were also a number of MDMA dealers who emerged to cater to a more recklessly recreational clientele, and who were primarily motivated by money. In the Bay Area, Maria Mangini, a nurse practitioner and midwife who first got involved in the psychedelics scene in the 1960s, recalled "the Moon Man": an almost certainly autistic, "congenitally rebellious" chemist from a conservative family in the Midwest who became a major MDMA producer in the 1980s. Mangini knew another dealer, too, a domineering man who synthesized "a roomful of MDMA," she said, and who always referred to his henchmen as "dumbfucks." Exasperated, Mangini once asked him, "In your business, why do you think you'd find any smartfucks?"

Echoing disagreements among LSD distributors two decades before, tension flared between those who wanted to limit access to MDMA to "intelligent, responsible, educated" users, as Beck and Rosenbaum wrote, and those who thought it should be "spread to the masses."

"The difference between 'us and them' is that in our camp, you were usually initiated by a friend or your therapist: someone who cared about you and with whom you had an ongoing relationship," Harlow said. "It was a slowly growing social network of friends sitting for friends."

But that changed, she said, "with Texas"—more specifically, when a man named Michael Clegg got involved with MDMA.

The Texas Group, as Clegg's international Ecstasy business came to be known, was almost certainly the world's largest MDMA producer from the early 1980s to the early 1990s. Clegg and his colleagues dominated not only in the sheer quantity of MDMA they churned out but also in the flagrancy with which Clegg operated. As Harlow said, "Our group of therapeutic, spiritual, and quieter recreational users was at odds with Michael Clegg's vision, which was to 'go big' and build an empire."

Clegg turned down my request for an interview, replying by email, "I am about interviewed out. In the past six months I have spent countless days and hours in interviews for 3 books, 3 documentaries and 2 movies about my life." He did, however, reply to some limited questions for fact checking I sent him. In his response, he called one former colleague a "pathological liar" and outright denied even knowing another close former associate he most certainly *did* know, given that he assisted the government in indicting the man in the 1990s.

Clegg's responses weren't surprising; I'd been warned ahead of time that I should take anything out of his mouth with "a full shaker of salt, not a mere grain," as one person put it. "Pathological liar," "self-aggrandized," "delusional," and "idiot" were among the words that six former colleagues and acquaintances used to describe him to me.

"Seeker" was the word Clegg once used to describe himself, which he defined as "someone who is searching for the ultimate meaning of life." Raised in an Irish Catholic family in Chicago, Clegg decided in the eighth grade that he "wanted to somehow find God." In pursuit of this mission, he went into the Catholic seminary to live a life "of celibacy, poverty and obedience," as he would later recount to a federal judge. When God didn't appear to him in the seminary, he dropped out at the age of twenty-six.

Clegg claimed to have made a few million dollars when he was in his thirties on a security company venture. But he had a knack for spending money as quickly as he accrued it, and according to court records, he also earned two convictions for wire and securities fraud. Still seeking answers, he got into yoga and meditation. Clegg claims to have tried MDMA for the first time in 1978 or 1979, when he was forty years old. "My eyes opened up in a way I never imagined possible on the earth," Clegg later recalled of that first experience. "It was like Moses on the mountain, with the revelation."

Clegg sensed an opportunity—an altruistic one, he would later aver in court: "I finally had a way to help the whole world, and I was absolutely committed to doing that."

But he'd need assistance in seeing that vision through.

In 1983 a knock came to the door of a Mendocino County, California, resident named Bob McMillen. McMillen had "a bit of a reputation" in the area, as he explained to me. For one, he lived in a castle overlooking the ocean. He had also formerly run a major marijuana smuggling and distribution ring that brought billions of dollars' worth of weed into the United States, first from Mexico and then from Thailand.

The man at McMillen's door was Clegg. He told McMillen he'd moved to Mendocino three months earlier. He'd heard of Bob, and he was here to pitch him on a new drug he called Therapy. McMillen was immediately repulsed. He was hooked on cocaine at the time, and the last thing he needed, he told Clegg, was another drug. But Clegg kept pushing. He even claimed that Therapy could sever McMillen's relationship with coke. McMillen rolled his eyes and shooed Clegg off his property. But he did accept some reading material Clegg gave him about the drug.

Eventually McMillen wound up agreeing to Clegg's offer, partly because he seemed so sincere—and also because he just wouldn't leave McMillen alone. Clegg and his wife, Pauline, arrived at five o'clock one evening in a white BMW. The couple put on a new Deuter album called *Ecstasy* and draped a blanket over McMillen, who lay on the couch. "I was extremely dubious," he said. "I didn't take pills."

After about twenty minutes, McMillen felt a chill. Suddenly the music "lit up like nothing I'd imagined," he recalled. "I floated off in a wonderful euphoria for a while, then I threw the sheet off, sat up and said, 'Sold! How much can I get?' "

As McMillen came down, he told the Cleggs that he wanted to share this new drug with everyone he knew. "I hope you guys have a lot of it," he said. "You're gonna need a lot."

The next day, he experienced no urge to do cocaine—nor the following day, or the day after that. "I never touched cocaine again," McMillen said. "MDMA cured about twenty of my smuggling buddies who were all strung out on coke, too."

McMillen agreed to help put the new drug out on the street. "We sold billions of dollars of pot, so I already had the infrastructure," he said. But the first order of business, he insisted, was changing the drug's name. "'Therapy' will never sell," he told Clegg. He suggested Ecstasy, after the Deuter album. Clegg at first pooh-poohed the idea: he'd already printed labels for bottles of Therapy. But when McMillen sold five thousand pills in four days under the name Ecstasy, Clegg came around. So much so, in fact, that he would later claim that *he* was the one who came up with the name Ecstasy.

As he told *Playboy*, "It came to me: It was pure ecstasy." (When I told McMillen about Clegg trying to take credit for the name, McMillen just started laughing; when I asked Clegg about McMillen coming up with the name, Clegg insisted that he'd called it Ecstasy from the beginning, adding, "Bob McMillen was the biggest liar I ever knew.")

For a short time Clegg linked up with the Boston Group as their Southwest distributor. But he wasn't happy with how the Boston chemists were prone to falling off the radar, or how they wouldn't supply him with the massive quantities of MDMA that he wanted to sell. After he got his hands on the drug's chemical formula (he claimed to various people to have been given it or to have bought it; in fact, it was published in the scientific literature), he found his own chemists to produce the drug in California. Within weeks McMillen had distributed MDMA "coast to coast," he said. "This took off like an explosion."

When McMillen handed Clegg seventy-five thousand dollars after clearing twenty-five thousand pills in a week, "that's when I first noticed the avarice in his eyes," McMillen said. "He just kept playing with the money, like he was playing with Legos."

As Clegg would later state in court, "This was the happiest period of my life."

McMillen set up a beeper with the number 1-800-ECSTASY for taking orders, and within a couple of months, he said, demand had soared to a hundred thousand pills per week. McMillen's guy in Hollywood distributed it among movie stars. Others passed it out to people in the music industry, who "just gobbled it up," McMillen said. "I got one testimonial after another, people were just unbelievably happy."

After McMillen introduced MDMA to one of the world's foremost cocaine dealers (alias "The Devil"), the man told McMillen that he wanted to get out of the coke business and start distributing Ecstasy. McMillen hated cocaine, and when he heard that, "I felt really, really, really good," he said. "I felt like I was doing something positive."

The Devil put in an order for one million pills, which Clegg told McMillen he could have by the first of the next month. But when the Devil arrived by private jet in Santa Rosa to collect his order, Clegg didn't show up. McMillen drove to Clegg's place, only to find he'd sold everything he'd made that month to Bhagwan Shree Rajneesh and his cultish Sanyassin followers in Oregon (the subject of Netflix's *Wild Wild Country*). Ecstasy "was discreetly slipped into rich Sanyassins' drinks just before fund-raising interviews," Rajneesh's former bodyguard, Hugh Milne, later wrote.

The Sanyassins' score meant problems for McMillen, though, who had to explain the situation to the Devil. "It was tough dealing with Michael, because he would always promise a lot more than he could produce, and in the drug business, that's a no-no," McMillen said. "All kinds of bad things can happen."

Despite the hiccups, Clegg's Ecstasy business grew to around twenty-five people. He started referring to them as the Texas Group, since his main partners were from there, and Dallas was becoming a major hub.

Although Ecstasy was still legal, McMillen knew enough about the government's zero-tolerance approach to drugs to urge his associates to proceed with caution. (One member of the crew would regularly fly to Texas with a bag of twenty thousand Ecstasy pills marked "Rabbit Food.") McMillen gave Clegg similar advice. "From now on, Michael, you've got to tip toe through the tulips," he said. "You'll be cannon fodder for the cops if they get wind of this."

Discretion was not Clegg's strong suit, however. He and Pauline spread MDMA throughout the Dallas community by throwing Tupperware-style "XTC" parties at their Dallas condo and in lavish hotel suites. Guests would listen to a lecture about MDMA and be given a 100- to 125-milligram dose. Clegg reverentially referred to the MDMA tablets as wafers, as though they were a sacrament. "Their lives were totally touched," Clegg said of his guests in an interview with Peter Jennings. "They'd walk out of there wanting to share it with their friends." He and Pauline would invite their blissed-out attendees to send new recruits their way, and Clegg also began putting MDMA out on consignment.

Based on his guests' tendencies to want to dance while high, Clegg struck on another brilliant idea: introduce MDMA to the clubs. As Torsten Passie said, "He brought it to the discotheque, and then it became great." Michael recruited distributors to hand out brochures advertising the new drug at the Starck Club and other venues.

It wasn't just customers whose eye Clegg caught, though. The police began getting complaints about "this hippy-type atmosphere that existed with the introduction of Ecstasy into the Dallas metroplex," Phil Jordan, the director of drug intelligence at the DEA at the time, told Cain in an unpublished interview. Ecstasy also came to the attention of then U.S. senator from Texas Lloyd Bentsen. The Democratic congressman contacted the DEA in 1985, urging them to schedule MDMA and put a stop to what he saw as a growing epidemic.

The DEA's Texas office was primarily focused on methamphetamine, cocaine, and heroin. But when officers began looking into "that kiddie drug," as some agents called Ecstasy, they realized that Dallas had become a major hub. And Clegg, they learned, was right at the center. "In DEA terminology, he was a godfather of the drug trade—in this case, Ecstasy," Jordan said. "The reason we made the Starck Club a priority, and also Michael Clegg a target, is because of the multi-thousand lot quantities of Ecstasy that was being sold."

Seeing the writing on the wall in terms of MDMA's impending illegality, McMillen gave Clegg six months' notice that he'd be parting ways with the Texas Group. It was more than just the future threat of arrest that made McMillen want to leave, though—it was also Clegg. On top of all the lies and false promises, Clegg had sold Ecstasy to the notorious Marcello gang in New Orleans, which crossed McMillen's ethical line. (Clegg denied this, telling me he'd "never even heard of this gang.")

"I was very proud to do what I was doing with Ecstasy, and still feel it's one of the best things I've ever done," McMillen said. "But as things progressed, it became apparent that Michael's only motivation was money. He showed his true colors."

*

THESE DEVELOPMENTS WERE not lost on the Shulgins and Leo Zeff, who had been keeping tabs on the recreational situation in Texas, New York City, and elsewhere. As the party grew, so did their awareness that MDMA's days of legality would soon come to an end. Sure enough, Sasha Shulgin—with his ties to the DEA and his friendship with Bob Sager—caught early rumors of an impending federal move to place MDMA into Schedule I, which would mean an abrupt halt to virtually all medical and scientific work with the drug. Even without the insider information, though, no one in Shulgin's circle was surprised. "Everybody knew that it was inevitable at some point that it would become a controlled substance, because it felt good," George Greer said. "Drugs like that, people wanna take."

Unlike the late 1960s, though—when many researchers who worked with LSD simply resigned themselves to its loss—this time the therapeutic community decided to organize and fight back. They would get ahead of the scheduling by conducting safety research on MDMA and by petitioning, when the time came, that MDMA should be placed in Schedule III rather than the much more restrictive Schedule I. If successful, this would permit medical use of MDMA and research on it to continue, while making recreational use illegal.

To take the lead on coordinating these efforts, the Shulgins reached out to two young women: therapist-in-training Debby Harlow and Alise Agar, who held a master's degree in dance therapy and was a gifted networker and psychedelic sitter. (Agar passed away in 2001.) Harlow and Agar knew that even if MDMA was scheduled, their small group would probably always have access to it for personal use. But scheduling would severely curtail their ability to do research and to share it with others who could benefit, such as those with PTSD or trauma.

The two friends were excited to helm a cause they fervently believed in, but they also faced a daunting road ahead. They needed to recruit scientists and therapists to submit testimony about MDMA's medicinal value, efficacy, and safety; find an attorney to help organize the group's legal strategy and file a lawsuit against the DEA; try to balance the one-sided, alarmist coverage in the press that was emerging as a result of the scene in Texas; and raise funds to fly witnesses to hearings to speak on MDMA's behalf. It was a lot for a couple of twentysomethings to take on by themselves. They could use another partner.

"Do you know anybody else who has time and enthusiasm?" Agar asked Harlow in a brainstorming session one day.

Harlow thought for a moment. "There is this young guy, Rick Doblin, who's gung-ho. I bet he'd be helpful."

# 4
# RICK KEPT GOING

THE MORNING AFTER his bar mitzvah, thirteen-year-old Rick Doblin woke up disappointed. God had not come to him in his dreams or waking life, and he felt exactly the same as he had the day before.

"He's just busy," Doblin rationalized of the Creator's schedule. "He must have a lot of people going through bar and bat mitzvahs, and He's just taking a while."

But as days continued to pass, God still did not show up, and Doblin did not miraculously transform into a spiritually enlightened adult man. After a week's worth of additional bar and bat mitzvahs had taken place, Doblin quietly accepted that he must have fallen off God's list.

Looking back more than fifty years later, Doblin thinks his bar mitzvah experience in fact could have been life-changing, if only it had included one key ingredient: MDMA.

"If I could have done MDMA when I was thirteen, I could have been opened up a bit to emotions, and I would have had a vastly better time in high school," Doblin said. "That's what my bar mitzvah should have been."

\*

BORN IN 1953, Doblin uses words like *shy, political,* and *unemotional* to describe his younger self. His pediatrician father and teacher mother were progressive liberals who sometimes talked to their four children about the Holocaust at the dinner table. These conversations left a deep impression on Doblin, who lived with a creeping sense of dread that everyone around him, at any moment, could break out into genocidal mania.

After the Cuban missile crisis, Doblin became obsessed with the process of "how we other-ize people," as he put it, so naturally he chose to study Russian in high school. In 1970 his parents gave him permission to spend the summer between his junior and senior year studying abroad in the Soviet Union. Despite it being the height of the Cold War, Doblin discovered that Russian high schoolers were interested in anything that looked American, from decorative buttons to blue jeans. With his language skills, Doblin became the black market conduit between his American classmates and the Russian kids who wanted to purchase their gear. He made a killing on commissions but decided to donate his share to a synagogue in Moscow, along with a couple of Jewish prayer books—forbidden in the Soviet Union—that his parents had sent with him for this purpose. This small first taste of nonviolent resistance made Doblin hungry for more opportunities to effect positive change. "What I learned from my parents is that there are big, big systems going on in the world, but you can make tiny individual differences," Doblin said. "You can't open up Judaism in Russia, but you can bring two prayer books."

Doblin returned home with a new conviction that oppressive rules are made to be broken. He also came away with an important lesson about love. While on the trip he'd started a relationship—his first ever—with a girl from Seattle. He was devastated when, midway through the summer, she decided to break it off because she was afraid of the inevitable pain of the goodbye at the end. But there was a silver lining: he had finally experienced for himself the heavenly highs and abysmal lows of human emotion. "I realized how unbalanced I had been," he said of his former single-minded focus on logic and rationality. He came to see his own emotional immaturity as a microcosm of the sorry state of the world. "We're overdeveloped intellectually, with nuclear weapons and all sorts of miraculous technology, but we lag behind in our emotional and spiritual development," he thought.

Doblin had resolved not to register for the Vietnam War draft, and fully expected to be arrested at any moment after graduating high school in 1972.

Meanwhile, though, he moved on with his life and enrolled at New College, an experimental school in Sarasota, Florida. New College had no grades and allowed students to design their own curriculums. To Doblin, it seemed like an ideal place to unpack his hang-ups about himself and the world—and to channel those revelations into something worthwhile.

What Doblin had missed on the campus tour with his dad was the fact that the New College student body regularly threw all-night psychedelics-fueled parties, and that the outdoor Olympic swimming pool was clothing optional. "It felt like this oasis of sanity from the real world, where we're bringing out things that are suppressed, like sex and drugs, and trying to do them in a healthier way," Doblin said. "I'd just wandered into this place."

Doblin had never done drugs before, but he dove right in. He'd loved *One Flew Over the Cuckoo's Nest* and had been astonished to learn that Ken Kesey had written parts of the book while high on LSD, so he decided to start there. His first experience on acid was revelatory—as first experiences with psychedelics are wont to be—revealing to him the connectedness of every being across the sweep of time and space. "I started to understand that the real reason for the backlash against psychedelics was not because they went wrong, but because they went right," Doblin said. "People had these experiences and thought, 'Why should I go kill these Vietnamese who are essentially similar to me?' "

Under the influence of LSD, Doblin also grappled with existentially challenging questions about who he was and what purpose his life served. But his lack of emotional maturity, as he interpreted it, would not permit him to fully let go and explore the expanses that lay beyond the tethers of his limited ego. He kept trying, though, repeatedly taking LSD, mescaline, and magic mushrooms (which "grew all over the place in Florida," he noted). As Doblin said, "I had the delusion that the more drugs you take, the faster you evolve. If only that were true."

By the end of his first semester, psychedelics were starting to take precedence over Doblin's studies, and "I just got all messed up," he said. In a testament to how open-minded New College was, Doblin visited the guidance counselor to talk about the difficulties he was having with his trips. Rather than lecture Doblin about the perils of drugs, the counselor handed him an unpublished manuscript. It was of *Realms of the Human Unconscious:*

*Observations from LSD Research* by Stanislav Grof, who had personally sent the guidance counselor an early copy.

Through a scientific lens, Grof's book delved into everything from Freudian psychodynamics to birth trauma and transpersonal experience. Most important of all, though, Grof wrote about psychedelic-assisted therapy using LSD—something Doblin had never heard of before—and described how the government had shut it down. Grof proposed that such treatment could not only produce healing but also nudge humanity toward a more connected, tolerant, and loving place. "Reading that book pulled it all together for me," Doblin said. "That was the epiphany, you can say, that really solidified my life forty-nine years ago. I decided to focus on psychedelic therapy, and bringing psychedelics back."

Doblin got Grof's address from the guidance counselor and wrote the famed psychiatrist a letter. Incredibly, Grof not only replied, but also invited Doblin to come join him at a workshop that he and his then wife, Christina, were hosting at the Esalen Institute. Somehow Doblin convinced his parents to let him drop out of college to go study LSD and even persuaded them to pay for it. He hitchhiked out to California, eager to learn all he could from Grof. Doblin was disappointed to find, however, that even under Grof's mentorship—and the influence of a whole host of therapies he tried—he still could not find the answers he was seeking. Enlightenment continued to evade him. He moved back in with his parents, feeling like a failure.

Eventually Doblin decided he had undervalued the process of integration of psychedelic experiences and was so ungrounded in his head, he should try to make something with his hands. He moved back to Sarasota, not to be a student but to build a handball court at New College (he'd been the handball champion of his high school). He enjoyed the process so much that he wound up getting his contractor license and building a house—a lost boys' paradise in the woods, designed to be the perfect place to trip. Doblin settled into life. He grew a bushy mustache to match his curls, and got a girlfriend and a pet timber wolf named Phaedrus (a rescue from the Humane Society). He launched a construction company, spent most of his time shirtless, and did lots and lots of drugs.

A decade after dropping out of school, Doblin decided it was time to reenroll and get his degree. He had not forgotten his dream of becoming a psychedelic-assisted therapist—something he felt compelled to pursue, but wasn't at all sure was the right decision. "Am I crazy to devote my life to psychedelics?" he asked his therapist at the time. "Am I not just on the edge, but over the edge?"

In 1982 Doblin received another invitation from Grof to attend a mystical quest workshop at Esalen. Doblin was only just beginning school again, but he couldn't turn down a personal invite from Grof and a chance to return to Esalen and all the promise it held. He got permission to do an off-campus study and headed back to the West Coast.

*

DEBBY HARLOW HAD two thoughts the first time she did MDMA. Number one: this medicine would make her future job as a clinician so much easier. And number two: she really wanted to share the experience with select friends. It was 1980, and MDMA was still fairly difficult to find. So if Harlow wanted others she knew to try the drug, she'd have to source it for them herself. She linked up with a few small producers in the Bay Area, mostly university-affiliated chemists, and became the connect for all of her friends. As an unofficial service to the community, about once a month she also drove down to Esalen—where she'd been an intern for Stan and Christina Grof—to see if anyone there wanted any MDMA. Indeed, people did.

"There was something about Esalen and MDMA that was in resonance," said Howard Kornfeld, a doctor in San Francisco who became a visiting physician in residence at Esalen in the early 1980s. "MDMA would allow people to drop their armor, so to speak, and feel what they were really feeling and feel safe, and there was something about Esalen that was also like that."

Doblin was one of the many people who first found his way to MDMA through Esalen and Harlow. "He seemed like a really enthusiastic, bright young man," Harlow recalled of her initial meeting with Doblin.

Doblin, for his part, remembered Harlow—blond, petite, and friendly—"talking about this drug that made you feel more love, more connected and self-accepting," he said. Harlow offered to sell him some for five dollars a pill, but he told her he was already in love and already accepted himself. "I wasn't impressed, initially," he recalled. When he later saw some people on MDMA sitting around in a circle, just casually chatting, "I was even less impressed," he said. "I was like, 'How profound can this be? If you can still talk and know who you are, it can't be very important.'"

Doblin now likes to say that he was stupid enough to underestimate MDMA, but smart enough to buy some. He purchased a few pills from Harlow and then forgot about them while he focused on training to be a psychedelic therapist. During his month at Esalen, he became somewhat smitten with a fellow student who asked him to sit with her while she tripped on LSD—an intimate and beautiful experience for them both. After the trip, as a token of thanks, the woman gave Doblin a gold chain necklace. Nothing physical ever happened between them, but when Doblin got back to Florida, his girlfriend immediately noticed the necklace. Doblin said something about sitting with someone through a trip, and then changed the subject. "You can imagine, it was a little bit of a delicate situation," he said.

A few days later, Doblin remembered the MDMA and suggested that he and his girlfriend try it. Like so many other couples before them, they were astounded by how easily they could communicate on MDMA about an otherwise difficult subject: the necklace. "I could explain in a very careful way how I was attracted to this woman and what we did together, and we were able to really work through it," Doblin said. His girlfriend, who would be moving away soon for graduate school, said it was a good thing for Doblin to connect with other women. To show her understanding, she even held the necklace and blessed it. "It was kind of astonishing to me," Doblin said, "how we were able to talk gracefully about something that could have been very fraught."

The other thing that stood out to him about the experience, he added, was "just how much love we felt for each other, and how much we could express that." At one point Doblin and his girlfriend questioned whether what they were feeling was just a product of the drug. But they decided, no, the drug simply brought to the surface what they already felt.

Harlow had explained to Doblin that she was collecting stories about people's experiences on MDMA, and had asked him to let her know how it went. Most people just wrote her a letter, but Doblin called her. "It was amazing!" he boisterously declared as soon as she picked up the phone.

Harlow became Doblin's MDMA hookup, and he distributed the then-legal drug to all of his friends at New College. On long phone calls, he and Harlow compared notes about their shared goals of becoming psychedelic-assisted therapists and talked about all the research they planned to do. Harlow and Doblin agreed on the importance of turning certain movers and shakers on to MDMA. At Esalen, for example, they gave MDMA to Albert Hofmann, the creator of LSD. The next day, whistling and grinning, Hofmann declared, "I feel like a young boy again!" His wife did not like LSD, he said, but he was convinced she would love MDMA. Harlow and Doblin gave him a little baggie to take back to Switzerland.

The two friends did disagree, though, about the extent to which they should spread the word about MDMA. "Rick was more in the Tim Leary camp of 'turn on the world,' " Harlow said. "I was more in the Aldous Huxley camp of doing this mindfully."

Indeed, Doblin wasted no time trying to effect global-level positive change with MDMA. Also at Esalen, he met Carol Rosin, the founder of the Institute for Security and Cooperation in Outer Space, a nonprofit group that advocates for peace in space, and gave her five hundred doses of MDMA to distribute among Soviet scientists and defense personnel that she knew. "That was one of those things you do, knowing you'll never hear back anything," Doblin said. "All I can say is the Soviets later signed an arms control agreement!"

Doblin also sent MDMA to Buddhist, Jewish, and Catholic thought leaders, echoing an idea put forward decades before by psychiatrist Humphry Osmond and LSD proponent Alfred Hubbard (and later by Paul McCartney) to send world leaders LSD to enlighten them. Sometime after Doblin mailed out his samples, a Benedictine monk named Brother David Steindl-Rast told *Newsweek* that MDMA delivers in an afternoon a feeling that otherwise takes twenty years of meditation to achieve.

*

"HERE'S THE SITUATION," Harlow told Doblin. "We need to raise money."

It was 1984, and Harlow and Alise Agar were organizing invitation-only conferences at Esalen to strategize for the coming DEA crackdown on

MDMA. The conference attendees included key people in the scientific and medical community, and together the group called themselves ARUPA— short for Association for the Responsible Use of Psychedelic Agents. *Arupa* also happened to be the Sanskrit word for "shapeless" or "ill-formed," which Dick Price, Esalen's cofounder, "teasingly said suggested our organizational structure at the time," Harlow recalled.

Harlow had extended a conference invite to Doblin, and when she asked if he'd like to get more directly involved in ARUPA, he emphatically agreed. Immediately, Doblin had an idea. A friend of his in Sarasota had a nonprofit organization, Earth Metabolic Design Laboratories, that he hadn't done anything with in years. The nonprofit's mission was geared toward alternative energy, and Doblin felt that alternative mental energy from psychedelics would fit in nicely with that overall goal. Doblin asked his friend if he could take over the nonprofit to sue the DEA, and his friend agreed.

Grof, the Shulgins, Leo Zeff, George Greer, and several other senior figures agreed to serve on the Earth Metabolic Design Laboratories board of advisors, and Agar, Doblin, and Harlow assumed the title of codirectors. It was up to the three of them to do the heavy lifting on getting the overall effort underway. Doblin stepped up as chief organizer and the "guy with the big vision," Harlow said. He set up meetings with FDA officials, coordinated planning sessions at Esalen, and commissioned animal toxicity studies of MDMA with a scientific facility in Arkansas. The ever-charming Agar served as the main networker and chief fundraiser, while Harlow, who was currently enrolled as a graduate student at Harvard University, focused on recruiting respected scientists to testify on MDMA's behalf. "Some I gave MDMA to, others I just talked to a lot," Harlow said.

To put together their legal case, alternative medicine doctor Andy Weil called up a friend from college, Rick Cotton, who was working for a big law firm in D.C. Cotton, who now heads the Port Authority of New York and New Jersey, agreed to represent the MDMA campaign pro bono. The plaintiffs were Greer and three professors, including Lester Grinspoon, a psychiatrist at Harvard Medical School whose graduate students had all done Harlow's MDMA.

In July 1984 the DEA quietly announced in the *Federal Register* its intention to place MDMA into Schedule I. Doblin, Harlow, and Agar responded by getting more than a dozen experts to write letters protesting the decision in order to have legal standing to stop the scheduling. Shulgin stated in his letter that MDMA "has unquestioned medical utility." Greer pointed out that his small business as a psychiatrist "will suffer both professionally and economically if MDMA is placed into Schedule I." On Purdue University letterhead, David Nichols stated that it is "very naive indeed" to expect that placing MDMA in Schedule I would not stifle research of a material "that could prove to be a major advance" for therapy.

Just before the thirty-day public comment period was up, Doblin traveled to DEA headquarters to file the letters and legal documents requesting a hearing. Cotton also officially informed the DEA that he had been retained by several physicians and professors, and that a scheduling hearing was now required by law. This was something the DEA had not seen coming.

"We were surprised, really, because initially, we didn't know anything about the medical use," said Frank Sapienza, the former DEA chemist who put together the documentation for MDMA's scheduling. "We started getting all this pushback from a number of psychiatrists who said that they were using MDMA to treat patients."

Dates for hearings were set in courtrooms in Los Angeles, Kansas City, and Washington, D.C.

Remembering what happened with LSD, some clinicians also decided it was time to more boldly share MDMA with other colleagues. Torsten Passie recalled Ralph Metzner and several other leading psychedelic researchers from the United States arriving at a conference in the Black Forest in Germany with bags packed full of bottles of MDMA. The plan was to show the European conference attendees what MDMA taken in a therapeutic context could do. Passie and around thirty or forty other mental health professionals were able to "participate in the ritual" firsthand, he said—that is, get high together on MDMA. The Europeans were just as impressed as their American colleagues had been, and afterward they helped spread the word throughout Germany, Switzerland, and beyond.

"It became quite obvious that a lot of anxieties, distrust, inner tensions, and all your kind of neurotic behavioral patterns are gone during an MDMA trip," Passie said. "We immediately realized that this is a therapeutic drug with enormous potential."

*

IN EARLY 1985 Harlow and Doblin found themselves facing yet another challenge: running interference on Michael Clegg. After Clegg had heard the news about the impending scheduling, he'd responded by upping operations, cranking out an estimated two million pills in just a few months. At a conference in Boston, he had even marched up to Sasha Shulgin and boasted about being "Mr. Texas," the biggest manufacturer of Ecstasy in the world. Shulgin took the news coolly, but as soon as he had a moment, he called Agar.

"We've got a problem," he said. He asked Agar if she and Harlow would pay Clegg a visit and try to convince him to "chill his jets," as Harlow put it.

Agar and Harlow agreed "to do that for the cause," Harlow said, and by dropping Shulgin's name, they secured an invite to Clegg's home in Mendocino County. When Agar had to cancel at the last minute, however, Doblin took her place.

At five P.M., Doblin and Harlow pulled up at a beautiful, expensive-looking home surrounded by forest. "It looked like something you might see in *Architectural Digest* or a magazine on interior design," Harlow said. "It was the kind of house that would have been nice for tripping in small groups."

Harlow quickly got to the point of why she and Doblin were there. "Please, there's therapists working with MDMA," she told Clegg. "We're conducting research affiliated with Harvard, and there's other studies planned. It's gonna be made illegal if you keep this up. Can you please just be more discreet?"

Clegg listened politely, but he didn't seem to really be hearing her. He told Harlow and Doblin that he was saving the world and launched into a monologue about consciousness. He bragged about producing millions of doses of Ecstasy a month.

The back-and-forth went on for ten hours. Finally, at three A.M., Clegg looked Harlow straight in the eye and brought the conversation to a close: "Frankly, Debby, if it's made illegal, I'll just make more money."

In a way, Harlow was grateful for Clegg's candor. "I knew, OK, that's the bottom line right there."

As Harlow and Doblin prepared to go, Doblin suggested to Clegg that since he was ruining everything for all the therapists and making millions of dollars in the process, he should at least consider "paying a tax to our efforts to try to fight the DEA." In other words, he could make a donation.

Clegg said he wouldn't be giving their nonprofit any money, but he would be happy to donate MDMA so they could sell it and use the proceeds to fund the campaign. "The guy was ready to load up our car," Harlow said—and Doblin was ready to take him up on the offer.

Harlow, however, put her foot down. She didn't have a problem with the idea of selling MDMA in general to raise funds, but she did have a problem with selling *Michael Clegg's* MDMA. He was the only distributor at the time selling pressed pills rather than powder or capsules, so "it isn't just a product, it's a product with his name on it," Harlow pointed out to Doblin. "Everyone will think that Earth Metabolic Design Laboratories is just a front for the biggest drug manufacturer in the country. It's about the integrity of the mission."

The disagreement wound up hanging heavily over the two friends, especially after Doblin decided to accept Clegg's offer anyway. Clegg donated twenty thousand pills for free and sold Doblin another nineteen thousand pills for three dollars each. Doblin sold the then-legal pills to his contacts, mostly in the therapeutic community, and used the proceeds to fund the animal toxicity studies of MDMA, among other activities in service to the cause. "The ends justified the means," Doblin said. "I also didn't have real ethical issues with what Michael was doing, other than the fact that he was putting all the therapy work at risk by doing it in such a public way."

The internal friction among Doblin and his colleagues only worsened in the coming weeks, however, as publicity about the scheduling case ramped up. Most of the scientists and therapists fighting to keep MDMA out of Schedule I did not welcome media attention. Shulgin, for his part, "hated the term 'Ecstasy,' " said Paul Daley, a chemist who now heads the Alexander Shulgin Research Institute. "He hated being identified as 'Dr. Ecstasy' or 'Grandfather Ecstasy.' " Doblin, on the other hand, was willing to be in the spotlight, and he and Harlow began butting heads over whether this was appropriate. Harlow believed that senior experts should be the ones speaking to the media, while Doblin thought otherwise—and more often than not got his way. "Rick is charming but extremely pushy," Harlow said. "He gets his idea and vision and just goes with it."

Problematically for the group, Doblin would frequently stray from the message that he and his colleagues' sole aim was to ensure MDMA's availability for research and therapy. When the interviewer would inevitably ask him what he thought of recreational use, Doblin couldn't contain himself. "I'd say, 'Well, it shouldn't be illegal! Prohibition doesn't work, it's counterproductive, it's stupid,' " Doblin said.

Another issue, Harlow added, was that Doblin insisted on stating publicly that millions of doses of MDMA had been safely consumed over the years, so there was no cause for alarm. But the DEA's guidelines for putting a drug into Schedule I specifically included high levels of nonmedical use of any drug, regardless of safety, so Doblin was effectively shooting the campaign in the foot.

"Everyone wanted Rick's help," Harlow said. "But in the early days, people frankly wanted him to shut the fuck up." At one point, she said, Cotton called her in exasperation about Doblin and asked her "to cut this guy off at the knees."

"I was elected as the best person to 'rein Rick in.' " Harlow sighed. "Not a job I enjoyed, believe me."

In April 1985, things reached a head when Phil Donahue devoted an episode of his popular talk show to MDMA. "Well, guess what, we've got another drug," Donahue announced to hundreds of thousands of viewers. "It is synthetic. And it makes you love everybody." One woman in the audience said that MDMA-assisted therapy had allowed her to resolve her marital problems, while another spoke about how it had helped her deal with the fear, anger, and emotional pain of her recent terminal cancer diagnosis. "MDMA is not an ecstasy drug," she said. "It allows you to see the world more clearly and to heal yourself. You realize that you don't need negative emotions . . . and you can let them go."

Things seemed to be going well, until the camera switched to Charles Schuster, the founder and director of the University of Chicago's Drug Abuse Research Center. Doblin had met Schuster at a World Health Organization

(WHO) meeting about MDMA in Geneva. The scheduling hearings had slowed the DEA down in their effort to ban MDMA in the United States, so DEA officials had started pushing for WHO to criminalize the drug internationally. The United States would then have to follow suit because of international treaty obligations. Schuster was the lead scientific consultant to the WHO committee that was reviewing the evidence about MDMA. He happened to mention to Doblin that a graduate student of his had just conducted research with the related drug MDA suggesting that that substance could harm the brain. But he also shared with Doblin his opinion that MDMA should be in Schedule III, not Schedule I. Because of Schuster's view about MDMA's scheduling, Doblin recommended that he be on the Donahue show.

While on the show, Schuster did state his support for placing MDMA into Schedule III. But then he unexpectedly started talking about the study his student had just wrapped up showing that MDA, when administered in large, repeated doses in rats, causes brain damage. While MDA is not MDMA, Schuster said, there was "a 99 percent chance" of the same results being replicated for MDMA.

"That was the first time the DEA heard about MDMA and neurotoxicity," Doblin said. "Now the DEA could say, 'This is a crisis, MDMA is causing brain damage.'"

Doblin had turned down an opportunity to be on the *Phil Donahue Show* himself, precisely because he was trying to be a better team player. But because he had recruited Schuster to be on the panel, he bore much of the blame for the problematic turn of events. His commitment to sharing his views about drug policy reform and the counterproductive nature of the war on drugs had also clearly become more of a hindrance than a help for his colleagues' core mission. Rather than cause more internal problems, Doblin resigned from Earth Metabolic Design Laboratories.

Doblin's devotion to the overall MDMA cause remained steadfast, however, and was reaffirmed during a solo camping trip at the beach at Big Sur. He took MDMA in the evening, and with the moonlit waves melodically crashing in front of him and the mountains looming behind him, he began to feel so small and insignificant in the expanse of eternity that he thought he would simply disappear. But he became aware of the force tethering him to the world—gravity. "I felt that gravity was like the arms of a lover," he said. "I was cradled in gravity and it was so palpably loving."

If everyone was able to experience the same mystical sense of benevolence and safety, he thought, this revelation could help discourage prejudice, genocide, and environmental destruction. MDMA-assisted therapy, he realized, could be a strategy for a larger mission: mass mental health in the service of world peace.

As the sun's rays broke through the morning mist, Doblin left the beach resolved to make that lofty vision a reality—whatever it took.

*

ON JULY 1, 1985, shortly after the *Donahue Show* aired, the DEA invoked emergency measures to temporarily place MDMA into Schedule I—a power Congress had granted the year before in response to problems caused by "synthetic heroin," or fentanyl. In justifying its decision, the DEA pointed to Schuster's rat study showing that large doses of MDA were neurotoxic—specifically, that the drug "selectively destroys" the ends of certain nerves that play a key role in regulating serotonin, a chemical messenger in the brain. The United Nations also fell in line, announcing in the same month that the WHO had decided to place MDMA into Schedule I.

There was more than just Schuster's study at play, though. As Harlow said, "Michael Clegg was the real reason we went into emergency scheduling."

MDMA, after all, had been associated with just eight emergency room admissions from 1972 to 1984, and one death in 1979 (with significant controversy over whether the drug responsible was indeed MDMA). And MDA, while chemically related to MDMA, was not the same drug. That had been apparent back in the 1950s, when the University of Michigan researchers found that it took nearly twice as much MDMA as MDA to reach doses that killed 50 percent of the rats it was administered to. The Schuster paper itself also notes that the equivalent doses of MDA required to produce neurotoxicity in rats were roughly three to five times higher than what a person would normally ingest. Additionally, the drug had been injected into the rats rather than taken orally, as a person would, and had been given to the animals every twelve hours for four days, a punishing schedule. "Given differences in species, dose, frequency and route of administration, as well as differences in the way in which rats and humans metabolize amphetamine, it would be premature to extrapolate our findings to humans," Schuster and his coauthors stated in their study.

But these subtleties were seemingly lost on those speaking on behalf of the DEA. "MDMA abuse has become a nationwide problem and it poses a serious health threat," John Lawn, the DEA's administrator at the time, stated in a press conference. Adding to the hype, Ron Siegel, a psychopharmacologist at the UCLA School of Medicine who was working with the DEA, told *New York* magazine that people who took MDMA became disoriented for days. "We've had people locked in fetal positions for as long as seventy-two hours," Siegel said. "We had a psychotherapist that took it, disappeared, and turned up a week later directing traffic."

This wasn't an isolated incident of the media getting it wrong. As Nichols recalled, "There were articles written in *Time*, *Newsweek*, and probably every magazine and newspaper in the country talking about the scourge of this new designer drug, MDMA."

The public reacted with panic. At the Haight Ashbury Free Clinics in San Francisco, staff began fielding calls from concerned East Coasters asking about the "epidemic of MDMA abuse" on the West Coast, and from concerned West Coasters asking about the same epidemic taking place on the East Coast. Some people had heard about a "nation-wide cult of Ecstasy users who wear sandals that leave 'X' shaped tan lines on their feet" and that members of this cult carry their Ecstasy supply in water bottles strung around their necks, reported Richard Seymour, the clinics' director of education programs. Others called in to report seeing *X*s painted on walls and other random places—signs, they thought, that the drug was taking over society.

For those selling Ecstasy to a recreational clientele, however, it turned out that any publicity was good publicity. "The illegality and all the press was like a big advertisement," said a chemist who worked with Michael Clegg, who asked that his real name not be revealed. "Demand for MDMA began to skyrocket."

Meanwhile, the MDMA scheduling hearings had begun. Sixteen witnesses—twelve of whom were psychiatrists—testified that MDMA did not belong in Schedule I. June Riedlinger, a licensed pharmacist, challenged the

DEA's assertion that MDMA "is guilty by association" with MDA, as she put it. Comparing MDMA and MDA based on their similar molecular structures alone would be like comparing quinidine, a cardiac suppressant, to quinine, a treatment for malaria, she said. The DEA itself acknowledged key differences between MDA and MDMA in its scheduling recommendation—and then just ignored them, she pointed out.

Seymour countered the DEA's assertion that MDMA has a high potential for abuse. Of the four hundred clients he and his colleagues regularly saw at the Haight Ashbury Free Clinics per month for drug-related problems, MDMA, he said, represented less than 1 percent. MDMA "was kind of a nonissue," Seymour recently recalled. "But the DEA was hot to get it scheduled."

Testifying on behalf of MDMA's medical use, Philip Wolfson, a psychiatrist in San Francisco, described using the drug clinically "in cases of severe emotional distress where prognosis was poor." Having seen positive outcomes in patients "who might otherwise be doomed," he said, "it is my experience that MDMA is a potentially valuable therapeutic agent that should not be lost to the psychiatric profession or to human beings."

In one of the most passionate and eloquent arguments, Lester Grinspoon pleaded with the DEA not to repeat the mistakes of policymakers two decades before, who caused scientists and doctors to prematurely abandon research on LSD. "In rejecting the absurd notion promoted by some that these drugs were a panacea, we have chosen to treat them as entirely worthless and extraordinarily dangerous," Grinspoon said. "The time has come to find an intermediate position."

The DEA's seven witnesses, however, presented ample evidence that MDMA is abused—which, by their definition, meant any nonmedical use. Siegel stated that the street use of MDMA had escalated from an estimated ten thousand doses distributed in all of 1976 to thirty thousand doses distributed per month in 1985. Robert Chester Jr., a DEA special agent, added that "those trafficking 'Ecstasy' in the Dallas area are operating in a manner which is similar to most structured illicit drug trafficking organizations."

Ultimately, though, the case really boiled down to what "currently accepted medical use" meant. The DEA decided to take the stance that "currently accepted medical use" could only pertain to drugs with FDA approval. As

Sapienza stated in his testimony, "MDMA has no currently accepted medical use in treatment in the United States since there are no approved new drug applications or exemptions for MDMA as determined by the FDA." This also meant that there was no accepted safety data for MDMA, because such data could only be determined by the FDA. "Thus, MDMA satisfies the criteria for Schedule I control under the [Controlled Substances Act]," Sapienza concluded.

Francis Young, the administrative law judge overseeing the case, listened attentively to all of the arguments and seemed to take very seriously how the outcome would affect future research. "You know, I just want to see to it that people do not look back at us a hundred years or so down the road in the same way that we now look back at the Holy Inquisition in Spain," he remarked at one point. After a couple of rounds of rebuttal testimony, plus more letters, sixty-two documentary exhibits, and eight cross-examination sessions— generating more than a thousand pages of transcripts—Young was finally ready to make a determination. It took him three months to issue his seventy-one-page ruling on May 22, 1986: MDMA, he'd concluded, should be placed into Schedule III, not Schedule I.

Young carefully laid out his reasoning. On the one hand, he wrote, he could understand why the DEA would turn to the FDA as the arbiter of what "currently accepted medical use" meant. Relying on the FDA "would greatly simplify the scheduling task of the DEA staff," Young wrote, and provide "a quick solution to the problem." But this strategy, he rebutted, "is wrong."

Young went on to exhaustively outline the legislative and regulatory authority granted to the FDA, even pointing to an FDA directive stating that good medical practice requires "that physicians be free to use drugs according to their best knowledge and judgment." He also concluded that, prior to its emergency scheduling the summer before, MDMA *did* have "a currently accepted medical use in treatment in the United States." It was being medically used by doctors—and that use was legitimate.

Sapienza and his colleagues at the DEA were gobsmacked. As Sapienza told me, "We thought the data we provided was sufficient to show the criteria for Schedule I."

The plaintiffs, on the other hand, were elated.

"This opinion represents an extraordinary vindication of every position we took in this matter," Rick Cotton wrote in a letter to the witnesses who had spoken on behalf of MDMA. "Congratulations to us all!"

"We won!" cheered George Greer in a note he wrote to David Nichols on the day of what he called Young's "landmark" ruling. "I want to thank you again for all the time and energy you put into the hearings. It certainly paid off."

The celebrations were short-lived. Three weeks later, the DEA's counsel responded by implying that Young had been willfully negligent in his ruling. "The Administrative Law Judge has systematically disregarded the evidence and arguments presented by the Government," the DEA's counsel wrote. Moreover, because of legal technicalities, rulings by administrative law judges are only advisory. The DEA didn't have to listen to Young at all. So Lawn, the DEA administrator, did what he had apparently planned to do all along: permanently place MDMA into Schedule I.

Grinspoon appealed, however, and in one final reprieve, a Boston court ruled that the DEA could not use FDA approval as the basis for arguing that MDMA had no proven medical use. In what became known as "the Grinspoon window," for three months—from December 22, 1987, to March 22, 1988—MDMA once again became legal.

"As a consequence of this, a few people were released from prison and many had MDMA charges against them dropped," Grinspoon said in a 2002 interview. (Grinspoon died in 2020.) "I received a couple of delightful thank-you notes from some of these people."

Just as quickly as it had opened, the window slammed shut. On March 23 Lawn once again ignored the latest ruling and placed MDMA into Schedule I. "Of course, the DEA came up with new criteria acceptable to the court, and bang, the window is closed," Grinspoon said.

Nearly forty years later, Sapienza still stands by the DEA's decision. Whether MDMA had an accepted medical use or not, it's still always a balancing act between potential harm and good, he said. "In my mind, there was no question that MDMA was a drug that was abusable and was causing harm to the public.

"I think sometimes DEA gets a bad rap," he added. "There are very good people at DEA that are focused on enforcing the laws that really help society. They're not trying to take decent medicines away from people."

*

FOR THOSE WHO had spent the last three years trying to make the case that MDMA *was* a decent medicine, the DEA's decision delivered a crushing blow. "This was our baby, our love," said Harlow, who had given up her graduate studies at Harvard to devote herself to the cause, and had been sleeping on her mom's couch in California. "It was truly devastating."

"It was dreadful," Ann Shulgin agreed. "That was a very bad day in history."

"Oh god, it was horrible," echoed Requa Greer. She had recently quit her job in order to conduct MDMA-assisted therapy full time, but she and George decided that, for them, it wasn't worth the risk to practice underground. Most other therapists quit, too, although a few did continue working with the molecule in secrecy. "We knew that people who were brave enough to have a quiet underground practice would always use [MDMA]," Requa said. "I guess we all just thought, 'That's the way it's gonna be.' "

Ever the outlier, Doblin, however, did not accept that this was just the way it would be. He was as disappointed with the case's outcome as everyone else, but he was still as committed as ever to making MDMA the mainstream medicine and mass mental health tool he was convinced it was destined to be. And he already had a blueprint for doing so—one given to him directly by Sapienza.

"When my boss and I first met with Rick Doblin, we said, 'You know, this all sounds interesting and there may be something to it, but until and unless you go through the FDA process, you're not going to have a drug that's considered to be in mainstream medicine,' " Sapienza recalled. " 'It's never going to be accepted, except maybe in a fringe group of people.' "

FDA approval, then, it would be.

After formally stepping down from Earth Metabolic Design Laboratories, Doblin at first thought about founding a for-profit company, Orphan Pharmaceuticals Inc., to "facilitat[e] MDMA research right now," as he eagerly wrote in his original proposal. He soon changed his mind, though, and decided that a nonprofit was the better way to go. The Multidisciplinary Association for Psychedelic Studies (MAPS), as he called his newly founded organization, would work within the scientific and policy system to bring MDMA back into the light of respectability, he decided, first for medical use and eventually for social awakening. Unlike typical for-profit pharmaceutical companies, MAPS would also make the entirety of its data available for free to all researchers looking to advance MDMA-related science, eliminating the need to spend time and money duplicating safety studies.

Remembering the schism created by the disagreement with Harlow over whether to take Michael Clegg's MDMA, as well as his frustration at having to be answerable to a board for everything he said publicly, Doblin decided that this time, he would be the boss. "I felt like I was credible enough to start MAPS without an illustrious board of advisors," Doblin said. "MAPS, to this day, does not have an advisory board."

Harlow and others watched these developments from the sidelines and quietly shook their heads. There was no doubt in their minds that it was only a matter of time before Doblin finally faced reality: MDMA was not coming back, and MAPS would prove to be just another futile waste of time, money, and energy. "Nobody believed MDMA would ever get to the point of being a medicine," Harlow said. "Only Rick—and not a single person believed that he could accomplish it."

For Doblin, though, believing in the MDMA mission had become one and the same as believing in himself. And he was certainly not going to give up on himself. As Harlow said, "Rick kept going. And for that, I forgive him for everything he's ever done, or will do."

Another thing that kept going? The party.

# GOOD CHEMISTRY

ON A PRISTINE February afternoon, Carina Leveriza-Franz—a hiking guide sporting a colorful Cotopaxi backpack, a crystal pendant, and a visor with a palm tree motif—led two guests to one of her favorite spots in Sedona, Arizona. Situated along the wooded banks of the Oak Creek, the area is referred to by believers as a "vortex," a swirling center of natural energy thought to be conducive to healing and personal growth.

The trio breezed past a group of white people performing a ceremony with drums, feathers, and burning sage, and gave a wide berth to a newlywed couple swigging White Claws and taking photos. Stopping at a quiet spot on a bed of red rock, Carina directed her guests' attention to the big reveal directly behind them: an unbroken view of the towering burnt-orange steeples of Cathedral Rock.

"Three hundred million years ago, there were no red rocks here," Carina explained with a smile. "When the oceans retreated and then came back, you can see they formed geological layers—fifteen layers of striated sandstone deposits in different colors on Cathedral Rock."

Carina has given hundreds of these tours. But she never tires of sharing Sedona's natural beauty and special energy with others—many of whom are repeat guests at the luxury hotel she works for, and who always request her for their hikes. Almost certainly, though, none of her clients would ever guess what their bubbly, sixty-seven-year-old guide used to do for a living.

For years, Carina was one of the world's most prolific underground MDMA chemists.

Carina formerly worked behind the scenes for Michael Clegg, who knew nothing about how to make MDMA. From the mid-1980s to the early 1990s, she was the perfectionist chemist who oversaw much of the production for the Texas Group. She herself was responsible for cranking out at least a thousand pounds of the drug. The pharmaceutical-grade Ecstasy she made helped to catalyze nothing short of a global cultural phenomenon. Carina wound up paying dearly for her involvement, yet she has no regrets. "We touched millions of people," she said. "This had a huge effect on humanity."

*

BORN AND RAISED in the Philippines, Carina got into politics as a teenager. She skipped a family vacation to the United States to teach remote mountain communities about government rights they were entitled to. With her Catholic high school friends, she marched in Manilla to protest the country's Marxist regime. "I was idealistic in the sense of always wanting to make a difference," she said.

Carina's parents feared their daughter's politics would get her in trouble, so they sent her to the States. Eventually, the whole family followed. Carina joined them in California and enrolled in college there. She especially excelled at chemistry and in 1979 took a job at Intel in Santa Clara. In November 1981 her boss—apparently impressed with her work—asked if she'd like to do some consulting on a side project he was involved with. "I was like, 'Of course, I can do anything!' " Carina said.

Carina was tasked with scaling up a chemical synthesis from the gram to kilogram level. Her boss didn't tell her what exactly she was working on; he just gave her some materials and handed her a 1980 paper, coauthored by Alexander Shulgin, describing the synthesis for a molecule with a mouthful of a name Carina had never heard of. The sparkling white end product had a melting point of 151°C—spot on, her boss told her. Carina already knew that would be the case. As she said, "When I did work, it had to be outstanding."

Several months later, in April 1982, Carina's boss approached her once again. "We're scaling up," he said. "Would you assist?"

She agreed—although this time she negotiated for a higher fee.

Her boss set her up at a foundry, where she had to teach a man with no chemistry background how to work his way around the lab. He was one of three brothers who had been in the seminary with Michael Clegg, whom she also briefly met. She was told that the product they were making was intended for industrial use. Carina got things going and then didn't think much about it. "I just did what was in front of me," she said. "I had other irons in the fire."

In March 1985 Clegg called Carina at Intel and asked her to meet him at the Santa Clara airfield. He wanted to interview her for an even bigger job, he said.

It was a warm day, and Carina arrived wearing a white-and-teal polka-dot sundress and open-toed blue pumps. She was ushered up the steps of a Cessna jet. Inside sat Clegg and his wife, Pauline, who were both conspicuously dressed in all white: a suit for Clegg and a tight, short leather dress for Pauline. "I think they were trying to demonstrate the purity of their intent," Carina said.

There was also another man with them, Walter Franz, a lanky New Yorker of German descent whose piercing blue eyes locked onto Carina's. "Why are you so beautiful?" he abruptly asked.

"What kind of a thing is that to say?" she shot back, flustered. Walt was not conventionally handsome, but there was something about him that made her feel like he was looking straight through her—"a soul recognition," she later called it.

Clegg had brought along clippings of media stories about Ecstasy to share with Carina. The "interview" wasn't actually an interview at all, but an offer. "We have a task for you," Clegg said. "We'd like to move forward."

The timing was perfect. Carina had become bored and burned out at Intel, where she never got to conduct her own research, yet was expected, she said, "to live and breathe and sleep at the lab." What she really wanted to do was launch a company and make something of her own on a commercial scale. Clegg's offer, she realized, could be a stepping stone for reaching that goal.

Carina left the meeting feeling like she was floating. She wasn't sure if the sensation was tied to the new job or to the blue-eyed man on the plane. He contacted her days later to negotiate her contract. They settled on a hundred thousand dollars per year for five years and began working on plans for large-scale MDMA production.

Walt, she learned, served alongside Clegg as one of the three executives of the mysterious group she was now working for. "It was an entirely male organization," Carina said. "But I was used to that environment at Intel, almost always surrounded by men who were trying to take advantage of me." She sensed that Walt was different, though. Eloquent, confident, and erudite, he had worked at the IRS and at the accounting firm Arthur Andersen, specializing in mergers and acquisitions and international tax.

The day after Carina signed her contract, the third Texas Group partner approached her. "It's time to know what you're making," he said. He handed her a 125-milligram pressed pill. Carina took it in a hotel room with him and two other colleagues. Half an hour later, she felt her chest tighten. She didn't necessarily like this new feeling. As she sat there on the bed, she realized that she was apprehensive about the people she was with, and unsure of what she was getting herself into. "The dominant emotion was fear," she said.

Shortly after, she tried MDMA for a second time and found it to be totally different. Most likely, it was because this time, she was with Walt. She describes the sensation as "heart opening"—a relaxed yet almost explosively energetic outpouring of love. "That's when we came to be," she said of her and Walt's relationship. "That was the start of our romance."

Before taking MDMA with Walt, Carina had been motivated solely by money and opportunity. But now she felt strongly compelled to share MDMA with others and became convinced that this was her destiny. "After I ingested the substance, I felt that I'm playing one small part in something that is far bigger than me," she said. "I knew I had to take this as far as I could, for as long as I possibly could. I was fulfilling a need, and that need was greater than me."

*

JUST AS CARINA was sampling MDMA for the first time, the Dallas police were making the nation's first Ecstasy-related arrest under the newly instated emergency scheduling. (Charges were later dropped, however, because the police report misspelled the full chemical name of MDMA.) The hearing to determine MDMA's fate was still underway, but for the Texas Group, the message was clear: the days of legal recreational use were over. In light of these developments, Carina and Walt decided it would be safer to move production from California to Mexico.

Walt found a former vulcanizing facility in Aguascalientes, and Carina hired a handful of retired engineers who spoke English. She ordered bulk shipments of chemical precursors from a company in the United States, and sourced lab supplies after her truckload of gear was confiscated at the Mexican border. "That year I was on sixty-five flights to and from Mexico," she said.

Within six months the Mexico plant had produced more than three hundred pounds (150 kilograms) of MDMA, or enough 125-milligram doses to reach 1.2 million people. "I put something very pure out there," Carina said. "There was so much empathy in the manufacturing of it, so much emotion. Every good cook will tell you, you gotta put the love in it."

The decision to exit the States had been a good one. With Ecstasy all over the news and now allegedly linked to brain damage, the DEA was taking the "kiddie drug" much more seriously. On August 8, 1986, officers in Dallas raided the Starck Club, characterized by the DEA's Phil Jordan as "the Mecca of the drug Ecstasy." Panicked patrons emptied their pockets, leading to the seizure of 274 tablets of MDMA, 13.5 grams of cocaine, 8 LSD papers, 5 grams of marijuana, 9 Percocet tablets, 3.5 Ritalin tablets, and various unknown pills. "The floor of the place looked like a pharmacy," one witness recalled.

The raid, and Ecstasy's subsequent scheduling, dealt a devastating blow to the club, which never fully recovered. At the same time the AIDS epidemic was sending shock waves through the community, and the collapse of oil prices put a damper on Dallasites' desire to spend. After just five years of business, the Starck's owners decided to close their doors for good. Grace Jones, who had performed on opening night, flew in for the occasion. "Where there's an ending, there's always a beginning," she declared to a cheering crowd. "Y'all gonna stick together and find another party, right?"

Indeed, for MDMA, the party had only gotten started—but its epicenter was shifting. Just as quickly as the Dallas scene had come and gone, Ecstasy culture was taken up across the pond, where young Brits transformed it into something entirely new and, arguably, world-changing.

"Early British dance culture detonated a huge explosion of musical creativity that continued to resonate for decades afterward," said journalist Matthew Collin, author of *Altered State* and *Rave On*. "Its open-access, do-it-yourself ideas also proved to be an enduring inspiration for musicians and cultural activists. And it made MDMA very, very popular indeed."

MDMA found its way to the United Kingdom by at least the early 1980s. Bob McMillen was regularly shipping pills in bottles labeled "Herbal Essence" to a contact there, and British citizens returning from trips to New York City and Dallas sometimes brought Ecstasy tablets back home. Some cultural ripples were already being felt. After Soft Cell's Marc Almond and Dave Ball scored MDMA from an enigmatic Brooklyn dealer called Cindy Ecstasy, for example, the drug helped inspire their hit 1981 debut album, *Non-Stop Erotic Cabaret*. "It became a whole album that was done all around Ecstasy and done on Ecstasy," Almond told Collin.

Still, MDMA was not exceptionally popular in the United Kingdom in the early to mid-1980s, and was mostly just taken at in-home parties. The pivotal moment for Ecstasy culture there came in August 1987, when now-superstar DJ Paul Oakenfold traveled to Ibiza with three mates to celebrate his twenty-fourth birthday. The Spanish island—whose name is derived from Bes, the Phoenician god of music and dance—had recently become an annual summer pilgrimage destination for thousands of British working-class youths.

By the time Oakenfold and his crew arrived, the party was well underway, and Ibiza was soon to take on yet another name: "XTC island." As in Britain, MDMA had arrived there in the early 1980s through visiting tourists and travelers coming from the United States. Evidence also indicates that Ecstasy was peddled across Ibiza by expat devotees of Bhagwan Shree Rajneesh, who had first gotten their Ecstasy from Michael Clegg and had relocated to Ibiza after their commune in Oregon collapsed.

In Ibiza, Ecstasy found an ideal setting. The drug's effects were enhanced by the island's warmth and beauty and by the mesmerizing rhythms of Balearic beat, a subgenre of house music with a bohemian and anything-goes twist. House had first emerged in Chicago's gay Black underground club scene in the early 1980s, and the DJs behind the new music genre defined it as a stripped-down and technologically updated version of disco. Their music soon inspired other DJs in the gay Black scene to create their own subgenres, including acid house in Chicago—characterized by the presence of bass synthesizers—and garage house in New York City and Newark, which included gospel-like vocals and R&B influences.

Whatever the particular subgenre, house music perfectly paired with dancing on Ecstasy. The average heart rate while on the drug is 120 beats per minute—the beat rate of early house tunes (and much contemporary dance music as well). "Some claim this was by design, but it's more likely it emerged naturally as DJs started taking Ecstasy and intuitively, creatively selecting tunes and turntable speeds which approximated 120 bpm, plus or minus 10," said Russell Newcombe, a Liverpool-based educator and researcher who specializes in "drug use, drinking and deviancy." House's repetitive musical structure also complemented the effects of Ecstasy, which, like all amphetamine-based drugs, encourages stereotypy: repetitive actions such as rocking movements, tapping, mechanically chewing gum—or dancing. "Repetitive action is more pleasurable under the influence of stimulants like methamphetamine and Ecstasy, and dancing on Ecstasy is a classic cultural expression of this," Newcombe said.

Oakenfold and his friends concurred. Johnny Walker, one of the DJs on the trip, later described their first encounter with Ecstasy in this setting as "almost like a religious experience."

"All four of us changed that night," agreed DJ Danny Rampling in a 2007 interview. "I can remember saying I think we may be on to something here."

The four friends spent the next week taking more Ecstasy and dancing under the stars to Balearic beat. When they returned home, they searched for a way to re-create their E-fueled glory nights, but found there was no venue for doing so. Clubs closed early and catered to a snobby, alcohol-guzzling crowd, and house music was derided by insecure, mainstream males as "homo shit." The four friends decided to change that.

"There's this kind of mythical boys' holiday to Ibiza," said Peder Clark, a historian of modern Britain at the University of Strathclyde in Glasgow. "All these DJs go there and want to bring that culture and its attendant intoxicants back to rainy Britain."

Oakenfold and his friends set about launching their own underground movement centered around Ecstasy and house music. As Oakenfold later said, "Ecstasy makes you think: 'I could do this, I'm going to do it.' And you do it."

In the United Kingdom, MDMA had been an illegal Class A drug since 1977, when the 1971 Misuse of Drugs Act was amended to include "other ring-substituted phenethylamines." But in 1987 most people there had never heard of Ecstasy and just assumed it was legal. And it certainly was not on the police's radar.

That winter Rampling and his wife, Jenni, started hosting Shoom, a free, invite-only, all-night weekly dance party, named for the feeling of coming up on Ecstasy. The Ramplings initially staged the party in a strobe-lit fitness center filled with strawberry-flavored smoke. Things started small, with just fifty guests. Twelve weeks later, two thousand people were lined up outside.

Loved up on Ecstasy, regular attendees ("Shoomers") regarded themselves as a family. They developed their own terminology ("Acieed," an expression of excitement that some clubbers would shout on the dance floor; "toppy top," slang for "very good"; and "shooming") and pioneered new styles of fashion. Some went for the casual Ibiza beach look, while others channeled cuteness, wearing oversize shirts and clip-on hearts and even carrying teddy bears. They also revived the yellow smiley face from the hippie era, which began appearing on rave clothes and paraphernalia. "I love you" was a common refrain on the dance floor, and hugs were given out in the thousands.

In April 1988 Oakenfold launched his own party at a popular gay club called Heaven, and in June DJ Nicky Holloway followed suit with another weekly event at the Astoria in London's West End. As at Shoom, these parties started small but soon ballooned to thousands of attendees.

What united all three parties was Ecstasy and the all-house soundtrack, including songs imported from Chicago, New York City, and Ibiza. The British DJs also created their own unique subgenre of acid house, at first emulating what was coming out of Chicago but then adding elements from dub reggae, hip-hop, and postpunk electronic music, Collin said.

"The combination of the drugs and the music, it becomes almost indivisible. It's this combination of going together like fish and chips—a very British combination," Clark added, paraphrasing journalist Sarah Champion.

As these and other parties grew, the scene quickly spread to additional clubs in London and to British cities beyond. By the summer of 1988, Ecstasy and house music were everywhere. "Ecstasy was the evangelical force that turned British youth on to the joys of raving to repetitive electronic beats and transformed 'underground' dance music culture into popular nocturnal entertainment in the UK," Collin said. Known as the "Second Summer of Love," this cultural tidal wave evolved into what he described as "the most vibrant, diverse and long-lasting youth movement that Britain had ever seen."

"The Ecstasy phenomenon literally exploded from maybe a handful of people using MDMA in 1987 to millions of pills being used the next year," said Steve Rolles, a senior policy analyst at the Transform Drug Policy Foundation in the United Kingdom. "It was a full-blown cultural phenomenon that went from underground to mainstream youth culture at an astonishing speed."

Former music journalist Mandi James remembers visiting Manchester's Haçienda club in 1988 and sensing that something was off. "I'd literally be one of the only people drinking alcohol," she said. Everyone else was on the dance floor, making fluid, repetitive movements, their pupils the size of saucers and some "pulling weird faces," completely unselfconsciously, she recalled. "I'm like, 'Why are all these people dancing like that? *What* is going on?' "

Mandi soon discovered the answer for herself. She had zero interest in "getting off my face" or exploring strange realms of consciousness, but in Ecstasy she found a frame of mind she loved. "What it is to be human—the way we're trapped in our heads all the time, thinking and cogitating and ruminating—when you're on MDMA, it just wipes the slate clean and you're completely in the moment," she said. "You're not reactive, you're not in pain, you're not in doubt. You just are."

The superhuman ability to dance all night was another major perk for Mandi and so many others, as was the sense of camaraderie and connection that Ecstasy sparked. "Even if it's fueled by a drug, it really is a beautiful thing," Mandi said. "A lot of people spend most of their lives seeking that connection."

Applied across hundreds of thousands of Ecstasy users, this sense of connection began to subtly reshape British social norms. "I don't want to suggest for one moment that Ecstasy was some kind of wonder drug that solved all the social ills of British society," Clark said. "But I do think there is a case for saying that it changed some emotional sensibilities."

People reported seeing men hugging in public for the first time, and class structures seemed to disappear on the dance floor. "You'd get working-class lads who go to football matches mixing with students, mixing with upper classes," Mandi said. "It really was a grand leveler in that respect."

According to popular lore, Ecstasy even seemed to play a role in reducing violence at British football matches—a problem that had plagued the sport since at least the 1950s. Geoff Pearson, a professor of law at the University of Manchester who specializes in football and hooliganism, pointed out that significant changes in stadium infrastructure, policing, and policy were also underway in the late 1980s and no doubt contributed to the reduction in violence. But quite a few hooligans did begin prioritizing clubbing over engaging in football violence, he added, particularly when going to an out-of-town match would interfere logistically with going to a favorite club on a Saturday night. And some, too, did experience a more profound revelation. "They realized, 'Why am I putting my career and possibly life on the line every Saturday when actually I could be doing this—and this is what it's all about,'" Pearson said.

In the late 1980s British youth further solidified their place in cultural history by inventing a new entertainment form, raves, in response to restrictive laws that required nightclubs to close at two to three A.M. "You go to a club and take a pill at eleven or midnight, and by the time you're being thrown out, you're still high as a kite," Clark said. As a solution, DIY illegal parties began popping up in warehouses, fields, deserted airport hangars, abandoned buildings, and empty lots off London's M25. Finding the parties was often an adventure in itself. "You'd just jump in a car with some people who had heard something from someone else, and off you'd go," Mandi recalled. "The police were always sort of three steps behind."

Ken Tappenden, a police chief tasked with finding and breaking up these parties, came to admire his youthful quarries' organizational abilities. As he told Collin, "If they were lieutenants in a military outfit they'd be brilliant at it because of the way they could move people."

The colossal cost of sending police out weekend after weekend wound up further reshaping Britain's legal nightlife landscape by encouraging policymakers to relax licensing laws and permit clubs to stay open later.

"Certainly there's clubs today that stay open until six A.M. and onward, and Ecstasy kicks off that process," Clark said.

MDMA additionally caused some nightclubs to start taking health and safety more seriously. When Newcombe—who had formerly specialized in heroin harm reduction—visited a popular Liverpool club in 1988, the first thing he noticed from a researcher's perspective was that people were not taking breaks. Instead, "it was wall-to-wall dancing, nonstop for six hours," he said. "It was like New Year's Eve every weekend. I'd never seen anything like it."

In one club packed with two thousand gyrating bodies, it got so hot that "clouds would form and it would rain on people," Newcombe recalled. He knew this was a recipe for heatstroke, so he helped to develop leaflets featuring humorous cartoons to educate Ecstasy users about the importance of drinking water and taking breaks. Newcombe and his colleagues at the "Rave Research Bureau" also worked directly with club owners to develop a ten-point harm reduction strategy, which included having "chill-out rooms," making sure water was available, and providing additional training for security staff who were used to dealing with aggressive drunks. "In the beginning, bouncers would come to us and say 'We know you're doing research, but there's this bloke sitting under a table crying and he won't come out and he's freaking us out,' " Newcombe said. "They'd never seen people tripping before."

By 1991 Newcombe and his colleagues' research at several major Liverpool clubs showed that if owners implemented their harm reduction points, they could keep drug-related problems to a minimum. Building on this success, Newcombe worked with Manchester's city council to produce the country's first safer clubbing strategy, adopted by more than one hundred nightclubs as a condition for their licensing. He also helped several clubs save their licenses from being revoked, a move that he ultimately saw as practical. "If you shut clubs, you'll just have illegal raves that are far more dangerous and risky," he explained.

As Ecstasy disrupted the social, political, and regulatory fabric of the United Kingdom, it was also spreading across Europe. In the Netherlands it was introduced in a more therapeutic context in 1986 by another former Bhagwan Shree Rajneesh follower who brought a thousand Ecstasy tablets with him from the United States—possibly made in Carina's lab. "He was traveling around with a bunch of pills in his trunk and a manual with instructions on how to use Ecstasy," said Dutch journalist Philippus Zandstra, coauthor of *XTC*. "He was the first one to actually sell it here."

It wasn't until 1988, though, that Ecstasy really exploded into the Dutch party scene. Other former Bhagwan followers had been pushing it on the dance floor at a nightclub they ran in Amsterdam, Zorba the Buddha, and it caught on. As in Britain, the drug shook up social norms. "Before, we had this heterotypical thing going on of girls dancing and men just standing on the side, drinking shit tons of beer," Zandstra said. "Ecstasy was used by men to get over their boundaries, to say, 'Fuck it, let's go have a good time!' "

In 1989 Berlin became a third major center of Ecstasy culture. After the wall fell, Berliners adopted techno—a genre invented by Black DJs in post-industrial Detroit—as the soundtrack for the city's reunification. Most young people in East Germany had never had the opportunity to experience drugs of any kind, and they were especially curious about psychedelics and Ecstasy. When Timothy Leary was invited to East Germany's Humboldt University to deliver a lecture, youths packed the room. "We listened intensely and hung onto his every word," said Mark Reeder, who founded Berlin's first trance label, in an interview with Collin. A Berlin-based DJ duo called System 01 even sampled snippets of Leary's lecture in tracks titled "Drugs Work" and "Any Reality Is an Opinion."

In addition to fueling marathon techno parties, Ecstasy also became a staple of Berlin's annual Love Parade, which favored house music. At its height, up to a million participants marched down Strasse des 17. Juni—Berlin's long central boulevard, which the Nazis once used for their demonstrations—beaming and blowing kisses on MDMA.

Whether in Britain, Berlin, or Amsterdam, many of the youths who participated in Europe's Ecstasy scene over these years felt, like Carina, that they were a part of something far bigger than themselves. As with LSD in the 1960s, Ecstasy seemed to hint at the possibility of a different kind of future, one in which love, empathy, and unity were paramount. As Mandi said, "Those were innocent times, when anything seemed possible."

*

AS CARINA'S MEXICO-MADE MDMA launched countless trips in the United States, Europe, and probably elsewhere, back in California she was having her own life-changing experiences on the drug. As a bonus for her work, Pauline had gifted her two bottles of MDMA, each containing a thousand pressed pills. "Those two thousand doses?" Carina said. "Walt and I took them all, every single one."

Walt, by this time, had divorced his wife and married Carina. They tried MDMA in every situation they could think of: out on their boat, cross-country skiing, sitting by the fire, and hiking in nature. They even took it while scuba diving. "All your fears are gone, all your inhibitions are gone, and you're just being one with the fish," Carina said.

Carina also used MDMA for her work in Silicon Valley. She once gave a conference talk about electron beams and polymers to an audience of two hundred technologists while high on half a tab of MDMA. "You had them eating out of the palm of your hand," the moderator marveled afterward.

"Oh yeah, you just don't know!" Carina giggled.

In 1988 Syn Labs, a startup Carina had launched, was awarded a patent for a new technology useful for developing superior memory chips for computers. Carina credited the achievement to MDMA. "Using the substance or just being near the substance, you could accomplish great things," she said. "I found my way through the most difficult problems."

Carina kept up the balancing act of living two very different lives, and both were marked with "huge successes," she said. She and Walt had made a few million dollars on MDMA, plus more on their legitimate business pursuits. In addition to the money, Carina felt invigorated by the scientific process of discovery, the thrill of breaking the law, and the conviction that she was doing meaningful work.

By the end of the year, however, Carina and Walt had started to hit some waves. Carina's small company had gotten into a costly lawsuit after a large tech consortium allegedly stole ideas from a proposal she had been invited to submit to them. The couple had also had a falling-out with Clegg, who was late on payments (if they came at all) and seemed to be growing increasingly jealous of them. He would try to convince Carina to travel alone with him and would make childish jabs at Walt in front of her. Behind the scenes, he complained to associates, "Walt stole my fucking chemist and then married her!"

"Michael had no idea how to run a company, and he didn't know how to run people," Carina said. "There was just no discipline."

For a time, Carina and Walt sold MDMA directly to Pauline Clegg. But in late 1989 they discovered that Pauline had broken her promise to sell MDMA from the Mexico lab only in Europe, and had in fact been importing it into the United States. They decided to sever their ties with Pauline and take a break from both the tech industry and MDMA. In early 1991, however, the two couples' lives intersected once again, when Clegg contacted Carina with a request for her help. He'd hired another chemist, Karl Janssen,‡ to set up a lab in Brazil, but Clegg claimed that Karl hadn't produced a milligram of product in three years. He offered to give Carina three million dollars if she'd go sort things out in Brazil.

Carina should have known better than to get caught up in another Michael Clegg plot. But she'd grown bored with semi-retirement, and she was flattered to feel like she was the only person who could save the operation. Clegg also assured Carina that whatever she produced in Brazil would be sent to the European market, where MDMA use was skyrocketing. So from a legal standpoint, she'd have nothing to worry about.

As Carina boarded the flight to Brazil, in the back of her mind, she kept repeating a single line: "I'm gonna be safe, I'm gonna be safe."

*

THE BRAZILIAN LAB Carina would be working in had been set up in a former textile factory outside Blumenau, a southern city surrounded by verdant jungle and populated with the blond-haired, blue-eyed descendants of German immigrants. It was a thematically appropriate location for MDMA production: it was sassafras country.

Sassafras trees have long been recognized for their medicinal properties. In seventeenth-century England, people drank sassafras tonic and tea as a cure-all for a host of ailments, including signs of aging. A popular drinking

---

‡ This is a pseudonym. Karl asked that his real name not be used because he's trying to move on with his life.

song, quoted by Jack London in an 1899 short story, hints at a more recreational use: "All drink of the sassafras root; . . . It's the juice of the forbidden fruit."

The song was right to call out sassafras roots in particular, because they contain the highest concentration of safrole, a root-beer-smelling essential oil that can also be derived from nutmeg, mace, and half a dozen other plant species. Chemists can transform safrole into piperonyl acetone, which can then be converted with the addition of a reducing agent and methylamine to MDMA. Of the three species of sassafras trees, the Brazilian one contains an especially high concentration of safrole.

Carina and Karl—who had been introduced to MDMA by none other than Rick Doblin, when they were both living in Florida—initially butted heads over chemistry- and production-related issues. But they soon got over their initial misgivings about each other. "I asked if she wanted to do some MDMA, she said yes, and suddenly we were allies," Karl said. Sitting by the pool, they talked late into the night about how many people's consciousnesses they had helped to change. They also compared notes on their experiences with Clegg. "We realized that the problem was Michael, and that Michael had to go," Karl said.

Carina didn't know it then, but Brazil would be the last time she'd take MDMA. The Texas Group's days were numbered—as were her days of freedom.

The DEA had been aware of Clegg's involvement in the MDMA business since the early 1980s. But in 1991 they caught a break in actually taking him down when one of Clegg's Ecstasy dealers, a man in the Fort Myers area named Peter Weber, was identified by a confidential informant. Weber incriminated himself by selling a large quantity of MDMA to an undercover DEA agent, and after he was taken into custody, he agreed to cooperate. "It was through Weber that we broke into this group you're calling the Texas Group," said James Klindt, a U.S. magistrate judge for the Middle District of Florida, who prosecuted the case when he was an assistant U.S. attorney. "He really nailed this whole thing from the government's perspective."

Klindt had never heard of Ecstasy or MDMA before, but over the next few years, he would learn all about the drug, the controversy over its scheduling, and the individuals at the heart of its trafficking. "It was a long time ago, but it was a memorable case because there were a lot of unique characters involved in it, and a lot of really smart people," Klindt said. The MDMA trade also captured his interest because it was different from other types of drug networks he'd dealt with as a prosecutor. Gangs were not involved, and the kingpins in this case claimed to be motivated by more than just money. "These guys like Peter Weber, Michael Clegg and Walter Franz, I really think they genuinely had a viewpoint that this MDMA or Ecstasy was—I don't want to say a miracle drug—but that it was capable of expanding a person's spirituality, that they were serving a greater social good," Klindt said. Even so, he added, "I also think that at some point the money got so good, they couldn't resist it."

Weber made recorded phone calls to Texas Group members, including Clegg, who readily discussed details about prices, quantities, and locations of MDMA labs in both Mexico and Brazil. He talked about his ties to Costa Rica and bragged that he planned for his labs to soon be able to produce more than 2,200 pounds of MDMA. That was more than enough for the DEA. Agents nabbed Clegg on March 11, 1992, at an airport in San Jose, California, where he'd dropped in on his Piper Arrow aircraft. As DEA special agent Eric Fowler noted in court proceedings, "he would use that airplane like you and I would use a car." Among the possessions Clegg was carrying was a fake ID identifying him as an ordained minister in the state of California.

Once in custody, Clegg "almost immediately" began cooperating with the government, according to court records. He agreed to turn on his colleagues in exchange for saving Pauline from prosecution, getting to keep his property in Costa Rica, and softening the sentence for the charges he faced, which carried a maximum of twenty years behind bars. Clegg "agreed to cooperate against everyone else in his indictment, including Franz and Leveriza [-Franz]," Klindt told me. "He also really helped us in terms of making new cases and bringing in new defendants."

The new defendants included Karl as well as Clegg's former distributor, Bob McMillen. Clegg told the government that Karl was probably sending MDMA to the United States from Brazil, and that McMillen had been purchasing MDMA from another Brazilian lab at twenty thousand dollars per kilogram.

"He turned in everybody he knew and a bunch of people he didn't know," said McMillen, who claimed to personally know about sixty people Clegg had named. "The federal prosecutor showed me Michael Clegg's complete plea bargain transcript when they were trying to get me to plead guilty. I knew he was a crook, but I didn't know he was so spineless."

Because of Clegg's tip-off, McMillen himself wound up serving nearly seven years in prison, even though he insists that he had ceased all involvement with Ecstasy in the United States six months before it was scheduled by the DEA. In terms of how many people were eventually indicted because of Clegg, Klindt said it wasn't anywhere close to sixty. "But we did feel like Michael Clegg told us about everything that he did, and with whom he was involved," he added.

After word got out about Clegg's arrest, Walt went to stay at the Hyatt Regency at Lake Tahoe, where he checked in under an assumed name. When agents finally caught up to him on March 20, 1992, he refused to disclose his wife's location. Carina, who was pregnant, had gone on the run and ended up hiding out at her parents' house. She was finally arrested on January 12, 1993, when Bruce Savell, the DEA agent who had undertaken the undercover work in Florida, was out in California for another case and, on a whim, stopped by Carina's parents' house to ask if they'd seen her. "Her dad got a look on his face like 'Oh my god,' " Klindt said. "Her father indicated that she was inside the residence."

According to Klindt, Savell and another agent found Carina in a bedroom, hiding under a blanket next to her infant daughter's crib. Carina recalls a more dramatic scene, with around thirty DEA officers surrounding the house and one gloating, "You are our prize!" as he marched her away.

"If you ever create a molecule that's legal, I'll be happy to buy it," she remembered another telling her.

"Up yours," she shot back.

Whatever exchanges were made, Klindt said that in fact it was just the two agents, plus two unmarked DEA cars, that showed up at Carina's parents' place. "But in her mind, a couple cars might have seemed like a SWAT team," he allowed.

Karl had moved back to California, and ten days after Carina's arrest, he was pulled over while driving through Petaluma and brought in for booking.

When the charges were read against him, the judge, he remembered, couldn't even pronounce the word *methylenedioxymethamphetamine*, throwing up his hands after several attempts: "Oh, hell, you know what it is!"

"They can charge me for something but they can't even read what it is," Karl noted with disdain. Karl was also flabbergasted over the fact that he'd been arrested at all. Like Carina, he had been under the impression that the product he made in Brazil would never be smuggled into the United States. When he found out that Clegg had turned him in, he especially couldn't believe it. "I don't blame him for cooperating, but there was no reason to lie and testify that I was part of a plan to smuggle MDMA into the U.S.," he said.

Klindt noted, however, that this interpretation overlooks the breadth of federal drug conspiracy law. "Once the government is able to prove that there's a conspiracy to manufacture, import and distribute MDMA, people can join that overall conspiracy by aiding and abetting without doing any specific act related to, say, Jacksonville, or Florida, or maybe even the United States," he said. "[Janssen] may not have specifically known where all of these tablets were going, but once you join a conspiracy, you're responsible for the actions of your coconspirators."

Clegg, Carina, Walt, and Karl all wound up in Jacksonville, where their case was being prosecuted thanks to Weber's original involvement. Clegg, during his sentencing proceedings, was in true form, and subjected Judge Harvey Schlesinger to a lecture about how MDMA "open[s] up the channel" between the right and left sides of the brain, among other things. "I really feel that this was a vision, and I was doing what I was compelled to do," Clegg said. "Someday we'll remember that I was too early."

Judge Schlesinger pointed out to Clegg that it's the law—not a person's intentions or a drug's particular merits—that reigns supreme in the courtroom. "I can't answer truthfully to a bunch of high school students when they come visit who want to ask, what's the difference between smoking marijuana or drinking alcohol—why is one ok and one isn't from an end result," Judge Schlesinger said. "Those are policy decisions that elected officials make."

There were more practical reasons for Judge Schlesinger to treat Clegg favorably, though. As Klindt noted during Clegg's sentencing proceedings, "Mr. Clegg took this case in great part himself from a narrow conspiracy that was done on the basis of undercover work and gave us the historical perspective that allowed us to find other evidence and other witnesses and expand the charge and expand the scope of the investigation and the prosecution. I think he should be rewarded for that."

Clegg's reward for his cooperation was a sentence of eighty-seven months in prison, significantly less than he could have been given. After being assured they would maintain their right to appeal, Carina, Karl, and Walt also pleaded guilty to their assortment of charges. Carina was sentenced to 78 months; Karl to 70 months; and Walt, the most of anyone, to 108 months.

The three of them spent their first few years behind bars putting together a joint appeal. Among other things, they contended that MDMA was not validly scheduled, so the charges against them were, by default, not valid either. They cited the administrative law judge Francis Young's ruling that MDMA should be placed into Schedule III, as well as Lester Grinspoon's appeal that resulted in the temporary removal of MDMA from Schedule I. In evaluating this argument, judges of the Eleventh Circuit Court of Appeals pointed to a 1990 case in which another defendant who was busted for MDMA in Dallas tried to make the same case to a Texas judge, who rejected it. "We agree," they wrote of the Texas judge's decision. The convictions were upheld.

*

FOR A FEW years the rave scene in the United Kingdom, as though paralleling Carina's life, had been spectacular. But by 1990 things had begun to sour for some participants. The early focus on peace, love, and creative entrepreneurialism was being displaced by people looking to capitalize on the novel social phenomenon—often with little regard for the safety of those whose money they were after. In Manchester especially, gangs got involved in distributing Ecstasy. The quality of the drugs decreased, and violence increased. "Clubs were getting ram-raided by cars, guns were going off inside," Mandi said. "It just got really dark and kind of spiraled out of control really quickly."

The health risks that can accompany Ecstasy use in the club environment were also being revealed, occasionally with tragic results. Novice users sometimes accidentally took too many pills, while some veteran users— seeking to maintain their high amid diminishing returns from having hammered their brains with too much MDMA too frequently—began taking even more Ecstasy. Still others began adding additional drugs to the mix, like speed and cocaine. "It got to the point where you'd be at the club at three or four in the morning, and it felt like being in a mental hospital," Mandi said. "People would be sweating and doing strange, repetitive movements, because they'd just done too much Ecstasy."

Britain saw its first Ecstasy-related death in June 1988, when twenty-one-year-old Ian Larcombe swallowed a bag of eighteen tablets in an effort to hide them from the police, and then died of a heart attack. More deaths sporadically followed, including two in 1989, five in 1991, twelve in 1993, and nineteen in 1994, according to official British statistics. Most of the deaths were attributed to hyperthermia, or extreme overheating caused by "sustained physical exertion, high ambient temperatures and inadequate fluid replacement," as one researcher put it.

"There were instances of clubs that would turn off the taps to sell bottled water, but if you're selling bottled water for three or four pounds, people wouldn't buy it and get dehydrated," Rolles said. "Or there would be clubs that weren't adequately ventilated and people would get overheated."

Given the number of Brits taking Ecstasy, deaths attributed to the drug were in fact exceedingly rare. But they often made headlines, and the media attention increased the perception that "taking Ecstasy is like playing Russian roulette," according to one oft-repeated catchphrase. A 1992 *Daily Star* story titled STOP THIS HELL FOR OUR KIDS captured the sentiment of the day surrounding "evil" Ecstasy. "There is now firm evidence that this stupid sensation-giving pill—especially when mixed with alcohol—is a KILLER," the story hysterically claimed.

It wasn't just health and safety, though, that concerned the mainstream British public about Ecstasy. "As it got bigger and bigger, there was a sense that it was a threat to social norms, to the fabric of society and to authority," Rolles said. Ecstasy seemed to be everywhere: in a 1992 poll conducted for the BBC of 693 regular clubgoers between the ages of sixteen and twenty-five, 31 percent said they had taken Ecstasy, and 67 percent said that their friends had. Extrapolating from these findings, sociologist Andrew Thompson calculated that some 1.7 to 3.5 million British youths had taken Ecstasy, with the total figure nationally for all age groups adding up to perhaps as high as five million. The press, meanwhile, regularly reported that in any given weekend, 500,000 to 1 million young people took Ecstasy. Based on the number of clubs and raves operating in the early 1990s, Newcombe, however, thinks the number was more likely on the order of 100,000 to 250,000 people taking Ecstasy per weekend. "It's all sophisticated guesswork in the end," he said.

Whatever the exact figure, Ecstasy's presence loomed large, and "politicians sought to exploit this threat by hyping it up and putting themselves forward as the answer to it," Rolles said. This created a political situation, he added, in which "you had two things moving in opposite directions." On the one hand, the government had started funding harm reduction efforts of the sort put forward by Newcombe. At the same time, though, the Home Office—the branch of government responsible for national security and law and order—decided it was time for a crackdown.

In response to the moral panic over Ecstasy and raves, in 1990 British lawmakers raised penalties to twenty thousand pounds and up to six months in prison for failing to secure the proper license for events where music and dancing takes place. The new legislation did not stop those who rejected the commodified club experience from continuing to throw illegal outdoor raves, however, so in 1994 lawmakers responded with the Criminal Justice and Public Order Act. This latest bill sought to stamp raves out once and for all by giving police the power to remove "persons attending or preparing for a rave," which they defined as "a gathering on land in the open air of 100 or more persons at which amplified music is played during the night." Music, the bill went on to clarify, means "sounds wholly or predominantly characterized by the emission of a succession of repetitive beats." The bill also made it a criminal rather than civil offense to trespass on someone else's property; removed the right to silence for anyone arrested; and granted the police the power to take intimate body samples. "They were trying to ban not just a drug, because the drug's already illegal, but a type of social gathering where people dance to music, which is absurd," Rolles said.

On May Day an estimated twenty thousand ravers and civil rights advocates showed up in London's Trafalgar Square to protest the bill. Nevertheless, it passed a few months later—and is still British law today. By mid-1996 police had made more than a thousand arrests using the powers granted by the new law, and large-scale outdoor raves had effectively been eradicated.

In a 2000 report, the Police Foundation, an independent think tank focused on improving policing in the United Kingdom, revealed that the longest sentences were given not for "hard drugs" like heroin, crack, or fentanyl, but for MDMA. David Nutt, a neuropsychopharmacologist who was then chairing the British government's Advisory Council on the Misuse of Drugs, remembers puzzling over this seemingly nonsensical finding and speculating that it must have something to do with a cultural disdain for pleasure. "If you're selling heroin, people think therefore you're an addict so you're compelled to do it," Nutt said. "But if you sell Ecstasy, it's for people having fun. People here hate other people having fun—it's part of this British thing."

Seeking an escape from the increasingly draconian situation in Britain, some party collectives moved to Paris, Berlin, Prague, or other European destinations. They established hundreds of "outlaw sound systems" across western Europe and the former Communist East, Collin wrote, where they often continued to come into conflict with the law. But most early participants in Britain's rave scene were not so hardcore as to be willing to uproot their lives to keep the party going. They simply accepted that dance culture had irrevocably shifted, and moved on to other things. "I was a little bit heartbroken, because as naive as it sounds, we really thought this had the potential to change everything," Mandi said. "But it didn't, because it just got swallowed up by commercialization, money, and all the rest of it."

Mandi still regards her experiences in the early rave scene as some of the most precious of her life, though. And although most of the connections she forged on the dance floor did not stand up to the sober light of day, three of the women Mandi used to party with are still her good friends.

"I just had such a blast, it was such a brilliant time," she said. "For this little country bumpkin girl to suddenly be involved in this huge groundswell and movement—it changed my life. It just opened my eyes to what could be possible."

*

MANDI AND CARINA both played parts in building early Ecstasy culture, and both women exited the scene around the same time. But while Mandi left by choice, Carina left by force of the U.S. criminal justice system.

While in "camp" (Carina's preferred term for prison), she and Walt wrote letters to each other every day. She also recalled receiving a memorable note from Rick Doblin. He sent her a MAPS newsletter and informed her that he'd had one of her pills analyzed: "99.99% pure!" she remembered him writing. "Well done!"

"Wow, that's better than gold!" Carina thought. "Little things like that kept me going."

According to Carina, Walt spent his time working on cases for other inmates, ultimately helping to free fourteen women. "My husband continued to be the legal beagle inside," she said. "We always did something good, no matter what."

Likewise, Karl helped a young man named Sticks—who had been busted for selling Texas Group MDMA—get out of prison eighteen months early by spotting an error in his sentencing.

Clegg also put his prison time to use. As he stated on a talk show in 1997, "I had a tremendous breakthrough that I call an awakening." In transitioning from "a life of extreme luxury and wealth to one of total deprivation," he was freed, he said, from "all the limitations of the third dimension." While behind bars, Clegg wrote a book about his "deliverance" from "the preconditioned ego personality," as he puts it on his website, and he also denounced drugs as a false path. He assumed a new name, Satyam Nadeen, and following his release, Clegg/Nadeen became a consultant for people "who want to explore what it's like to live with one foot in the third dimension and one foot in the fourth dimension." There was one precondition, though: "For me to talk to a group of people, the requirement is that they have to read [my] book." Clegg wound up dropping the guru thing after a few years and now runs yoga retreats in Costa Rica and Georgia.

Karl said he got through prison by imagining the hundreds of thousands of people who had likely taken his MDMA. "I knew it changed peoples' lives, and assumed most of it was for the better," he said. After his release, he launched a small, successful company. But more than twenty years later, he still suffers from insomnia and nightmares about his time behind bars. "One of the weird ironies is that MDMA is used for trauma, but I have trauma from MDMA," he said.

Carina and Walt were released a year early as a reward, Carina said, for attending a drug abuse education program. They made a huge bonfire of all the letters they'd written each other in prison. Walt got a job as the chief financial officer of a software company, and Carina worked for a tax office. "We appeared to be normal to everyone else, but little did they know," Carina chuckled.

After visiting Sedona as tourists, in 2011 the couple decided to move there. They planned to spend their golden years playing tennis in the high desert's sun. But in 2014 Walt died from cancer. "I lost him, and I had to reinvent myself," Carina said. She swore off all mind-altering substances, including alcohol, and began hiking the town's four-hundred-plus miles of trails with another widow. Eventually, she decided to convert her hobby into a full-time job as a hiking guide. Out in nature, "I have the opportunity to turn people on without any substance," she said. "I'm the living MDMA—it is within me, it's part of me, cellularly."

Despite all the lows, Carina is at peace with her past. "If I'd just gone for the Intel stock, my life would not have been exciting," she said. She's even enjoyed sharing some of her MDMA stories with her daughter, who is pursuing her master's degree in psychology with a specialty in addiction. "When *Breaking Bad* came out, I told my daughter, 'That's the male me!' " Carina laughed. "Except I didn't go so much into mobile homes.' "

# 6
# THE NEUROTOXICITY PUZZLE

IN A 1987 lecture to first-semester pharmacology students, Alexander Shulgin argued that in the broadest sense, we can define a drug as anything that "modifies the expected state of a living thing." Based on this reasoning, almost everything can count as a drug, from the endorphin rush of vigorous exercise to the energetic blast of radiation therapy given to a cancer patient. Drugs, Shulgin pointed out, are also a full-body experience, things that affect the entire organism rather than just a relatively small handful of that organism's billions of brain cells, also called neurons.

Narrowing that definition down, psychedelic drugs like MDMA, at the most obvious level, are "mind manifesting"—that is, they affect the brain. They primarily do this by imperfectly imitating the structure of natural signaling chemicals that communicate with neurons—the biological hardware of consciousness, memory, mood, and behavior. Rather than act in isolation, neurotransmitters and other chemicals, like the ingredients in a fine cocktail, combine to produce the complex internal landscapes and subjective experiences that define us as individuals. As Shulgin explained to his students, "all affective states, from emotion to stimulation to depression to curiosity, are somehow functionally explainable (if not today, at least someday) by the tracing of the neuronal pathways, and all these pathways are glued together by the magic of neurotransmitters."

In the case of MDMA, the drug's structure primarily mimics serotonin—a jack-of-all-trades neurotransmitter that scientists first discovered in the 1940s. Those early researchers only identified serotonin's effects on the constriction and dilation of the body's blood vessels; experts later learned that serotonin can also be found in the brain, where it helps to regulate mood, sleep, appetite, temperature, and more. Serotonin is moved into neurons by specialized proteins called reuptake transporters, which are located on the ends of neurons. These transporters serve to regulate the amount of serotonin available in synapses, the small spaces between neurons where chemical signals are conveyed. Like tiny vacuums, the transporters recapture serotonin within a millisecond or so of the chemical's release into a synapse.

MDMA specifically exerts its effect by binding to serotonin transporters and causing a novel action: it makes the vacuum-like transporters operate in reverse, dumping up to 80 percent of their stored serotonin into synapses rather than recapturing it. This burst of serotonin activates a subset of up to fourteen different serotonin receptors, which in turn triggers the brain to release a flurry of other neurotransmitters and hormones, including oxytocin. Sometimes called "the love hormone," oxytocin is implicated in interpersonal bonding and feelings of closeness and connection. As oxytocin, serotonin, and other natural chemicals ramp up under the influence of MDMA, activity is reduced in the amygdala—the brain's fear center—and increases in the prefrontal cortex, where information processing takes place.

Much of the knowledge about how MDMA works in the brain was originally pieced together not to understand why the drug seems to be such an effective therapeutic catalyst, however—or why it's become the darling of ravers—but to figure out whether and how it *damages* the brain. Whether it is neurotoxic, in other words. This is the question that obsessed mainstream scientists throughout the 1990s and 2000s, and that drove almost all MDMA-related research at the time.

At MAPS, Rick Doblin also turned his attention to neurotoxicity because he knew it was key for determining whether or not MDMA had an above-ground future. In particular, Doblin wanted answers to what he saw as the two fundamental questions of the neurotoxicity puzzle: If neuron damage does occur, is it permanent or temporary? And when MDMA is given to humans in therapeutic doses, does any damage occur at all?

One of the first things Doblin did after selling Michael Clegg's Ecstasy was commission animal toxicity studies of MDMA—a requirement for any drug undergoing FDA approval. In experiments with forty rats given increasing amounts of MDMA over thirteen days, researchers found that when the drug was administered at doses 100 to 150 times the equivalent of what a therapist would give to a patient, it resulted in "adverse clinical reactions," including death. But the researchers did not find any evidence of brain damage in the autopsied animals. Dogs given daily MDMA doses for twenty-eight consecutive days likewise showed no brain, heart, or liver damage.

This data conflicted, however, with several other studies that looked more closely at the brains of rats given MDMA. Those studies indicated that the drug did in fact seem to damage or destroy certain axon terminals—the button-like endings of nerve fibers that carry signals from one neuron to another. In particular, MDMA seemed to impact axon terminals involved in serotonin regulation.

Doblin knew that more definitive answers were needed, but to get those answers, he had to find a scientist. David Nichols at Purdue strongly encouraged Doblin to collaborate with George Ricaurte, a neurologist at Johns Hopkins–Bayview Medical Center, in the hope that primate data Ricaurte could produce in his lab would help clarify whether MDMA could advance to clinical trials. In a way, this seemed like an odd choice. Ricaurte was a protégé of Charles Schuster, the psychiatrist who had conflated MDA's and MDMA's neurotoxicity on the *Donahue Show*, and Ricaurte was the lead author on the study in question. Doblin took Nichols up on his suggestion, though, because he was willing to work with anyone so long as it served the MDMA cause. "The fears of neurotoxicity were used to justify the emergency scheduling, and the same fears were used by the FDA to justify blocking MDMA research," Doblin said. "The only way forward was to foster Ricaurte's research, to help all of us better understand the actual risks of neurotoxicity."

The two got along well, and Doblin even went to Ricaurte's wedding to Una McCann, a psychiatrist also at Johns Hopkins with whom Ricaurte often coauthored papers. In 1988 Doblin used MAPS funding to purchase and donate fifteen squirrel monkeys to Ricaurte for use in MDMA toxicity trials.

Doblin didn't know it then, but Ricaurte would soon become "famous for using government grants to find everything possible that is dangerous about MDMA," as Ann Shulgin put it. Ricaurte would also go on to frequently claim that "even one dose of MDMA can lead to permanent brain damage." In the beginning, though, Doblin didn't see any reason to doubt Ricaurte's commitment to objectivity, but his opinion later changed. "Initially, I felt George was an impartial scientist," he said. "Over time, I saw that was not the case."

Neither Ricaurte nor McCann, both of whom still work at Johns Hopkins, responded to multiple interview requests I sent them. Other researchers I contacted who might have been able to lend perspective on the MDMA neurotoxicity investigations of the 1990s and 2000s—including one whose lab also heavily focused on this question, and another who was Ricaurte's former graduate student and coauthor of several major papers—did not respond to repeated interview requests, either. Given how politicized this line of investigation wound up becoming, though, it did not surprise me that the people formerly at the helm of it did not care to revisit the past with a journalist.

Ricaurte gave the monkeys donated by MAPS a single oral dose of 5 milligrams per kilogram (mg/kg) of body weight of MDMA, the upper range of what a committed, veteran recreational user might take at a rave (for comparison, therapeutic doses are usually around 1.7 mg/kg). The monkeys' behavior seemed normal after they came down from their forced high, but when Ricaurte examined the animals' brains two weeks later, he found reduced concentrations of serotonin in various regions. In the study reporting the results, Ricaurte ventured that humans might be more sensitive than monkeys to toxic effects caused by MDMA, including "when ingesting a typical 'moderate' oral dose." This message was widely disseminated by the media, generating headlines such as NEW DATA INTENSIFY THE AGONY OVER ECSTASY.

Disturbed by the way the study's findings were being spun, Doblin implored Ricaurte to conduct additional tests with doses of MDMA more in line with those given in therapy or taken by most recreational users. Ricaurte accepted more monkeys from Doblin and gave them 2.5 mg/kg of MDMA once every two weeks for four months (a dose still higher and more frequent than would ever be given in therapy). This time, Ricaurte found no detectable effect on serotonin. He balked at publishing the results, however, reportedly telling Doblin that a single new data point didn't justify an entire paper. Doblin convinced Ricaurte to send his findings to the FDA, at least, but this incident made Doblin question whether Ricaurte was actually committed to reporting the data as it was.

Doblin was still determined to get to the bottom of the neurotoxicity issue, though, and he realized there was something even better than monkeys that he could offer Ricaurte, and something that would surely warrant a publication: human subjects. Ricaurte and McCann couldn't dose people with an illegal drug and then kill them and cut out their brains, but they could use samples of volunteers' cerebrospinal fluid to indirectly measure brain serotonin levels based on the presence of metabolites that break the neurotransmitter down. Doblin volunteered for the first spinal tap, and he convinced twenty-nine other MDMA users to undergo the painful procedure in the name of science as well.

Compared to thirty participants who had never taken MDMA, the drug-using group had 32 percent lower levels of the serotonin metabolite. "The present results indicate that MDMA neurotoxicity, heretofore only documented in animals, may generalize to humans," Ricaurte, McMann, and their colleagues concluded in a paper describing their results. Importantly, though, the researchers had not proven that MDMA caused serotonin depletion—and they had glossed over some key caveats. For one, most of the Ecstasy users also dabbled in other drugs that could affect serotonin. Additionally, they did not disclose that the thirty control participants had been chronic pain patients—and chronic pain is known to *increase* serotonin levels. An unrelated study published around the same time also found a correlation between lower serotonin levels and risk-taking behaviors. "Since drug taking is generally perceived as a risky behavior, it would follow that the low serotonin levels could have led to MDMA use rather than the other way around," journalist Tom Shroder pointed out in *Acid Test*.

The National Institute on Drug Abuse (NIDA), which had awarded Ricaurte a $161,416 grant for the spinal tap study, also seemed uninterested in the caveats. The government agency went on to provide Ricaurte with $14.6 million in grants for various other MDMA-related research from 1989 to 2002, making his lab one of the most influential and well funded in the world for studying the molecule. Ricaurte's papers, often coauthored with McCann, addressed everything from MDMA's effect on sleep, mood, and neuroendocrine responses to its impact on the carnal behavior of "sexually vigorous" male rats. Ultimately, though, all of this research was done in service of exploring one key hypothesis: "That MDMA neurotoxicity generalizes to humans, and that toxicity has functional consequences," as Ricaurte wrote in a NIDA application.

The government's support of labs like Ricaurte's—ones that are focused on proving the harm of drugs—was not surprising, as it built on years of escalating efforts in service of the war on drugs. In the 1980s Ronald Reagan had scaled up global military actions in drug-producing nations and established mandatory minimum prison sentences for drug offenses through the Anti-Drug Abuse Act. George H. W. Bush doubled down on Reagan's efforts—stating in 1989 that drugs are "the gravest domestic threat facing our nation"—and Bill Clinton carried the torch from there. From 1980 to 1997, the number of people behind bars for nonviolent drug offenses octupled from fifty thousand to more than four hundred thousand. Nancy Reagan's message of "Just Say No" was also being taught in DARE classes in schools around the country, and the public messaging worked. In 1985, just 2 to 6 percent of Americans ranked drug abuse as the nation's "number one problem," but by 1989, 64 percent did.

In 1994 Sasha Shulgin even became a target of the war on drugs when around thirty DEA agents raided his laboratory. Shulgin was fined twenty-five thousand dollars for "anonymous drug samples" that people had sent him unsolicited, hoping he'd test them, and the DEA terminated his Schedule I license. Given that two previous inspections had turned up no such infractions—and that Shulgin had collaborated with the DEA for some thirty years—he and Ann could only conclude that the raid was retribution for the detailed synthesis instructions they'd recently published for 179 different psychedelics in *PIHKAL*.

"Dr. Shulgin apparently was a pretty good chemist, but he was always on the line between what's legal and what's not legal," said Frank Sapienza, formerly of the DEA. "He would push the envelope in terms of personal freedoms with drugs."

Among the many negative outcomes created by the war on drugs was a stifling of legitimate scientific research on any aspect of controlled substances other than their abuse. NIDA was not interested, for example, in funding another ethnographic study of MDMA users to follow up on the one Jerome Beck and Marsha Rosenbaum conducted in the late 1980s, even though that data could have helped reveal important information about how people's relationship with the drug changes over time. "The problem was, we didn't find that many problems," Rosenbaum said. "These were not sad stories, which is probably why NIDA didn't give us any more money." She and Beck never did get to do a second study, because alternative grant sources did not exist.

NIDA funds nearly 90 percent of world's drug research, and it generally does not support studies that seek, for example, to investigate the positive or medical aspects of scheduled drugs, the cost-benefit analysis of drug policy, the consequences of harsh criminal penalties for drugs, harm reduction efforts that could make drug taking safer, or how and why people use drugs. "Those questions just aren't asked," said Ethan Nadelmann, the founder and former executive director of the Drug Policy Alliance.

The end result has been a chilling effect on the entire field, and ultimately on the type and amount of knowledge generated about drugs. "As an academic, if you can't get grants, your career is over," Nichols said. "There wasn't money for research for psychedelics, so no matter how interested people were, they thought, 'I can't go into that field.' "

*

IN 1990 SASHA Shulgin mailed Doblin a letter published in the *Archives of General Psychiatry* by three doctors at UC Irvine. In their letter, the doctors criticized some of Ricaurte and his colleagues' methods. More fundamentally, they questioned whether "concerns over long-term neuropsychiatric damage" caused by MDMA "have been overstated."

Doblin immediately reached out to the lead author, psychiatrist Charles Grob.

"I'm sitting in my office and I get a call," Grob recently recalled. "This guy's like, 'Hi, you don't know me, but my name's Rick Doblin. Sasha Shulgin showed me your letter to the editor and I thought it was great. I'm interested in funding human research and I'll be in L.A. next week, can we meet?' "

"Okay, come on down," Grob replied.

Grob had developed an interest in psychedelics after trying LSD in 1969 as an undergraduate at Oberlin College. A few years later, while working overnight shifts at a dream lab in Brooklyn, he discovered an office library with virtually every journal article and book written to date on psychedelics. In between monitoring EEGs of sleeping study participants, Grob devoured the collection. "One morning, at three or four A.M., it just hit me: I wanted to study psychedelics," Grob said. He called his dad on the spot, waking him from a deep sleep to announce that he'd had a career epiphany.

Grob's dad, an internal medicine doctor, replied with some practical advice: "Okay son, there may be something to what you say, but no one will listen to you unless you get your credentials."

So Grob enrolled in medical school. Every month, almost ritually, he would head to the library and comb through the new scientific literature for mentions of LSD. But he never found anything, because research "was all off the board." As he worked his way through a specialty in child psychiatry, he struggled to connect with anyone else who shared his interests. At Johns Hopkins, the conservative chairman of Grob's department "basically said, 'Not on my watch. These are dangerous drugs.' I was warned off that this would be a career killer."

After Grob was recruited for a position at UC Irvine, for the first time, he met a handful of colleagues who shared his fascination with psychedelics. The four doctors collaborated on a study evaluating the subjective experience of twenty psychiatrists who had taken MDMA, and found that 40 to 50 percent credited the drug with long-term positive changes such as improved interpersonal relationships, better performance at work, or favorable shifts in their outlook on religious, spiritual, or life priorities. By this time, though, the MDMA neurotoxicity issue was gaining momentum, and other research groups had tried and failed to get approval from the FDA to study various psychedelic substances in a clinical setting. Research on psychedelic-assisted therapy seemed like a dead end.

When Doblin showed up at Grob's office, though, he had some good news to share. He had inside information from the FDA indicating that clinical research of psychedelics might be possible after all.

After finally graduating from New College sixteen years after enrolling, Doblin had decided that he could best serve the MDMA mission by becoming a public policy whiz. His GRE score—in the top one tenth of 1 percent—apparently helped offset his meandering undergraduate record, and he gained admission into a master's program at the John F. Kennedy School of Government at Harvard University. "I was absorbing the establishment vibe, learning the system," Doblin said of his time at Harvard.

Following graduate school, Doblin was selected as a presidential management intern at the White House Office of Personnel Management, a program intended for young people who want careers in the federal government. Doblin was open to this, thinking that a job with the feds could be an opportunity to work from the inside out to change MDMA policy. He interviewed with the CIA but was denied an offer when he insisted that his sole goal as an agent would be ending the war on drugs. He got further along in interviews with the FDA, but after months of meetings the DEA stepped in and said they would refuse to work with Doblin because he had previously sued them. "I like to say the DEA saved me from giving up drugs and having to wear a suit and tie to work," Doblin quipped. He decided a job in government wasn't for him, after all, and that he would be better served by pursuing a PhD at the Kennedy School.

Although Doblin's time on the inside hadn't ended in a federal job, it had given him important insight on how the system works. "The masterstroke was Rick enrolling at the Harvard Kennedy School of Government and essentially using that platform to be able to go to the top folks in D.C., especially at the DEA and FDA," Beck said. "All of them would be saying 'Of course it's possible to research these drugs,' and Rick would say, 'Well, how would you go about that, exactly?' No one had ever really done that before and then, step by step, did it."

Doblin learned that previously, the responsibility for reviewing psychedelic protocols—essentially, research proposals submitted to the FDA—was handled by Paul Leber, director of the administration's Division of Neuropharmacological Drug Products. Leber had been notoriously opposed to psychedelic research of any kind since the early 1970s. True to his reputation, after MDMA's scheduling, Leber declined a request from George Greer for compassionate use of MDMA-assisted therapy for a terminal cancer patient, and he also nixed a plea put in by Doblin for doing the same for his dying, depressed grandmother. Any application on mind-altering substances that wound up on Leber's desk would mean "certain death," as Doblin put it.

In March 1989, however, the FDA transferred authority for research involving Schedule I drugs to a new group, the Pilot Drug Evaluation Staff, headed by long-time FDA official John Harter. One of Harter's deputies was a doctor named Curtis Wright, who set about combing through all the old Investigative New Drug applications. Wright found project proposals for marijuana, LSD, MDMA, and DMT, but all had been put on a clinical hold— FDA-speak for an indefinite delay, considered by researchers to be "the kiss of death." There was no information about why these applications had been put on hold, however, or what needed to be done to address the issues upon which the holds were based. The implications seemed clear: someone at the top did not want these studies to get done. Wright was disturbed to see this apparent bias, later noting that "it is invidious to prevent research, even if it will produce results you don't want."

Under Harter's leadership, in 1990 the Pilot Drug Evaluation Staff approved the first new psychedelic research application in about two decades: a study of DMT led by Rick Strassman at the University of New Mexico. Two more applications for small LSD studies were approved after that.

Explaining all of these developments to Grob, Doblin thought the time was ripe for submitting an MDMA protocol to the FDA. "What do you think?" he asked.

Doblin struck Grob as "bubbling with optimism" and in a hurry to get things done, but Grob was also impressed with Doblin's knowledge. "One thing about Rick, he knew the FDA system inside and out, and he had cultivated rapport with many of the inside people," Grob said.

Case studies from the 1970s and early 1980s suggested that MDMA-assisted therapy could help alleviate worries about death in people with terminal illnesses and redirect their attention to enjoying the life they had left, so Grob and Doblin agreed to move forward on a protocol to test the treatment in terminal pancreatic cancer patients. It took two years, but "like persistent turtles," as Doblin put it, in 1992 he and Grob finally had a protocol to submit to the FDA. Rather than evaluate it outright, though, the FDA decided to convene a meeting to discuss the agency's general policies regarding psychedelic research. For the first time in fourteen years, NIDA also agreed to review their approach toward "hallucinogen" research. Grob and Doblin traveled to Rockville, Maryland, to attend the NIDA and FDA meetings, as did other experts from around the country, including Shulgin, Ricaurte, and Nichols.

In the NIDA meeting, things seemed to go well. Shulgin made the room laugh by asking how researchers would ever get rats to provide sufficient data on psychedelic experiences of a religious or mystical nature, and the NIDA official overseeing the session confirmed that her office is "interested in exploring therapeutic utility, if there is any, for hallucinogenic drugs."

The FDA meeting was a bit more dramatic. In front of TV crews and reporters, Wright told attendees about discovering all the indefinitely frozen psychedelic study applications. "I can think of nothing that has a more chilling effect in research," Wright said. He emphasized that the FDA "has a tremendous responsibility to take great care that the regulatory process does not become a major factor in the inhibition of needed research."

Reese Jones, a psychiatrist from UCSF, criticized alarmist interpretations of MDMA neurotoxicity data. He noted that since serotonin depletion didn't seem to harm lab animals and seemed to be enjoyed by so many human users—many of whom reported lasting positive changes—perhaps this effect was actually advantageous in some way rather than dangerous. If a pharmaceutical company created a drug that produced benefits tied to brain changes, he half joked, those brain changes would no doubt be a major selling point.

After Ricaurte gave a presentation about MDMA neurotoxicity, Jones pressed him to describe the functional consequences of those changes. Ricaurte admitted that functional consequences had yet to be identified—or perhaps might only happen over time. Wright asked Ricaurte to estimate the risk of MDMA to the subjects in Grob's proposed cancer study, and Ricaurte allowed that the dose probably would not pose a serious risk. After further discussion, the committee agreed that the risk could likely be controlled, and that the cancer study seemed to be warranted.

"It was very exciting," Grob recalled of the decision. "I felt we were making history."

At the end of the day, as Doblin and Grob were preparing to go their separate ways, Doblin pulled out a joint in the FDA parking lot. "A celebratory toke," Grob said. "Which by today's standards is perfectly normal, but back then it was taking a risk."

In November 1992 the FDA officially gave Grob the green light to conduct the first ever government-approved study administering MDMA to people. FDA trials take part in three phases, and this would be the first small Phase 1 trial on the journey toward possible clinical approval. There was just one hitch: rather than start with terminal cancer patients, Wright told Grob, he would have to first complete a safety study administering MDMA to healthy volunteers. This seemed like a reasonable request. At last things seemed to be moving in the right direction.

*

IN 1993 GROB moved from UC Irvine to Harbor-UCLA Medical Center, where he continued to work on the Phase 1 trial. Meanwhile, at Johns Hopkins, Ricaurte and McMann remained focused on MDMA neurotoxicity. Their research was often picked up by the media under headlines such as PROOF THAT ECSTASY DAMAGES THE BRAIN. Based on their findings, in 1998 NIDA launched a now-notorious messaging campaign suggesting that Ecstasy caused "holes in the brain." The "holes," in fact, were just normal computer-generated depictions of areas of lesser blood flow in the brain, but that detail was glossed over by Oprah, MTV, and other alarmist media.

Grob and other experts continued to point out problems associated with Ricaurte and McCann's studies, which Grob damningly characterized in a 2002 article as showing a "pattern of flawed research methodologies and deceptive practices of data analysis."

In a 1999 study, for example, the Johns Hopkins researchers reported "subtle, but significant, cognitive deficits" in MDMA users, including problems with short-term memory. But as usual, they had not taken into account confounding variables, such as the fact that people who take Ecstasy are almost always polydrug users—also using marijuana, cocaine, ketamine, methamphetamine, or other psychedelics—and that those substances could also potentially influence performance on a memory test. Additionally, compared to the control group (which were likely graduate students), Ecstasy users tend to be committed partiers who regularly miss meals and nights of sleep—which likewise could impact memory. These oversights alone make the claim that MDMA causes memory impairment "highly suspect," Grob wrote.

Grob and others' complaints about Ricaurte and McCann's work mostly fell on deaf ears, though. Rave culture had arrived in North America by the early 1990s, imported by British expats starting in San Francisco at the popular venue ToonTown and spreading from there. My husband, Paul, for example—a computer programmer in New York City in his mid-forties—fondly recalls attending illegal raves in Denver on most Saturdays from 1996 to 1998. He and his friends would find out about raves through paper flyers left on their cars' windshields, and on the day of the event they'd either call a phone number or go to a record shop on Capitol Hill to find out the location. "They wanted to check you out to make sure you weren't some narc that would get the party busted," Paul said.

The raves were always held in warehouses in seedy areas of town, far from any apartments or open businesses, and "you could hear the bass a block away," Paul said. Alcohol was never sold, but Ecstasy was easy to find. Certain raver kids doubled as runners for higher-level dealers who would never set foot on the premises, and attendees usually bought from the same salesperson every weekend. "There was this South African guy, James, who had a black belt in ken po, and Bill, a big teddy bear-looking dude," Paul recalled of his go-to Ecstasy dealers. "None of these were shady, scary-looking people. These were suburban kids there for a good time. Depending on when you caught them, they'd already be rolling."

The ages of attendees ranged from about fifteen to twenty-one, and 70 to 80 percent of the people there were on Ecstasy, Paul estimated. JNCO jeans were in—the bigger the bottoms, the better—as were skateboarder shoes and wallet chains. Alternatively, some people went for the candy raver look, dressing "like cute little kids," Paul said, complete with pacifiers, pigtails, and brightly colored beaded bracelets. Tickle Me Elmo, the must-have children's Christmas present of 1996, was also a hit in the scene. "When you tickled him, he'd vibrate—which felt really crazy when you're rolling—and he'd say little things like, 'Hahaha, love me!'" Paul recalled. "Soccer moms were competing with raver kids to acquire an Elmo."

Similar to early British Ecstasy culture's focus on camaraderie and connection, some U.S. ravers adopted a behavioral and ethical framework called

Peace, Love, Unity, and Respect (PLUR), meant to foster safety and inclusivity in the community. "PLUR was the motto for the rave scene," Paul said. "It's a beautiful message, but I was kind of cynical about it. Like, don't kid yourself about what's going on here—you're not changing the world, you're just a bunch of teenagers getting fucked up in a warehouse."

Raves and the associated PLUR culture might not have saved the world, but they definitely did shape some participants' outlooks on life. UCLA social neuroscientist Matthew Lieberman recalls attending warehouse parties in Los Angeles in the early 2000s as a young psychologist and being blown away by the openness, friendliness, and acceptance he experienced on the dance floor. "In some ways it was like being in preschool again, like, everybody is your friend!" he recalled. "It had a huge impact on me."

In particular, he said, he developed a lifelong tendency to give others the benefit of the doubt and to assume that "underneath all the pressures of society, people just want to connect and to feel positively connected to other people." Lieberman doesn't remember formal associations with PLUR at the raves he attended, but an ethos of camaraderie and warmth permeated the scene. He later realized this atmosphere was contingent not just on MDMA but also on the setting in which the drug was taken. When he and his friends traveled to Ibiza and attended a few raves there, for example, he felt like the style of dancing was more aggressive and the sense of connection with the strangers around him was lacking. "If that was where I had initially done MDMA, I wouldn't have had the same experience at all," he said. "It's not just about taking the drug, but about the experience and how that's curated."

No firm statistics exist quantifying just how many American kids took Ecstasy in the 1990s and early aughts, but evidence indicates that its use was widespread and growing. A 1993 NIDA survey estimated that 2 percent of U.S. college students took the drug over the last year, and in 1999, 8 percent of high school seniors were estimated to have done the same. According to another national survey, in 2001 alone, nearly two million Americans tried Ecstasy for the first time—bringing the total number who had tried the drug up to an estimated ten million.

Mirroring what happened in Britain a few years before, as more American youths discovered Ecstasy, mainstream public panic ensued. Some concerns were warranted. By the mid-1990s pill adulteration, for example, had become a serious problem. With the Texas Group out of the picture, more unscrupulous producers had stepped in. From at least 1997 until his arrest in 2000, Oded Tuito, a two-hundred-pound Israeli fugitive, was said to be the largest Ecstasy distributor in the world. The "Fat Man," as Tuito was nicknamed, had formerly dealt in heroin, cocaine, and marijuana, but Ecstasy proved to be more lucrative. He recruited strippers, Hasidic students, and intellectually disabled people to smuggle millions of pills from Europe to the United States and distributed them around the country, including to mobsters like John Gotti.

Although Tuito's signature "Tweety" pills were known for their high MDMA content, by the late 1990s only an estimated 40 percent of what was sold as Ecstasy in the United States tested positive for MDMA, according to the DEA. (Conflictingly, however, a DEA PowerPoint presentation from 1999 states that 80 percent of tested MDMA samples contained the drug.) Tablets were found cut with a wide variety of adulterants, from more benign substances like aspirin or caffeine to more dangerous ones such as methamphetamine, PCP, or even potentially lethal paramethoxyamphetamine (PMA). Ecstasy, by this time, was causing thirty to forty deaths per year in the United States. The fatalities followed the same patterns as seen in Britain: users at raves or clubs becoming hyperthermic; users taking excessive doses, either accidentally or intentionally (the latter is known as "macho ingestion syndrome"); and users unknowingly taking Ecstasy tablets tainted with dangerous substances. While the deaths were "all tragic, they were, for the most, part preventable," Grob pointed out. They also failed to point to any fatal neurotoxic effect of MDMA.

In addition to claiming that MDMA neurotoxicity was deadly, though, Ricaurte and other labs had also promoted the idea that the drug caused nonlethal brain damage. Yet millions of ravers around the world had so far escaped any severe mental impairment or extreme memory loss. While some were burned out from partying too hard, for the most part their brains, at least, seemed to be intact.

To buttress against what their critics regarded as an awkward lack of real-world evidence, Ricaurte and others created what came to be known as the "time bomb" theory of MDMA neurotoxicity. Echoing claims from the late 1960s that LSD damaged chromosomes, they warned of a coming host of problems for MDMA users later in life. "What we don't know is whether twenty or thirty years from now, at the age of 45, [MDMA users] may begin to be showing central nervous system degenerative signs that ordinarily would not be seen until they get to be 70 or 80," Schuster, Ricaurte's mentor, told the Associated Press. Ricaurte later went so far as to warn that MDMA users were putting themselves at risk for Parkinson's disease.

More than three decades have now passed since widespread recreational Ecstasy use first emerged, and for many early ravers, the proof is in the pudding that the "time bomb" worries were unwarranted. As one formerly heavy Ecstasy user told me, "If MDMA is as neurotoxic as the government alleged it is, I'd be brain dead."

"I've taken MDMA a hundred and thirty times over the last forty years," Doblin added. "I'd be less capable of speaking now, I guess, if I had all these holes in my brain."

Bay Area physician Howard Kornfeld, a leader in the field of opioid addiction, agreed with these anecdotal accounts. "There are people who say, 'During that period when I was taking too much MDMA, I wasn't right mentally,'" Kornfeld said. "But in my medical practice, I have not seen or had anyone tell me that they haven't recovered."

"MDMA neurotoxicity just hasn't happened to anything like the degree we had been given to expect in the early 1990s," agreed psychiatrist Ben Sessa, the chief medical officer at Awakn, a psychedelic medicine company in the United Kingdom. Sessa clarified, though, that that doesn't mean there aren't any repercussions for taking too much MDMA. "If you're a very heavy user, there's no doubt [MDMA] can cause damage to your brain," he said. "But there's also evidence that shows that when you stop, your brain returns to normal."

MDMA is not physically addicting, so overuse usually occurs in service of social and recreational motivations. This usually winds up being a self-correcting problem, though. "I've been in private practice since 1995, and I've never had a patient come into practice and say 'I'm currently abusing Ecstasy.' But I have had a few say 'There was a time I was using a lot of Ecstasy and I stopped,'" said psychiatrist Julie Holland, editor of *Ecstasy: The Complete Guide*. "If you're using too much MDMA, it doesn't feel good—it feels bad. You can't sustain an addiction because it just feels bad."

Beck and Rosenbaum likewise found in their interviews with a hundred MDMA users that when people did overuse the drug, within a few months most had tapered off. Relatedly, a 1999 study revealed that average ravers in Toronto had a "shelf-life" of just two years, while a 2001 study in Munich found that 80 percent of Ecstasy users gave the drug up sometime in their twenties. Young people frequently just outgrow the lifestyle—as was the case for Paul. "I always felt like a tourist in the party scene," he said. "I knew I had this limited window of time I can party on the weekends, and at some point, that time was gonna be up. I had goals and plans for my life."

MDMA also sometimes facilitates its own disuse. If taken too often and at too-high doses, the drug loses its magic, people often report. In an unpublished survey of six hundred MDMA users, neuroscientist Matthew Baggott found that 40 percent said the drug's effects changed over time. As the pleasurable parts of the experience diminish, users say they are left with more negative side effects: jaw clenching, wiggling eyes, speedy jitteriness, and a low mood in the days after. "Sadly, when I hit my fifties, the upside of MDMA became less and less and the downside became more and more," said Nadelmann, who formerly used the drug primarily for enhancing communication with romantic partners. Eventually he just gave up on MDMA. "That's been quite sad for me," he said.

Scientists still do not know the mechanisms behind this particular type of tolerance, why it occurs in some MDMA users but not others, and why some people who lose the Ecstasy high are able to recapture it after taking a break, while for others it seems to be gone forever. Ann Shulgin, for example, wrote all of her contributions to *PIHKAL* with the help of her "ally," MDMA. "It was my writing drug," she told me. Ann took MDMA every Monday for a year, and by the end of that time she was having to use 250 milligrams with a 150-milligram booster to achieve the same effects she once got on less than half that amount. Eventually the drug produced depression rather than euphoria.

Ann tried taking breaks—even waiting as long as ten years—but the magic continued to elude her. "I have lost one of my best friends," she lamented. She was ninety when I interviewed her, and she told me she still hadn't given up hope. "One of these days I'm going to try it again and see if it works," she said with a twinkle in her blue eyes. Ann passed away in July 2022. Whether she gave MDMA one more shot, we'll never know.

*

IN 1998 GROB published Phase 1 trial results showing that MDMA could be safely administered in a clinical setting. The eighteen volunteers—all of whom had prior experience taking Ecstasy, per the FDA's requirement—were randomly assigned doses ranging from 0.25 mg/kg to 2.5 mg/kg. Most volunteers had three sessions, two on different doses of MDMA and one on an inactive placebo.

The MDMA used in the trial had actually come courtesy of Doblin, who had arranged prior to the drug's scheduling for Nichols to synthesize a large batch at Purdue (which Doblin paid for with the proceeds from Michael Clegg's Ecstasy). "We made him about two kilograms of very pure MDMA, and I only charged for the cost of the starting materials," Nichols said. "It was beautiful stuff." Kept under lock and key, the Nichols MDMA would prove valuable for years to come for both MAPS-sponsored studies and for research conducted by other groups. Some of the original two kilograms is still left over today, and as Nichols noted, it's "still stable and good."

Grob's study using Nichols's MDMA produced valuable insights. For one, he learned that 2.5 mg/kg of MDMA is way too much for some subjects. Two of the participants who received that dose had hypertensive reactions that concerned Grob. (Gripped in the throes of the MDMA high, the participants themselves hadn't actually minded.) Several other participants experienced slightly elevated heart rates and blood pressure, but overall, MDMA did not produce any concerning mental or physical side effects. The only real complaint came from the charge nurse at the hospital, who was unhappy that her subordinates were neglecting their duties in favor of spending time with Grob's high study participants. "The subjects were so empathetic and so interested in the lives of the nurses that the nurses were really enjoying sitting in there," Grob said.

With these favorable findings in hand, all of the roadblocks seemed to be out of the way for MDMA-assisted therapy to finally be investigated in a controlled clinical setting. As Grob submitted the draft protocol to the FDA for the long-awaited terminal cancer patient study, he felt great satisfaction knowing that he'd helped to establish a precedent for other researchers. "If you're serious and you do a good enough job putting together your protocol, it's possible to do this kind of work," he said.

When he didn't hear back from the FDA immediately after submitting his proposal, he wrote it off as bureaucratic slowness. But as weeks turned into months and he continued to hear nothing, he and Doblin began to worry.

As it turned out, things had changed at the FDA since the meetings in 1992. The Pilot Drug Evaluation Staff had been dissolved in 1995. Most of the original members who shared Harter's favorable views about the scientific research process no longer worked there, and Wright was about to leave for a job in the pharmaceutical industry. Also working against Grob and Doblin's interests, "there was this incredible rise of even more of this paranoia from neurotoxicity fear," Doblin said. "It kept growing and growing and growing."

In March 1999 Grob finally received an answer: the FDA would not be giving their blessing to any more MDMA trials in humans until additional preclinical animal studies had been completed. Grob lodged a formal complaint, asking officials to elucidate why his protocol had not been approved.

As he awaited an answer, though, Grob began to realize just how weary he'd grown of the MDMA fight. The subject was too controversial, he thought, and too politically charged. He knew there were other psychedelics out there, ones that also seemed to hold therapeutic promise but were less fraught. He reached out to Nichols to talk things through. Nichols himself had given up on MDMA research years earlier, when support for his studies had dried up. "It became clear the only thing NIDA was interested in funding was understanding the neurotoxicity of MDMA," Nichols said. "That wasn't what I wanted to do."

In 1993 Nichols founded the Heffter Research Institute, a nonprofit group that supports studies predominantly of psilocybin, the main psychoactive ingredient in magic mushrooms. Nichols chose psilocybin specifically because it seemed to have the least amount of political and social baggage, and like MDMA, had a relatively short action. "Nowadays, most people have heard of psilocybin, but back then, the average Mr. Citizen hadn't."

After a long conversation with Nichols during a Heffter board meeting, Grob decided he would still pursue the cancer patient study. But he would use psilocybin rather than MDMA, and he would partner with the Heffter Research Institute rather than MAPS. Breaking the news to Doblin caused "a bit of a dispute," as Grob put it. "Rick yelled—he threw a tantrum."

Whereas both men's stubbornness had previously been aligned, now, Grob said, "we were pushing our stubbornness in different directions."

*

AS THE NEW millennium dawned, MDMA continued to be portrayed as a deadly drug by U.S. politicians and the media. A DEA presentation from around this time, for example, described the drug as "stripping bare" serotonin nerve terminals. Complications from taking recreational doses of MDMA, the administration claimed, include "immediate life-threatening events"; "HIV, AIDS, hepatitis and other communicable diseases"; Parkinson's and Alzheimer's diseases; and "drug dependence." "Ecstasy is neurotoxic in the dose-range experienced in Rave clubs," the DEA definitively stated. "There is no 'recovery' from cell damage."

In response to the fever pitch, in 2000 U.S. lawmakers passed the Ecstasy Anti-Proliferation Act, increasing sentences for trafficking MDMA by up to 300 percent. This made dealing in MDMA more heavily punished, dose by dose, than heroin. In 2002 then-senator Joe Biden, a preeminent crusader in the war on drugs, introduced the Reducing Americans' Vulnerability to Ecstasy (RAVE) Act. Among other things, the new legislation sought to prohibit any event at which Ecstasy was known to be taken, and the presence of pacifiers and glow sticks—labeled as "drug paraphernalia"—were enough to prove as much. After complaints arose that this violated the First Amendment right to freedom of assembly, a slightly tweaked version of the bill, renamed the Illicit Drug Anti-Proliferation Act, passed.

Vilification of Ecstasy from the scientific establishment was also at a boil. In 2002 Grob spotted a startling paper published in the prestigious journal *Science* that, at first glance, seemed to vindicate his decision to leave MDMA behind. It was another Ricaurte and McCann study. This time, they had injected ten squirrel monkeys and baboons with a dose of MDMA equivalent to what a recreational user would take. Alarmingly, two of the animals had died and two others collapsed from heatstroke. When the researchers conducted autopsies, they found not only that neurons involved with serotonin had been damaged, but also that 60 to 80 percent of those involved with dopamine had been destroyed, too. "The implication being that all these young ravers are going to come down with Parkinson's because they're blowing out their dopamine systems," Grob said. "It looked like MDMA neurotoxicity had won the field."

From the beginning, though, the findings were fishy, and even prior to publication, there had been some pushback by researchers who peer-reviewed the study. "When that paper was submitted saying MDMA use in clubs causes permanent brain damage, some scientists said, 'Well, hold on a second. I don't see people coming out of clubs with Parkinsonism,'" said David Nutt, director of the Neuropsychopharmacology Unit at Imperial College London. "Allegedly, [the paper] was initially rejected. But because *Science* is published by [the American Association for the Advancement of Science], and that gets funding from the U.S. government, there was pressure on the editor to get it published even though the referees said no."

The $1.3 million NIDA-funded study was widely reported in the news, including by the *New York Times*, the *Washington Post*, and the Associated Press. Throughout the media blitz, Doblin and a handful of scientists continued to raise concerns. Neuroscientist Matthew Baggott was working with MAPS at the time and recalls puzzling over Ricaurte and McCann's results, because they appeared to be typical findings from a methamphetamine study rather than some novel MDMA-caused syndrome. "It looks like their tech stole the MDMA and swapped it out for meth," Baggott half joked to his MAPS colleagues. For a year, letters to the editor flew back and forth about the *Science* paper's questionable findings. But confined to the professional literature, the dispute remained out of the public eye. For ordinary Americans, the message was clear: Ecstasy was a potentially deadly drug that caused serious brain damage.

But then, in September 2003, *Science* issued a startling retraction. Ricaurte, McCann, and their colleagues hadn't given the primates MDMA at all. Just as Baggott had suspected, they had used methamphetamine, aka crystal meth—a drug significantly more toxic than MDMA. This explained the animals' adverse reactions and also the finding about dopamine. What it didn't explain, though, was how on earth such a serious mix-up had happened. "Reporting on the wrong drug?" Grob said. "That's bizarre, really bizarre."

The media picked up on "the great retraction," as Grob and others came to refer to the incident, and other scientists sharply criticized the mistake. Schuster, castigating his former mentee, told the *New York Times* that the dead animals should have sent up a red flag, and "the better part of valor" would have been to hold off on publishing the results until they were repeated. Richard Wurtman, a clinician at Harvard and MIT, accused Ricaurte of "running a cottage industry showing that everything under the sun is neurotoxic." Even Nora Volkow, the notoriously antidrug director of NIDA, called the error "crying wolf and losing your credibility."

"I still talk about that study all the time, because I think it's one of the worst examples of politicization of science in my lifetime," Nutt told me.

Ricaurte, McCann, and their colleagues never provided a satisfactory explanation for what happened. In their retraction, they stated that the drug bottles had been mislabeled—an accusation that RTI, the chemical manufacturing company NIDA contracted with, insisted was not possible. "RTI duly audited their procedures, found no possible way they could have made this kind of mistake and sent out a letter saying as much to the research community," Baggott said. He still suspects that someone working in the lab, likely a technician, engaged in foul play. "It was easy to imagine a scenario where this was malevolent and was intended to hide the theft of more valued MDMA," he said. "I even knew of a case where one of the labs at UCSF had fired a technician for stealing drugs and then had to rethink all their security procedures."

The real scandal, though, was how long Ricaurte's team took to acknowledge their error, Baggott said, and how fervently they continued to promote their results even after multiple scientists raised legitimate questions about the findings. With the retraction, that finally ended. Ricaurte and McCann had been the preeminent scientists investigating the dangers of MDMA and "the darlings of the press" for anti-Ecstasy messaging, Grob said. But afterward they "just faded away. I don't think they wanted to touch this subject."

*

IN THE INTERVENING years since "the great retraction," scientists have confirmed that MDMA at some doses does cause an acute but temporary depletion of serotonin in the brain. There is also no question that MDMA, when given in high, repeated doses, can inflict major changes on the brain's serotonin system in lab animals. But no evidence has emerged that MDMA damages the human dopamine system, as the retracted study claimed. There's also evidence that damage to the serotonin system gradually repairs once a lab animal or a raver's brain stops being assaulted by too much MDMA.

Long-term heavy MDMA users do sometimes report problems with memory, and studies in the early aughts confirmed some modest but statistically significant deficiencies in this group's recall and other cognitive abilities. But researchers still struggled with the same methodological challenge that Ricaurte and McCann had long ignored: How to disentangle the effect of Ecstasy alone from the polydrug lifestyle of most heavy users?

Shortly after the Ricaurte retraction, Doblin received an email from a physics doctoral student in Salt Lake City informing him of a unique set of MDMA users who might get around the polydrug problem: Mormons. The student himself was Mormon and had done Ecstasy more than a thousand times, and he said he knew other Mormon ravers in the same position. Critically, none of them did other drugs—not even alcohol. Doblin put the student in touch with John Halpern, a psychiatrist at McLean Hospital and Harvard Medical School, who agreed to conduct a study. As Halpern said, "If I'm interested in the therapeutic effects of this substance, of course I want to know as a physician how these things may prove harmful."

Halpern managed to recruit fifty-two participants who regularly used Ecstasy but who took virtually no other drugs and didn't drink (as confirmed through hair, breath, and urine tests). Most identified as practicing Mormons, although some described themselves as having an evolving relationship with their faith. While MDMA is not explicitly mentioned in the church's *General Handbook*, the rules do state that members are to "avoid substances that are harmful, illegal, or addictive or that impair judgement." Halpern got the sense that, rather than some special carve-out existing for MDMA, some Mormon members of this unique Salt Lake City subculture were performing significant mental gymnastics to justify their use of the drug.

Halpern divided the Ecstasy users into two groups, "moderate" (22 to 50 times taking the drug) and "heavy" (60 to 250 times). He also recruited fifty-nine people who didn't use any drugs but who were part of the rave scene. "My control was raver kids doing all-night dancing, but they're straight-edgers," Halpern said. "That way, it wasn't like one group's sleep deprived and the other isn't."

Halpern compared the straight-edge and the Ecstasy-using ravers' performance on a wide range of tests that measured memory, verbal fluency, attention, processing speed, finger dexterity, and executive function. As he and his colleagues reported in the journal *Addiction*, on almost all test variables, they found no significant difference between the users and nonusers, or the moderate users and heavy users. Heavy Ecstasy users were slightly slower than nonusers when completing a puzzle using their nondominant hand, and Ecstasy users in general also had lower vocabulary scores than nonusers. But both of these differences were minor enough that they could have been due to chance. The most consistently significant finding was that heavy users seemed more predisposed toward impulsivity—a correlation also revealed in some previous studies. But again, impulsivity could be an existing factor that inclined people to take Ecstasy, rather than something *caused* by taking Ecstasy. As Halpern summarized of his findings, "There are some points that are statistically significant, but taken as a whole, it doesn't appear to be anything valuable or noticeable in everyday life."

Halpern's study provided an important reassurance to Doblin and to the FDA that MDMA did not seem to cause serious brain damage. Nearly twenty years since neurotoxicity was brought up on the *Donahue Show*, the issue seemed to be closed. And with it, an opening had finally arrived for MAPS to put MDMA-assisted therapy to the scientific test.

# A SPLINTER IN THE MIND

LORI TIPTON WOKE up on Monday feeling like something was wrong. She quickly put her finger on it: she hadn't heard from her mom all weekend.

Lori had visited her mom just a few days before, on Friday, to try to talk her down from a rage-filled manic episode. Her mom had been triggered by the discovery that her ex-girlfriend, who was still living with her, was dating someone new. Lori's attempted intervention had been unsuccessful, and she had departed on tense terms. But her mother always called over the weekend. Now it was Monday, and she wasn't even answering her phone.

With a sense of dread, Lori jumped in her car and headed to her mom's place in Chalmette, a low-lying blue-collar neighborhood on the banks of the Mississippi River, about half an hour from Lori's house in New Orleans. On the drive, she called a friend and said out loud what she felt in her gut to be true: "I know they're dead in the house."

"You're overreacting," her friend reassured her.

"No, I know what I'm going to find."

"Then why don't you just call the cops?"

"Because I have to find them. This is my family."

*

WHEN I ARRIVED at a café in New Orleans' Bywater neighborhood on Christmas Eve, I immediately recognized Lori's long red hair and warm, almost-maroon brown eyes from the photos I'd seen of her in news stories. It was a glorious morning, so we took our coffees to a table outside. Over the next two hours, Lori shared the story of her life.

She began with her mother, Trish, a woman who was "as beautiful as she was crazy," Lori said. Trish had little education, but with her eighteen-inch waistline, flowing brown hair, and dark eyes, she easily landed a job at the Playboy Club on Bourbon Street. Trish was a true New Orleans character. She drank only unsweetened ice tea with extra lemon, carried a loaded .38 handgun at all times, and was never seen in public without high heels. Except when showering, she always wore a gold body chain. "I'll know when I'm gaining or losing weight because my body chain fits me differently," she used to tell Lori.

When Trish met Lori's father, Billy—a gregarious French Quarter bartender who knew everyone and was twenty years Trish's senior—she jumped at the opportunity to be taken care of. "She was swept off her feet," Lori said. "It was very easy to be loved by my father."

As a child, Lori knew her mom was different from other mothers. She had obsessive-compulsive tendencies about cleaning—if the kids used the sink, they knew not to leave fingerprints—and was emotionally unpredictable. She got into explosive fights with Billy and regularly threatened to kill him. When Lori was in elementary school, Trish was institutionalized for what was then called manic depression (now called bipolar disorder). After her discharge, the family went on as though nothing had happened. As Lori said, "No one talked about mental illness, and you certainly didn't speak about your mother being institutionalized."

When Lori was ten her parents got divorced, and her dad settled in New Mexico. Trish began working as a house mom at strip clubs in the Quarter. The girls loved "Mama Trish" for her protective attitude and her willingness to happily spend hours just chatting with them in the dressing room. "To many of them, she was the only mama they ever had," one former colleague wrote on Trish's obituary page. "Mama had class, style and one of the richest personalities I ever had the pleasure of experiencing in my life."

While Trish spent time in the Quarter with her "extended family," Lori enrolled at Tulane University in the Garden District to study psychology. In 1999 her brother, Davin, came to stay at her apartment to celebrate his twenty-second birthday. Lori, Davin, and his friends partied all night, and before crashing, Davin took some pills. He never woke up. "This was 1999, when people were starting to fuck around with opioids," Lori said. "It was just devastating."

Trish had been closer to Davin than to Lori, and her son's death "set the ball rolling for her in a bad direction," Lori said. Lori swallowed her own grief so she could take care of her mother, who refused to get professional help. Trish's emotional, sometimes violent outbursts intensified, but as Lori pointed out, "the problem with dealing with a person suffering from mental illness is that their unpredictability becomes normalized over time." The murderous threats Trish sometimes made toward others were dismissed as "just how she lets off steam."

Trish, who was raised in a strict Catholic family, was also struggling with her sexuality. By the time she came out to her daughter, Lori had known for years that her mom was a lesbian.

"Aren't you ashamed?" Trish asked. "Aren't you afraid your friends will find out and will stop being your friends?"

"Mom, if anyone stopped being my friend because you're fucking a woman, then they're not my friend," Lori reassured her.

Lori was happy when her mom started dating Julie, a close friend of the family. But in 2005 Trish and Julie broke up, and Julie started dating a well-known local gay rights champion named Lark, famous around town for her pink poodle, Godiva. Julie was still living with Trish, and when Trish found out she holed up in their house, chain-smoking Virginia Slims, refusing to eat, and making her usual violent threats.

That Friday Lori dropped by to try to talk some sense into her mom. "You're not in love with Julie anymore, why do you give a fuck?" she asked in exasperation. But there was no getting through. "I remember feeling so frustrated and mad at her, and not even feeling compassion for her."

By the time Monday rolled around, though, Lori just felt worried. When she arrived at her mother's home that morning, she was all but resigned to what she would find inside. Sure enough, the three women were there, all dead. Trish was sitting in her favorite rocking chair, her back facing the entryway. Lark was slumped next to the back door, and Julie was on the floor next to the couch. There was no doubt in Lori's mind who was responsible for the double-murder-suicide. "My mom shot all three of them, one bullet each, each through the heart," Lori said. "That's how good a shot she was."

*

THE WORD TRAUMA derives from the Greek term for "wound," and in its original meaning, it refers to a physical injury. In the current usage, though, trauma has come to mean a deep emotional wounding triggered by a profoundly distressing event or events. If that emotional wound is not addressed, then like a physical injury, it can fester until it overwhelms a person's ability to cope, leading to the condition called post-traumatic stress disorder (PTSD).

Potentially traumatizing events are more commonplace than many of us realize or would like to know. Based on CDC data, one in five American children is sexually molested; one in three couples engage in physical violence; one in eight children witnesses their mother being hit; one in five women and one in thirty-eight men experience complete or attempted rape; and a quarter of the population grew up with an alcoholic relative. Untold numbers of people in the United States and beyond suffer from war, mass shootings, terrorism, natural disasters, and accidents. As I write this, the collective trauma of the Covid-19 pandemic is also ongoing. "Turn on the news, and almost everything that is reported on is a potential event that can trigger PTSD to many," said psychiatrist and neuroscientist Rachel Yehuda, who directs the Center for Psychedelic Psychotherapy and Trauma Research at the Icahn School of Medicine at Mount Sinai.

In the United States, an estimated 7 percent of the population experiences PTSD at some point in life, with around fifteen million people suffering from the condition in any given year. PTSD can stem from any event that threatens a person's life or physical integrity, or that otherwise makes them feel paralyzed by fear and helplessness. Although virtually every person will experience trauma or a traumatic event at least once in their lifetime, not all of them will go on to develop PTSD. Scientists have identified a complex set of risk factors that may increase the chance of PTSD developing, including whether someone had an early history of trauma; whether any of their family members have had PTSD; and, to a lesser extent, whether they have certain predisposing biological factors, such as low cortisol.

Although the symptoms of PTSD have long been recognized—including among late nineteenth-century women labeled "hysterical" and World War I soldiers diagnosed with "traumatic neuroses"—the condition was only officially defined in 1980. This was thanks to the efforts of a group of Vietnam War veterans who returned the medals they had received for bravery, spoke openly about the atrocities they had committed and witnessed overseas, and demanded help for what was then called "post-Vietnam syndrome." Responding to the veteran-led movement, lawmakers mandated that the Department of Veterans Affairs (VA) establish a psychological treatment program. The veterans' cause was further aided in 1980, when the American Psychiatric Association created a new diagnosis, PTSD, to explain what the former soldiers were experiencing.

PTSD's inclusion in the Diagnostic and Statistical Manual of Mental Disorders (DSM)—the so-called bible of psychiatry—finally legitimized a serious condition that society had for so long turned its back on. At first, though, PTSD was considered only to be a soldier's disorder. It took the women's liberation movement to raise awareness that violence and trauma are also staples of many women's and children's civilian lives. Feminist activists forced the medical establishment to acknowledge that rape, incest, childhood abuse, and domestic violence not only are prevalent but also could all cause long-term trauma that belonged under the umbrella of PTSD.

Scientists' understanding of trauma further deepened in 2007, when Robert Carter, a psychologist at Columbia University, published a landmark paper on racial trauma. As Carter defined it, racial trauma occurs when a person is subjected to a lifetime of direct discrimination and racism, as well as to more covert impacts from living in an oppressive society. "The experience of African Americans has been traumatic from the start," pointed out Joseph McCowan, a clinical psychologist and psychotherapist in Los Angeles. "So there's both historical trauma and also ongoing trauma which people are experiencing collectively on a daily basis."

That ongoing trauma takes the form of obvious harms like police violence against Black people, racially motivated acts of domestic terror against minorities (like mass shootings), and a racist system of mass incarceration. But it also extends to subtler traumas that nevertheless undermine a person's sense of identity and self-worth, such as feeling like their ideas are never heard or they are constantly overlooked because of the color of their skin.

While some experts think racial trauma is something separate from PTSD, others believe they are the same. "When people come to me with racial trauma, they have all the symptoms of PTSD," said clinical psychologist Monnica Williams, the Canada research chair in mental health disparities at the University of Ottawa. "They're desperate, and clearly they're suffering and struggling."

*

FOR YEARS AFTER PTSD was established as a formal diagnosis—and despite a growing body of scientific evidence—some doctors and Western culture at large continued to push back against the idea that trauma can't just be willed away, and that victims are credible. A 1993 op-ed published in the *Times* of London titled PLEASE KEEP YOUR TROUBLES TO YOURSELF clearly illustrates this pernicious attitude. The author, a doctor, compares the increasing number of claims of childhood abuse and incest to "the medieval atmosphere of a witch-hunt" and asserts that, even if someone is abused, "surely repression of painful memories may be in many cases desirable." "Will no one speak in favor of fortitude and overcoming one's difficulties oneself?" he whines.

Fortunately, the scientific establishment has moved beyond this damaging and flawed approach. Doctors today accept that PTSD is not only real but also a major public health crisis. "People who have been traumatized in whatever way are changed forever," said Stephen Xenakis, a psychiatrist and retired Brigadier General. "In really severe cases, they can't work, they can't live with anybody, and they think about suicide every day."

Mount Sinai's Rachel Yehuda and other experts have dedicated their careers to elucidating the biological mechanisms behind trauma's enduring shadow. In simplified terms, PTSD occurs when a person's nervous system becomes "stuck," as though they are still experiencing a threatening event in real time. Like a deeply buried splinter that becomes infected, it's the body's reaction to the trauma rather than the traumatic event itself that causes the most harm. "PTSD is about reorganization of your brain and mind so it becomes very hard to fully engage with the present," said Bessel van der Kolk, the founder and medical director of the Trauma Center in Brookline, Massachusetts, and author of *The Body Keeps the Score.* "The terror, the reactivity, the anger, and the threat live on inside your body."

People with PTSD see and experience the world differently than nontraumatized individuals because their nervous systems have been fundamentally altered. They often have higher levels of stress hormones like adrenaline, and after a perceived threat has passed, their bodies continue to secrete those hormones for longer than a nontraumatized person's would. This is thought to result from heightened activity in the amygdala, the brain region associated with processing fear and danger, and lower activity in regions like the medial prefrontal cortex that suppress fear after a threat has subsided.

When people with PTSD recall their trauma, activity decreases in Broca's area, a region of the brain responsible for speech. This could mean they are less able to put their thoughts and feelings into words. At the same time, activity lights up in parts of the visual cortex. People with PTSD, in other words, may be responding to the memory of their trauma as though it is actually happening to them again in real time.

PTSD is also frequently associated with significantly lower activity in self-sensing areas such as the anterior cingulate, the parietal cortex, and the insula. Shutting down activity in these areas allows a person to rid themselves of visceral feelings of terror and anger, but it also cuts them off from other emotions and a sense of feeling embodied. The clinical term for this is alexithymia—an inability to experience, talk about, or express emotion. Loss of activity in self-sensing brain regions also decreases a person's ability to self-regulate without the aid of crutches like alcohol or drugs. The earlier and more severe the trauma, the more ingrained these changes tend to become.

The stress and exhaustion caused by PTSD and the brain changes it entails can snowball into other physiological problems, too, including fibromyalgia, chronic fatigue and pain, migraines, irritable bowel syndrome, cancer, heart attacks, and autoimmune diseases. A 2019 study in *Cancer Research* conducted by scientists at Harvard University, for example, revealed that women with severe PTSD had twice the risk of developing ovarian cancer compared to women who had no trauma history, and that the aggressiveness of their cancer increased proportionately with the severity of their PTSD symptoms.

"There's a huge link between trauma and medical problems," said Gabor Maté, a physician and author in Vancouver who specializes in trauma and addiction. "Yet the average medical student never hears about those links, because the Western medical model separates the mind from the body, and the individual from the environment."

At the most basic level, some nervous system alterations seem to stem from epigenetic changes, or shifts in how a person's genes function. "If you think of your brain as a kind of a computer—the hardware—then epigenetics is the software," said Yehuda, who is at the forefront of research in this field. Genes contain our bodies' instruction manuals for making proteins—basic biological building blocks that perform crucial jobs ranging from transmitting signals to fighting diseases. But these instructions are not always expressed in the same way. They can be turned on or off by the addition or subtraction of certain molecules, altering the gene's function. Environmental triggers can influence how genes are expressed, and scientists suspect that traumatic exposures might be able to, too. As Maté wrote in *The Myth of Normal*, "far from being the arbiters of our destinies, genes answer to their environment."

The ability to flexibly respond to the environment "is fundamentally adaptive and the basis of human resilience," Yehuda wrote, so epigenetic plasticity can in itself be a good thing. Shifts in gene expression may help a soldier adapt to the conditions of war, for example, or a child to develop strategies to survive the hardships of an abusive household. But if genes don't reset to their normal expression after an environmental insult has passed, then these changes can become maladaptive and, over time, be deleterious to mental and physical health. "The reason these dynamics are so tenacious is because they had an adaptive purpose in the first place," Maté said. "Once you associate something with survival, you're not going to give it up that easily."

The consequences could extend from the individual to the next generation. In recent years, scientists have found that although epigenetic changes do not alter DNA, if they are present when a person's cells are dividing (including when they're making eggs or sperm), then they will be present in those new cells as well. This is one means of transmission for what researchers call multi- or intergenerational trauma: trauma that gets passed down from family members who directly lived through it to subsequent generations, like that which Naomi Fiske inherited from her Holocaust-survivor parents.

Intergenerational trauma can be caused by the behavioral repercussions of parents who suffer from trauma; by a mother's stress, delivered to her fetus in the womb; or by epigenetic changes. Researchers are turning up more and more evidence for this. Yehuda found, for example, that the adult children of Holocaust survivors were more likely to develop PTSD if their mothers had the condition. She and her colleagues also found that mothers who had been pregnant and in New York City during 9/11 and who went on to develop PTSD gave birth to babies who had lower cortisol levels—a measure that has been linked in other studies to PTSD vulnerability. This persistent form of trauma can also reach beyond individuals to impact entire peoples or nations. Colonialism, for example, has left a legacy of multigenerational trauma that continues to impact Native peoples across North America, as has slavery and racism for Black Americans.

Scientists are increasingly recognizing, too, that PTSD is not homogenous. PTSD caused by combat differs from PTSD triggered by surviving a discrete event such as a car crash or a hurricane, which does not compare, in turn, to deeply ingrained trauma stemming from chronic childhood abuse or neglect. "There's a very good paper that says there's 630,000 permutations of how you can put things together to diagnose PTSD," Xenakis said. "There's a really subjective aspect to it."

Even so, trauma affects many more people than qualify for a PTSD diagnosis according to the DSM. Childhood trauma in particular is so radically different from trauma incurred during adulthood that 82 percent of children who are seen by the National Child Traumatic Stress Network do not meet the diagnostic criteria for PTSD. Based on data collected from twenty thousand traumatized children, in 2009 van der Kolk and colleagues proposed a new diagnosis for this group, developmental trauma disorder, that would provide a single label capturing the full range of traumatized children's symptoms. This is important, van der Kolk wrote, because "if doctors can't agree on what ails their patients, there is no way they can provide proper treatment."

The American Psychiatric Association rejected van der Kolk and his colleagues' proposal, however, stating that no new diagnosis was required to fill a "missing diagnostic niche." That "niche," van der Kolk pointed out, represents one million children who are abused and neglected each year in the United States, and who make up the country's biggest and most costly public health issue, according to the Centers for Disease Control. Yet the oversight has not been amended, and even today, no diagnosis exists to represent traumatized children.

*

BY THE TIME Lori discovered the bodies, she had already been operating her entire life under the insidious weight of childhood trauma caused by being raised by a mother with her own unaddressed mental health struggles. And the world, as it turned out, wasn't finished sending major traumatic events Lori's way. A month and a half after her mom's funeral, Hurricane Katrina hit. Given the enormity of the suffering around her, Lori felt like she no longer had the right to grieve. "My grief was just a drop in a sea of grief," she said. "I didn't really feel like I had a place for it."

So Lori did what she had done when her brother died: "I didn't let myself feel things." She got a job at one of the same strip clubs her mom used to work at and "fell right into that world." She began "drinking like crazy" and developed a Xanax, Vicodin, and methamphetamine habit. Under the influence of alcohol, her sorrow, otherwise held in check, would overwhelm her. "I'd get drunk and want to die," she said. "I didn't try to take my life, but I'd engage in severe risk-taking behaviors, like driving blackout drunk. There were vodka-Xanax days where I'd wake up and know nothing that I did."

In 2006 Lori realized that she was going to lose her life if she didn't make some changes. She quit all drugs and cut back on drinking. Things seemed to be looking up, but then a co-worker she had walked home invited her inside and raped her. "It was so devastating, because it was someone I trusted," she said. Lori didn't see a point in reporting the rape to the police, and when she told friends what happened, they dismissed or even blamed her. "You've always been kind of slutty," one close friend chided.

Things only worsened from there: Lori became pregnant from the rape. When she had a bad reaction to the abortion pill she was prescribed, she ended up in a hospital where a pro-life nurse made her feel like "an abomination." As she lay there in pain, taking the woman's insults, she realized how completely and utterly alone she was. "I just remember being like, 'I want my mom,'" she recalled.

After the rape and abortion, Lori completely shut down. She focused on work, spoke to no one about her traumas, and told herself she was stronger than the sum of her experiences. But after evenings out drinking with friends, she would often consider shooting herself or overdosing on pills. As she got older, her mental health worsened. If someone surprised her, she would leap out of her chair, and her heart would pound for minutes after. She had terrible nightmares and was short with co-workers and friends. If a partner touched her a certain way during consensual sex, she would have a panic attack. She realized she needed help.

Lori saw a series of psychologists, psychiatrists, and even an endocrinologist, but it never occurred to any of them—or to her—that she might have PTSD. "I shit into bags, I spit into vials to test my hormones," she said. She tried acupuncture, meditation, and reiki. She changed her diet and became a certified yoga instructor. Still, she could not find relief for the nameless affliction torturing her; "There was something wrong with me, and no one knew what it was."

Finally, one of the psychologists told her he thought she had "pretty bad PTSD."

Lori brushed him off. "That's something that happens to soldiers, and those people are agoraphobic," she said. "I'm not that."

Eventually, though, she agreed to try cognitive behavioral therapy (CBT), the first treatment doctors usually recommend for PTSD. CBT is a type of talk therapy that seeks to identify and change underlying thought patterns—in the case of PTSD, through exposure therapy, an approach first developed to treat phobias. For those with PTSD, exposure therapy entails getting the person to retell the story of their trauma over and over again until they realize they are in fact safe, and the memory can be integrated and relegated to the past. But this requires actually being able to engage with the memory rather than disassociate from it, and then tolerate that engagement, which for many people can be extremely difficult.

When Lori tried CBT, she didn't get past the disassociation stage. "It was like I was telling a story that wasn't mine," she said. "It was like, 'This happened and that happened, and I'm gonna go to the store after this and get grapes or whatever.'"

Like at least one third of all PTSD patients, Lori dropped out of talk therapy. Even if she had stuck with it, though, there's no guarantee it would have helped: in studies of those with PTSD who do manage to get through a full round of CBT, only about one in three people show improvement, and just 15 percent no longer have major symptoms. "CBT alone is OK for the person who got into a car accident and then had trouble afterwards with driving," said Jennifer Mitchell, a neuroscientist at UCSF. "But when you're talking about people who survived the Holocaust or escaped a serial killer or had repeated sexual trauma or went into combat, it's often not enough."

For people who do not find relief through talk therapy, medications are the next line of defense. Zoloft and Paxil are the only two FDA-approved pharmaceuticals for PTSD. Both are selective serotonin reuptake inhibitors (SSRIs), a class of antidepressant drugs that includes Prozac. Like MDMA, SSRIs mimic serotonin and bind to serotonin reuptake transporters in neurons. They work by blocking reabsorption of the neurotransmitter, causing it to hang around in synapses longer and increasing its chemical signal. SSRIs can blunt certain symptoms of PTSD such as depression and insomnia, but they do not address the root of a person's trauma, and thus do not offer a cure. They also often come with unwanted side effects, ranging from sexual dysfunction and exhaustion to cognitive impairment and weight gain.

Lori tried Paxil and found that it was helpful for reducing suicidal ideation. But it also prevented her from mustering creative inspiration or motivation—an unacceptable trade-off, given that she'd started working as a professional writer. "It was like moving through Jell-O at all times," she said of the drug. She tried switching to Prozac and had a similar reaction, and she wound up staying on both drugs longer than she wanted to because weaning herself off caused bouts of dizziness and nausea.

In 2013 Lori had a son, Wilder. She and her partner, Andy, could not have children together, so they chose to coparent with a gay couple. Lori's dad had recently passed away, and she was excited about building and regaining a family. "My child has three dads," Lori said. "It's wonderful."

After Wilder's birth, though, Lori started having intrusive thoughts about how her son would die. She had to take a Xanax to calm her nerves enough just to bring Wilder to the park. Even then, her hands would shake as she took him out of the car, and while pushing him in his stroller, she was on constant alert for danger. "A dog's going to break off its leash and attack my baby," she'd think. "A tree is going to fall as I'm walking under it and squash him."

To Lori's distress, her suicidal urges also intensified. "I'd be sitting there with this beautiful baby, looking at him, and feeling nothing," she said. "What forced me to want to kill myself was the pure absence of joy. Not even a depression—it was like an emptiness of being."

Lori was scrolling through Facebook one night when she saw an ad someone had reposted. It was from a group called MAPS, and they were seeking participants to take part in a Phase 2 clinical trial of MDMA-assisted therapy to treat PTSD. Lori clicked the link. "Within thirty minutes of seeing it, I'd emailed them," she said.

*

AFTER THE CANCER study with Charles Grob collapsed, Rick Doblin took a step back to reevaluate. He needed to find a new researcher to partner with on clinical trials for MDMA-assisted therapy, and he was also thinking about switching his focus to PTSD. Doblin knew the need for effective treatments for PTSD was huge, and on a practical level, he suspected that it might be easier to rally public support for helping veterans than it would be for easing the death process for terminal cancer patients. "Even though we're all gonna die and have anxiety about facing death, it's something people don't want to talk about," he said.

This wasn't the first time Doblin had considered PTSD. Back in 1995, he had taken a stab at getting the VA involved in MDMA research after he met a neurobiologist and psychologist named David Presti at one of the Shulgins' Wednesday-night dinners. At the time, Presti was working at the VA in San Francisco, where he specialized in treating PTSD and substance abuse in Vietnam veterans. He was also familiar with the preprohibition literature on LSD therapy. So when the two met, Presti immediately understood what Doblin was trying to do. "I never doubted the vision that folks like Rick had way back then, that this would happen," he said.

Doblin told Presti that MAPS would pay for an MDMA-assisted therapy trial for veterans with PTSD, if only the VA would host it. But the VA director whom Presti approached thought the idea was ridiculous. "From what I know about MDMA, it opens you up and people become flooded with emotion," the director said. "It would make PTSD worse."

"That was the end of that," Presti said. "It went nowhere. The time was not yet right."

After the dead end in San Francisco, Doblin tried getting research started at other VAs, but all attempts were blocked by their respective directors. He also took a stab at doing the same in Israel, but likewise hit a wall there. Briefly, he had some success in Spain, but in 2002 the Madrid Anti-Drug Authority abruptly shut the trials down after George Ricaurte flew over and gave a talk about the risks of MDMA neurotoxicity.

By then, though, another avenue had opened up. In March 2000 a psychiatrist named Michael Mithoefer introduced himself to Doblin at an ayahuasca conference in San Francisco. Mithoefer had originally been an emergency medicine doctor, but after a decade working in the ER, he had noticed a pattern. People would come in at the brink of death from stab wounds, drug overdoses, or failed suicide attempts, and Mithoefer would do his best to patch them up. Even when he saved their lives, though, he didn't feel like he was actually *healing* them. "I was catching the tail end of much deeper problems," he said. "I became more interested in what was happening before they came into the ER."

Discovering Stan Grof's work about consciousness was the final push Mithoefer needed, and he went back to school to become a psychiatrist. He came into the field interested in partnering with patients to address the root of their problems, but he was disheartened to find that ever since Prozac hit the market in 1988, psychiatry had mostly abandoned therapy in favor of a pharmaceutical treatment paradigm. Mental health challenges had been "recast as 'disorders' that could be fixed by the administration of appropriate chemicals," as van der Kolk summarized of this shift.

Most psychiatrists welcomed the income and profits suddenly being generated for their profession by the pharmaceutical industry. Mithoefer, however, was not especially interested in prescribing what he saw as pharmaceutical Band-Aids. When he learned that talk therapy remained the gold standard for treating PTSD, he decided to specialize in that condition. Mithoefer and his wife, Annie, a registered nurse, also became certified in holotropic breathwork, a therapeutic method developed by Stan and Christina Grof that can allow people to reach nonordinary states of consciousness through breathing exercises.

For ten years, Mithoefer saw patients one-on-one for therapy, and he and Annie would work together with them doing solo or group breathwork at their Charleston office. Many patients had experienced sexual abuse or other forms of childhood trauma, and some also had dissociative disorders; the latter diagnosis sometimes accompanies and complicates PTSD, and is characterized by a lack of continuity between a person's thoughts, memories, and identity. Annie would sometimes even accompany psychotic clients to the grocery store. "It was a mom-and-pop business," Mithoefer said.

Frequently, though, they were distressed to find that they could only get so far with patients using therapy and breathwork. "It wasn't helping everyone, so we were always looking for something else," Mithoefer said. They tried various other cutting-edge methods—including eye movement desensitization and reprocessing, and neurofeedback therapy—but still, these things "didn't do it for everyone," Mithoefer said. "Like everything in medicine, we need different tools for different people."

The Mithoefers had both had personal experiences with MDMA and other psychedelics, and they were familiar with the old literature about psychedelic-assisted therapy. "It was foolish not to be looking into these tools that had some evidence of working," Mithoefer remembered thinking. He was driving home one day when he heard an interview on NPR with Deborah Mash, a neurologist and molecular and cellular pharmacologist at the University of Miami who had opened a legal ibogaine clinic in St. Kitts. He wound up accompanying one of his patients, a woman addicted to opioids, to St. Kitts, and got to see Mash's work firsthand.

The Mithoefers decided to look into doing something similar. First, though, they needed to find a suitable overseas location. At the ayahuasca conference in San Francisco, Mithoefer recognized Doblin from the MAPS bulletin. He asked Doblin if he had any pointers about which countries could be favorable to his and Annie's psychedelic-assisted practice.

Doblin's ears pricked up. "You don't need to leave the country," he told Mithoefer. "You can do psychedelic therapy here, and I'll help you. What do you want to study?"

"MDMA, ayahuasca, LSD, ibogaine, and psilocybin," Mithoefer enthusiastically replied.

"Me too, but we need to start somewhere," Doblin said. He proposed MDMA for treating PTSD, and told Mithoefer about his five-year, five-million-dollar plan for FDA approval.

Mithoefer wasn't interested in a career in research, but this sounded like a reasonable path for obtaining better outcomes for his patients. As soon as he got home, he started writing a draft protocol for a Phase 2 study using MDMA-assisted therapy to treat severe PTSD. In 2001 he and Annie attended a "State of Ecstasy" conference in San Francisco, where Mithoefer shared the protocol draft with George Greer, David Nichols, Charles Grob, Matthew Baggott, and other major players in the field for input. Then he crossed his fingers and submitted the protocol to the FDA. "On a rational level, I knew we might not get permission," Mithoefer said. "But on another level, I just felt like this is going to happen, this makes sense."

FDA approval arrived the very next month—a testament to the more than a decade's worth of work that Grob and Doblin had already done, as well as to the strength of the new protocol. But in keeping with the history of regulatory blockage around MDMA research (not to mention Doblin's tendency to be the loosest of loose cannons with his messaging to the press), there would still be a glut of additional challenges to overcome before the team could begin recruiting participants. For one, the FDA requires sign-off on clinical research from an institutional review board (IRB), a type of administrative body set up to "protect the rights and welfare of humans participating as subjects in research," as the FDA puts it.

Doblin and Mithoefer had hoped to go through the IRB at the Medical University of South Carolina, where Mithoefer was on the clinical faculty and had set up a meeting with the chairman of his department to discuss this. But on the day of the meeting, the *Wall Street Journal* published a story about "Ecstasy" being used to treat PTSD—and the story named the Medical University as the site where the clinical trials would be taking place. Doblin, it turned out, had gotten a bit ahead of himself when talking to the reporter. A friend from the university called the Mithoefers that morning to warn them that top brass were none too pleased: "It's a shit storm down here."

Later that day, Mithoefer was summoned to the provost's office. "They were going berserk, saying 'We have nothing to do with this!' " he recalled.

"That was a challenging time for me with Rick," Annie added. "The phone was just going off—there were so many reporters."

Needless to say, the Medical University of South Carolina did not agree to host the clinical trial or to grant the protocol IRB approval. Mithoefer, in fact, wound up losing his faculty position over the incident. "They wanted nothing to do with me for a while," he said. (He was reappointed in 2009, after delivering a standing-room-only talk to the faculty and residents about MAPS's results with MDMA-assisted therapy. The Medical University is also now launching its own psychedelic research center.)

Although the *Wall Street Journal* incident was unfortunate, the Mithoefers did not consider severing their relationship with Doblin or with MAPS. "Rick and I seemed to strike a chord with each other," Mithoefer said. "We're both so focused on doing this."

With the Medical University out, though, they still needed to find an IRB. In July 2002 the Western IRB in Olympia, Washington, the largest independent IRB in the country, approved the protocol. But two months later Mithoefer received a letter from the group's chair, William Jacobs, stating that he and his colleagues had reconsidered and decided to withdraw approval. One of the sources behind this sudden change of heart turned out to be Una McCann at Johns Hopkins, who a year later would issue the "great retraction" for giving monkeys meth instead of MDMA.

"Dr. McCann reiterated that MDMA, as an amphetamine derivative, is the only psychedelic with neurotoxic effects," Jacobs wrote in his withdrawal notice. "She further stated that there is no scientific evidence that MDMA has therapeutic effects—there are only unsubstantiated anecdotal reports." Jacobs also took a personal stab at Mithoefer and MAPS: "The Board concluded that both the sponsor and yourself appear to lack the scientific objectivity and rigor required to carry out this research."

After that, MAPS cycled through seven North American IRBs, all of which rejected the protocol. "That was a low point," Doblin recalled. He got so frustrated that he took a one-week break from everything MAPS-related to paint his house a dour shade of gray. "Painting the house gave me this sense that I can actually do something and the world changes," Doblin said. (The gray didn't last: Doblin's house is now an exuberant plum purple.)

Doblin had all but given up on finding an external IRB to sponsor the trial when he came across a reference to a North Carolina–based IRB called Copernicus Group. Copernicus, Doblin knew, was the Polish Renaissance astronomer who discovered that Earth is not the center of the universe; the Catholic Church banned his book outlining this theory for more than two hundred years. "An IRB that's called Copernicus would be sensitized to political and religious pressure against science," Doblin reasoned optimistically.

He was right. In September 2003 Copernicus approved MAPS's protocol—although only after MAPS purchased a million-dollar insurance policy to indemnify the group if anything went wrong. "We produced the world's longest consent form to protect the IRB, and we agreed to hire a board-certified emergency medicine physician and nurse to sit in the next room during treatment sessions," Doblin said. "We spent a hundred thousand dollars on this stuff, just to get Copernicus to say yes."

As the IRB drama was going on, Mithoefer was also engaged in a back-and-forth with the DEA to obtain a Schedule I license needed to handle MDMA. He'd first reached out to them in 2002, and now—countless phone calls, faxes, letters, and emails later—it was 2004. "There was just delay after delay after delay," Mithoefer said. "I had a chronology of pages and pages of all the phone calls."

The excuses were starting to get ridiculous. MAPS, for example, had to send five hard copies of the five-hundred-page application on three separate occasions, because the DEA's office kept saying they hadn't received it. Finally, Mithoefer reached out to a friend who worked in the State Department, who gave him contact information for someone at U.S. senator for South Carolina Fritz Hollings's office. "This is impending science," Mithoefer pleaded to the staff person.

Two weeks later, the DEA called Mithoefer to tell him the permission was in the mail, and the official even apologized to him for the delay. "It's a good ending, but if this turns out to be a treatment that saves lives, what about those people in those two-plus years who couldn't get the treatment?" Mithoefer said. "It's a travesty."

In April 2004 the Mithoefers finally welcomed their first study participant to their office. The woman had been raped seven years earlier, and she had struggled to feel connected to the world ever since. Medications, therapy, and alternative treatments like breathwork had all failed to bring relief.

"I never dreamed I'd take a drug like this, but I'm so desperate, I'll do anything that might help," she told the Mithoefers. "I'll go to Tibet if I have to."

They gave the woman a capsule—no one knew at the time if it was a placebo or MDMA—and invited her to recline on a bed in the middle of the room. She wore eyeshades and headphones playing ambient music. The Mithoefers sat on either side of her, waiting. About an hour in, the woman sat up, pulled the eyeshades off, and spoke for the first time: "I guess I'm not gonna have to go to Tibet."

Later that day, the woman told the Mithoefers that she felt love for the first time since the rape. "I know I have a lot to be grateful for, that my kids and husband love me, but I couldn't feel any of that," she said. In her second session with MDMA, held a month later, she revisited the memory of the rape and saw the exact moment when her break from reality began. In recognizing that, Annie said, "she could begin to heal."

*

LORI WAS HOPEFUL yet skeptical when she received confirmation that she'd made the cut for the MAPS study. She couldn't count the number of times over the past few years she'd been told, "This is the thing that's going to cure you," but as she'd learned time and time again, "it never fucking works. You've spent your money and time and you feel like there's something wrong with you because it worked for other people."

Lori was one of 107 people who took part in MAPS's Phase 2 trials, held at five sites in the United States, Canada, Switzerland, and Israel. The list of participants included combat veterans, first responders, sexual assault victims, and individuals with complex trauma from childhood. On average, they had been diagnosed with PTSD for nearly eighteen years, and all were considered to be "treatment resistant," based on existing interventions having failed them. Unlike most PTSD trials, participants were not excluded if they had previously attempted suicide. As Mithoefer noted of the selection criteria, "I thought it was important to see if we could treat the hardest people."

Lori had never tried MDMA before—"I was an alcoholic at the time Ecstasy was super popular," she noted—and she had no idea what to expect. Half an hour after taking the pill, lying on the couch in her therapists' office wearing eyeshades and headphones, she felt her heart rate increase slightly. Exquisitely vivid memories began to wash over her. She was back in New Mexico, playing with her brother in the snow—a recollection that summoned such an all-encompassing feeling of joy that it still brings tears to her eyes recounting it today. She remembered the bad times, too, including the fear and loneliness she felt as a kid living under the threat of her mom's temper. Instead of being afraid of the emotions—positive or negative—attached to these memories, for the first time in years Lori permitted herself to be fully present, to really *feel*.

Lori did not explore her trauma in that first session. Her therapists, Shari Taylor and Ray Worthy, simply sat with her as she worked through her memories and rediscovered what it is to experience emotion. "The thing that's so revolutionary and beautiful about psychedelic therapy is it's really completely client led," Lori said. "My therapists were just there for me, and that in itself was so healing and beautiful, like, 'Oh my god, these people are just going to take care of me.' And I'd felt so not taken care of for so long."

The MAPS protocol generally requires therapists to adhere to an inner-directed approach, but permits them to incorporate other types of therapy, too. There is no agenda for what needs to come up when. Some people jump straight into the trauma, while others take a more meandering path, revisiting long-buried childhood memories, unpacking their relationships, or analyzing their behaviors and motivations. Some prefer to spend the entire session talking, while others process things internally and remain virtually silent. Whatever a person's particular journey, though, the experience is not usually characterized by the blissed-out euphoria associated with taking MDMA recreationally. As Mithoefer noted, "People in our studies often say 'I don't know why they call this Ecstasy.' "

In the month after Lori's first session, she began to rediscover the simple joys of being. She'd comment to Andy about how good her morning coffee was, even as he amusedly reminded her that it was the same coffee they always drank. She'd gush about how beautiful the sound of the birds singing outside the window were, and Andy would gently point out that the birds were always there; "You're just more present than you've ever been."

Lori's second and third MDMA-assisted therapy sessions were more difficult than the first. In the second, she focused on "trying to understand what made me me." She allowed herself to grieve for what she saw as the missed opportunities of her life: for the neuroscientist she never became, for the emotional disconnection she experienced during her son's early years. Mostly, though, she grieved for the person who had lost so much, yet had never permitted herself to hold space for those losses. She allowed herself to cry harder and deeper than she had in years, and in between sobs, "I fucking talked so much, those poor therapists never got a break," Lori said. "I called my team the trauma doulas, because they're really just holding space for me to deliver the trauma."

When people talk about how MDMA-assisted therapy actually helps individuals overcome trauma, they often reference an "inner healer" or "inner healing intelligence" to which the drug allows access. These terms, originally coined by Stan Grof, sound "a little squishy," Mithoefer admitted. So he prefers to explain MDMA-assisted therapy using a metaphor from his time in the ER. As a doctor, he couldn't force a patient's body to heal a gunshot wound or a broken bone, but he could "remove the obstacles and create favorable conditions for this very complex and elegant process in the body to start the healing," he said. In the therapist's office, he likewise cannot force a patient's mind to heal. But he and his colleagues can use the tools at their disposal—in this case, talk therapy and MDMA—to stimulate the body's own restorative ability.

Lori appreciated and embraced this approach. "It was so beautiful and powerful and empowering to have therapists who weren't like, 'We're gonna fix you,' " Lori said. "Instead, they're like, 'We're gonna give you all the tools you need to do the work, because you innately know what you need.' "

By her third session, Lori felt that she had built up enough self-compassion and bravery to work on some of her deeper traumas. As she half-jokingly told her therapists, "Like in *Poltergeist*, tie a rope around me and jerk me out if it gets too bad."

She first revisited the memory of discovering the bodies of her mother, Lark, and Julie. Before, when she had dared to think about that day at all, she had felt like "a rat in a maze, where all you see is walls," and there were also stretches of memory that were just completely blank. Now she felt like she was peering down from above, with a bird's-eye view of the entire situation. She experienced empathy for her mother—for the mental anguish she had weathered her entire life, for her self-loathing about being gay—and she understood the external factors that had led her mother "to that moment, to that horrible decision she made," she said. She also felt profound compassion for herself. "My god, this poor child—to walk into that," she thought. "And all she could feel after was shame and anger, and there was no space to honor what she lost."

Lori also realized the depth of shame she had been carrying as a result of her rape—in particular, the silencing she had experienced afterward. Even under the influence of MDMA, she found herself struggling to talk about it. So her therapists suggested she try a yoga pose—Halasana, or plow—that she'd always avoided because it reminded her of her rape and would trigger a panic attack. Lori agreed, but the moment she went into Halasana, as usual, she began to panic.

Taylor, her female therapist, reached for Lori's hand. "What does the feeling need?"

"I just need to be heard, I need someone to hear me," Lori replied through tears. "I need you to hear and believe me."

"We're here," Taylor reassured her. "Just stay and breathe deep, know that you're held and you're loved and you're heard. You're not alone."

Taylor's words were like an elixir. Lori suddenly saw clearly that the rape was not her fault, and that she had done nothing wrong. More than that, her brother's death was not her fault, and neither was her mother's. Bad things happen in life, and she was not to blame. The narrative she'd been telling herself about herself was just a story—and one she could change, because she was the editor. "There's nothing wrong with me," she realized. "I just need to reintegrate these parts of myself that I have exiled, and say, 'It's OK.'"

Following the clinical trial, Lori's textbook PTSD symptoms—hypervigilance, mood swings, anxiety, poor sleep, sexual problems, suicidal ideation, and constant physical malaise—either disappeared or significantly declined. Her relationships with loved ones are now deeper; she's fully present when she's with her son; and she feels more compassion and connection toward others, including strangers. It's not that MDMA-assisted therapy made her life perfect, though, or that she doesn't still get overwhelmed. "The difference is, the perspective I gained in the trial never leaves me," she said. "I don't get lost in the maze as much, because I can pull up that bird's-eye view and be like, 'You're telling yourself the story again!' "

Lori's experience was not an outlier. Immediately following participation in the Phase 2 trials, 56 percent of the group that took MDMA no longer met the diagnostic criteria for PTSD, compared to 22 percent of the control group, which included people who received the same talk therapy paired with a placebo or a very low 40-milligram dose of MDMA§. The large effect size—a commonly used statistical measure of the magnitude of difference between

---

§ Double blinding is the practice by which both research participants and the scientists administering the study are prevented from knowing information that might influence them, such as which drug a participant received. Achieving true double blinding is an inherent challenge with most psychiatric studies, however, regardless of whether psychedelics are involved. Side effects can give away whether a participant received an active drug or a placebo, and blinding simply is not possible for testing something like talk therapy. Some researchers also argue that it is unethical to use placebos for trials in which evidence already exists that the treatment in question brings some benefits, and that the insistence on double blinding in psychiatric studies adheres to an outdated, reductionist mode of thinking about drugs as having stand-alone effects.

For now, though, double blinding is still the gold standard for clinical research. In the Phase 2 trials, Mithoefer and his colleagues tried to solve this problem by testing a wide range of MDMA doses in hopes of finding a lower dose that would fool participants into thinking they had received the drug, but that would be low enough not to be effective. This did not work out: the lower doses tended to make people feel anxious—to the point that the effectiveness of the therapy actually decreased compared to the completely inactive placebo—and, not surprisingly, people usually still seemed to be able to recognize whether they received the therapeutic-level dose. After extensive discussions following the Phase 2 trials, including with the FDA, the team decided that there is no complete solution to the blinding problem for a treatment like MDMA-assisted therapy, and that moving forward, they would use only placebos or full doses of MDMA. Encouragingly, the fact that the results have lasted more than one year in the majority of participants who received MDMA-assisted therapy suggest that the gains probably are not reflective of a placebo effect, which does not typically last that long. Eduardo Ekman Schenberg, "Who Is Blind in Psychedelic Research? Letter to the Editor Regarding 'Blinding and Expectancy Confounds in Psychedelic Randomized Controlled Trials,'" *Expert Review of Clinical Pharmacology* 14, no. 10 (August 2021): 1317–19, https://www.tandfonline.com/doi/full/10.1080/17512433.2021.1951473?src=recsys.

experimental conditions—of 0.8 reinforced confidence that MDMA did add a meaningful overall benefit. The MDMA treatment seemed to work equally well, too, regardless of a participant's age, sex, or race, the study site they visited, the cause or duration of their PTSD, or whether or not they had ever taken MDMA before. Most encouragingly, most participants continued to improve as time went on. Twelve months or more after completing the trial, 67 percent of ninety-one interviewed participants no longer qualified for PTSD. "MDMA is like aged cheese—it can get better over time," said Jennifer Mitchell, the UCSF neuroscientist. "The six- or twelve-month follow-up almost always looked better than the immediate results."

Not everyone has been able to maintain the gains they made in the trial, however. Lori was fortunate to have a supportive home environment, but as she pointed out, "there are some people who profit off others being sick." Participants whose mental health wound up deteriorating afterward tended to be individuals facing poverty, family instability, and other detrimental factors outside their control. "Some people can't get disability, and they don't have money to live," Annie Mithoefer said. "The way our society treats people, it's just a no-win situation."

Lori is doing her own part to try to change this. In 2018 she became the codirector of the Psychedelic Society of New Orleans, and her work includes striving to ensure that psychedelic-assisted therapy reaches the traditionally underserved communities that need it most, such as the one she grew up in. "I want to be a voice for people, specifically people in the South," she said. "We get so left behind."

She's also encouraging legalization and social acceptance of MDMA-assisted therapy by sharing her story—even if that story sometimes gets simplified in the retelling. "I do all these interviews, and my mother becomes the villain, because there needs to be a villain for me to get cured," Lori said. "But what if she'd had access to psychedelic therapy?"

*

IN RESPONSE TO the data from the Phase 2 studies, in 2017 the FDA permitted MAPS to move to Phase 3 research. The administration also designated MDMA-assisted therapy a "breakthrough therapy" for PTSD, a special classification that serves to expedite the development of promising drugs. By the time these landmarks arrived, though, sixteen years had passed since Mithoefer submitted his Phase 2 protocol. Regulatory hurdles had slowed the process down, as had the fact that MAPS was having to pay for the trials purely through donations that Doblin fundraised. Two Phase 3 studies—another multiyear process—also still needed to be conducted before the FDA could consider granting approval. For some people, it was simply too long to wait for relief.

Around 2006, a man from Florida named Zulfi Riza reached out to Doblin to ask for help finding an underground MDMA therapist. Riza told Doblin he suffered from PTSD, anxiety, depression, anger management issues, and multiple sclerosis, and that all means of conventional treatment had failed him. But he also had epileptic seizures, a condition that excluded him from enrolling in MAPS's clinical trial. Doblin knew that if a medical emergency happened while Riza was working with an underground therapist, it could risk not only Riza's life but also the therapist's license and, potentially, their freedom. So Doblin told Riza he couldn't help.

A couple of months later, Doblin received a phone call from a police officer. Riza had committed suicide the morning after his conversation with Doblin. Riza had left Doblin a note, and the police officer needed Doblin's address to send it to him.

"My last hope was through psychedelic therapy, but after our conversation yesterday . . . that hope also fizzled," Riza wrote to Doblin. He added that he understood "how your hands are tied" by the "damn DEA" and FDA, and thanked him for "your sincere desire to help." He granted Doblin permission to use the letter in efforts geared toward giving others the opportunity he had not had, concluding, "I may have been one life saved, had I had access to psychedelic therapy."

Reading Riza's note made Doblin painfully aware of the cost of saying no to desperate people. It also made him incredibly angry at the DEA for going against Judge Francis Young's ruling and scheduling MDMA in the first place. "It reminded me of the enormous amount of suffering that's happened in what's now thirty-six years since the DEA made MDMA illegal," Doblin recently reflected. "How many hundreds of thousands of people have committed suicide that might not have?"

Doblin's stance on whether therapists assisting with the clinical trials should engage in underground work changed after he read Riza's note. While Mithoefer still thinks it's best for them to refrain so as not to put the clinical trials at risk, Doblin thinks it should be up to them. "There's an enormous amount of suffering, and some people can't wait for this to become medicine," Doblin said. "People are committing suicide all the time."

Underground therapy is illegal, so not much is known about how many people offer these services; what their training or qualifications are, if any; or how many people they treat. I had the opportunity to meet an underground therapist, Xena (not her real name), a clinical psychologist in New York City who has been quietly administering MDMA-assisted therapy since 2016. She was recruited by one of her mentors, who had more people coming to him for MDMA-assisted therapy than he could treat. When I met Xena, her wait-list was about six months long.

Xena underwent MAPS's hundred-hour clinical training program for MDMA-assisted therapy (some two thousand clinicians have completed the initial part of the program), and she more or less follows the group's treatment protocol, which Doblin and his colleagues share for free online. Xena estimates she has seen thirty to forty people in total, some of whom she's worked with multiple times. She requires every client to attend at least three sober psychotherapy sessions before undertaking any work with MDMA, and she also strongly recommends at least one integration session afterward. She charges around $1,200 to $1,500 for the MDMA-assisted therapy session itself.

People come to Xena for all sorts of reasons. She treated one client with a severe eating disorder, for example, and another who was struggling with their trans identity. Basically, though, her clients are all seeking help with processing trauma. Sexual abuse—especially repressed childhood sexual abuse—is "extremely prevalent," she said.

While Xena has seen a few clients who were not helped by MDMA-assisted therapy at all, in most cases, she said, people do gain valuable insights. Their breakthroughs don't always sound dramatic, but for the individuals involved, they are significant. After an MDMA-assisted therapy session, a wife who hadn't touched her husband in years went home and hugged him. In another case, a young woman who couldn't stand the sight of her nose because it reminded her of an uncle who sexually abused her was able to look in the mirror and see not her abuser, but a cute nose on a pretty face. One man—a veteran who suffered sexual and physical abuse as a child—referred to himself as "the monster" or "the creature" during his first meeting with Xena. It took four sessions of MDMA-assisted therapy for him to finally stop seeing himself as an abomination.

MDMA-assisted therapy is not an instantaneous magic fix, Xena stressed, and sometimes the insights clients have during their sessions do not wind up sticking. "It's ten years of therapy in a day, I think that's true," she said. "However, it's so easy for people to slip back into old habits and patterns, which is why integration is just as important, if not more important, than the medicine itself."

*

PTSD CAUSED BY combat is not as prevalent as childhood trauma, but it looms largest in terms of public awareness about the condition. This is partly because of the surge in new diagnoses over the last two decades. When Michael Mithoefer submitted the first PTSD protocol to the FDA in 2001, he, Annie, and Doblin had no idea that they were on the cusp of a twenty-year conflict that would see two million U.S. service members deployed to Iraq and Afghanistan, significantly adding to the already high number of veterans who suffer from PTSD from the Vietnam War, the Gulf War, and more.

Studies reveal that 15 to 19 percent of soldiers who are exposed to combat will go on to develop PTSD, and the VA's National Center for PTSD estimates that anywhere from 11 to 20 percent of veterans have PTSD in a given year. Around one million U.S. veterans today qualify for the diagnosis, and about seventeen commit suicide per day. According to a 2021 report published by Brown University, more than thirty thousand U.S. active-duty personnel and veterans who served in global war on terror operations have committed suicide since 9/11—more than four times the number of service members killed in combat over the same time.

The VA offers a range of screening and treatment services for PTSD, but it sees low relative use of those services, particularly by the veterans who are most in need. "By and large, soldiers don't like to reveal that they have any problems, so they tend to minimize their symptoms," said Elspeth Cameron

Ritchie, the chair of psychiatry at MedStar Washington Hospital Center. "Many also don't seek treatment because they worry about being able to continue their military career."

Soldiers and veterans who do try to address PTSD with therapy tend to drop out. According to a 2010 study, fewer than one in ten of nearly fifty thousand veterans who sought help for PTSD from the VA actually completed the recommended treatment. Other studies reveal that at best half of veterans who try therapy experience a meaningful decline in symptoms, and two thirds retain their diagnosis afterward (almost the exact inverse of the Phase 2 MDMA trial results). "I have been working for twenty years with veterans, and many report numerous failures of exposure-based treatments," said Eric Vermetten, a professor of psychiatry at Leiden University Medical Center in the Netherlands. "We do our best, but have limited results."

The cost of all this suffering is huge. In 2020 the VA spent nearly ninety-nine billion dollars on disability payments to two million veterans. Although the VA does not break down what proportion of that amount goes specifically to veterans with PTSD, about a quarter of those who seek help from the VA do so because they are struggling from PTSD. Whatever the dollar figure, it should be considered "a lowball estimate," said Stephen Xenakis, the psychiatrist and retired Brigadier General, because "it doesn't look at how PTSD fundamentally impairs people's lives."

PTSD can already be difficult to address, but combat veterans often return from war with multiple problems that can further complicate treatment compared to their civilian counterparts. Between 2000 and 2019 nearly 414,000 American service members deployed in the Middle East suffered traumatic brain injury (TBI), mostly as a result of improvised explosive devices. TBI frequently occurs in the brain's frontal lobes, which can impact mood, personality, judgment, attention, social behavior, problem solving, and flexibility in thinking. Chronic pain from combat-related injuries is another common complication, impacting around 30 percent of veterans, according to the CDC. "We tend to drill in on one problem like PTSD, but all of these things interact with each other," Xenakis said.

Another serious condition that frequently co-occurs with PTSD in veterans is a phenomenon called moral injury. Sometimes described as "a wounding of the soul," moral injury occurs when a service member perpetrates an act, or fails to stop an act, that violates their deeply held values or beliefs. "Killing civilians, especially women and children, is a common trigger, and the result is often intense feelings of shame, self-recrimination, and guilt," said Robert Koffman, a psychiatrist and retired Navy Captain. "These are existential injuries that take years of therapy and are not necessarily mitigated by a round of prolonged exposure. Sometimes, they're made worse."

"The guilt, the shame, and the anger that veterans often feel after war is distinct from PTSD," added Rakesh Jetly, a retired Colonel and senior psychiatrist in the Canadian Forces. "Some of us have hypothesized that it's this guilt and shame that traditional treatments don't get access to that may explain some of the suicides that occur because of how people feel about themselves."

According to Vermetten, the great hope is that MDMA-assisted therapy could help veterans find relief not just from PTSD, but also moral injury. As he said, "acceptance and forgiveness need to come from within."

*

JOHN REISSENWEBER WAS about to start his senior year at the University of Michigan when he received a draft notice for the Vietnam War. John had never shot a gun, had never gotten into a fight, and had no interest in going into the military. But he did not consider trying to dodge the draft. "My grandfather had served in World War I, and my dad served on a minesweeper in World War II," he said. "I wasn't going to shirk my responsibility."

In 1969, barely two months into his tour in northern Vietnam, John was struck by a mortar round that knocked him unconscious. When he came to, he was covered in burns and bleeding from his chest, arms, and ears. Both of his eardrums were broken, but his injuries were not bad enough to get him sent home.

John managed to make it through the rest of the year without incurring further serious physical harm. But mentally, things got worse. One night, a mortar-based flare he fired to illuminate the perimeter of his base accidentally went off course and struck a village, killing a two-year-old boy. "When you get back to the States and everybody says you were a baby killer," he said, "yeah, you were."

Like many veterans, John returned from Vietnam "a very different person," he said. For one, he was now "a full blown alcoholic." His formerly happy-go-lucky personality had also turned dark. None of his friends had served in Vietnam, and they all struck him now as shallow. He also drifted apart from his brother, with whom he used to be close.

John never made it back to college and instead got a job at the Ford Motor Company. He made some work friends, he said, "but they just didn't understand what I'd been through, so we could only go so far." John would go to bars after his shift, drink until two in the morning, and then pass out in the grass in the backyard at his dad and stepmom's house. "Sleeping outside felt natural."

John spent the next thirty years drinking, keeping others at arm's length, and honing his skills at "controlling everything so nothing would hurt me." In work meetings, he would bully the room by loudly talking over his co-workers, ensuring that he always got his way, and he frequently lied to get out of responsibilities. If anyone ever tried calling him out, he would respond with "one of the most acid tongues there were." He also became expert at blocking out anything or anyone he didn't want to engage with. He lost everything in a divorce to his first wife because he didn't want to deal with the logistical and emotional hassle of negotiating, and his second marriage also ended in divorce—although it took him ten years to sign the papers. "If I could throw it out of my mind, it didn't exist," he said. "That goes right back to blocking out killing kids. If you blocked it out, it didn't matter."

John never considered that he might have any sort of problem, and he certainly never thought that he might have PTSD. "Oh, hell no! In order to have PTSD, you're weak," he said of his past mindset. He never even applied to the VA for benefits he was entitled to for his broken eardrums because "I didn't need any help from anybody," he said. "I didn't need anybody telling me I was disabled, because I came back with ten fingers and ten toes and others didn't."

In 2003 John's life changed for the better when he met Stacy Turner, his current wife. They had connected online, and the first time he saw her in person, he exclaimed, "My god, you are so beautiful!"

"How do you not love a man who says that to you with all this warmth in his eyes?" Stacy said. "John loved so much about me, and I felt that way about him, too."

Things were great for half a year or so, but then Stacy "started to see the cracks," as she put it. One beautiful afternoon, they were sitting on a blanket in a woodsy section of San Francisco's Glen Canyon Park, having a picnic, when John's demeanor suddenly changed. He started scanning the area and became "real cold and distant," Stacy recalled. "Then he starts talking about strategic and vulnerable positions and where you could worry about a fire-fight and where people could be hiding. I looked at him, and I was like, 'He is fucking back in Vietnam.' I just corked the wine, packed up, and said 'We're going home, this is not a good place for you to be.' "

Stacy loved John, but the stress and strain of tiptoeing around his temper worsened over the years. "No matter what I said or did, the chance of it being wrong was huge, and if it was wrong, the results were cata-strophic," she said.

Twice, she kicked him out, but they always got back together. Finally Stacy told John that he had to get professional help, or she was done. A psychia-trist diagnosed him with PTSD, but talk therapy wasn't improving things. One day his psychiatrist handed him a copy of Michael Pollan's *How to Change Your Mind* and told him about the MAPS MDMA trials. "I had a very strong aversion to mind-altering drugs, because by now, I knew I was wrapped pretty tightly," John said. "I was afraid if I did anything I'd really come undone."

Stacy and John's doctor convinced him to apply for the trial anyway. But when he took a PTSD evaluation to find out if he qualified, he reverted to his old habit of downplaying his symptoms. "I lied to myself again, like I did all my life since I came back from Vietnam," he said. It worked: shortly after taking the test, he received a polite letter stating that he did not meet the criteria for the study.

Stacy wasn't having it. She reached out to Gregory Wells, a psychologist coleading the San Francisco trials, and asked him to take a closer look at their evaluation process. "If you dismissed John for high blood pressure, I'd under-stand," she said. "But if you dismissed him because you thought he wasn't messed up enough, you just really missed the boat and he totally snowed you."

Stacy's letter did the trick. In August 2019 John arrived at Wells's office for his first session of MDMA-assisted therapy. "I felt a combination of scared shitless and determined," he said. "I'd gotten to the point where I had realized that maybe there is something to this, maybe I do have some PTSD. And maybe this can help."

As he reclined on the daybed with headphones and eyeshades on, it didn't take John long to "realize that something was going on," he said. He felt deeply affected by the music and ungrounded in his own body. Suddenly, a vision appeared in his mind. He was standing on a lunar plane reminiscent of the Apollo 10 "Earthrise" photo, with stars all around. In the lower lefthand corner there was a dark, foreboding hole, which John chose to ignore. He focused instead on a liquid-like drop of energy that appeared in front of him, which John realized represented his consciousness coalescing at the time of his birth. "Everything was nice, calm, serene," John said. "I felt a connection to everything."

However, when a second drop appeared and hit the ground, John heard helicopters, gunfire, and shouting—the disruption Vietnam had caused to his psyche. Although John's therapists were "really super," he said, he kept quiet. "I didn't want to talk about it with anybody," he said. "I was doing it on my own."

In the month after that first session, John felt more relaxed than he had in decades. He could take a walk outside and enjoy feeling the breeze on his skin. He could have a conversation with Stacy and imagine what she was thinking and feeling.

John began his second session of MDMA-assisted therapy eager to see what other gains it might bring. Immediately, his mind brought him back to the same lunar landscape. The fearful black pit was still there, but he focused solely on the first drop, and the second drop never came. All day he lay on the couch, hugging himself, rocking back and forth, and petting a dog that one of his therapists had brought along. "I was caring for that child self of me," he said.

Following his second session, for the first time, John started remembering his dreams. A few days before his third and final session, however, he had a terrible nightmare: he was in military clothing, deathly afraid, as the sounds of mortar blasts overwhelmed him. He was left with a sense of dread, and he went into the last MDMA session determined to engage with the black pit in the corner. "You can't shy away from it anymore," he told himself—and jumped straight in. He thought he would pass through it—"like Pollan's book said, 'passing into the light,'" he explained—but he got "completely and totally stuck." John spent the rest of the session trapped in the pit, unable to move.

The next morning, his entire body was sore. When he came by the therapists' office for his integration session, he was too terrified to go back into the room. He knew he needed more help than the limited clinical trial could provide, so he got a new therapist. With her guidance, he came to realize that the black pit represented the anger and hurt he had felt since Vietnam. That revelation permitted him to examine his life afresh, pulling out memories, one by one, like a series of file cards that he could rearrange into a coherent whole.

While the MDMA-assisted therapy on its own by no means healed John, it was "like an electric shock to the system," he said. It revealed his hurt and his fears, and more importantly, it showed him that he was entitled to feel that way. "It was like a complete and total rebirth," he said. "It gave me the ability to look at myself and say, 'You know, you don't have to be perfect, you don't have to be right, it's okay to be who you are.' Without it, I could have taken all the cognitive behavior therapy in the world and nothing would have happened."

John has continued traditional therapy and has also gotten involved at the VA, where he connected with other veterans. In October 2021 he began volunteering with a VA program aimed at rehabilitating veterans through golf. He no longer feels like he's "running at 100 percent" all the time, he said, and he isn't sent into a tailspin by the small, unavoidable obstacles that daily life throws his way. Most importantly, he's been able to connect more deeply with Stacy, whom he calls his guardian angel.

"I can talk to Stacy," he said. "I'm not afraid of doing that anymore."

*

ON MAY 10, 2021, MAPS and a team of thirty-plus expert coauthors reported in *Nature Medicine* the results of the first Phase 3 trial of MDMA-assisted therapy for PTSD—"the first-ever, late-stage clinical trial for a psychedelic," as Mitchell, the lead author of the study, pointed out in a feature story for *Scientific American*. And the findings, which I wrote about in the *New York Times*, were even more encouraging than the Phase 2 ones.

The ninety participants received treatment from seventy therapists at fifteen study sites spread across three countries. All had severe PTSD and had been diagnosed with the condition, on average, for fourteen years. Ninety percent reported a history of suicidal ideation or behavior, and the majority also had comorbidities like depression or a history of alcohol use disorder. Sixteen participants, including John, were combat veterans.

At the two-month follow-up mark after the participants completed their sessions, 67 percent of those who received MDMA no longer qualified for a PTSD diagnosis, compared to 32 percent who were in the placebo group. Scientists and therapists were especially excited about the large placebo-subtracted effect size of 0.91, a measure that emphasized the difference between "just getting good therapy and what MDMA adds," said van der Kolk, a coauthor on the study. The before-and-after effect size for those who received MDMA-assisted therapy compared to the placebo was a similarly impressive 2.1—a finding that Doblin called "remarkable."

Effect sizes like these are "unlike any I have seen in PTSD before," said Yehuda, who was not involved in the research. "This is not like someone being really good at statistics trying to get a headline. These data are very robust, and it has to do with the combination of the psychedelic and the psychotherapy."

There were also additional perks, all of which were statistically larger for the MDMA group. The researchers found that the 90 percent of participants who had depression experienced a clinically significant reduction in symptoms, as did the thirteen participants who had eating disorder scores in the clinical risk range. All told, MDMA-assisted therapy was just as effective for those with comorbidities, "a group of people previously considered to be somewhat treatment resistant," said Mitchell. "That opens up a possible path of recovery for a bunch of people who had been previously excluded."

Thomas Insel, a psychiatrist and neuroscientist who formerly directed the National Institute of Mental Health, and who was not involved in the research, noted that MAPS actually put itself at a disadvantage by seeking out participants who were suffering from the most severe cases of PTSD and who had additional comorbidities. Normally scientists exclude this group in favor of collecting more promising data. "But they pulled it off, and they did it well," Insel said. "When you look at the data, certainly the effects are remarkable."

Most other outside experts I spoke to were similarly encouraged by the results. "To finally have all the data from this multi-site, randomized, placebo-controlled trial in the books is very exciting for the field," said Albert Garcia Romeu, a psychopharmacologist at Johns Hopkins University School of Medicine. "The data are pretty clear that this is safe and works an order of magnitude better than talk therapy alone in the placebo group."

A few outside experts were more skeptical, however. "The study is well done on its own limited terms, but far from convincing that MDMA is ready for prime time widespread clinical use or deserving of enthusiastic hype that will likely lead to potentially dangerous street use," said Allen Francis, the chairman emeritus of psychiatry at Duke University. "It is far too soon to tell whether the benefits of MDMA-assisted therapy are worth its considerable risks."

Xenakis, who also was not involved in the research, noted, however, that resistance from more establishment doctors is to be fully expected. "This is really going to shake up many senior psychiatrists who for the past thirty to forty years have been working in the model of 'Oh, we've got the right drug,'" he said. "Doctors are pretty conservative and don't change the way they do things very easily."

Whether doctors welcome change or not, it's likely coming. At the time of writing, the final Phase 3 trial was well underway. If its results are in line with the first one, then FDA approval could arrive by the end of 2023.

In the United States, a second step will also be needed prior to the treatment becoming available: rescheduling of MDMA to a lesser category than strictly banned Schedule I. If the FDA approves the treatment, then the DEA will have to federally reschedule MDMA, because its status as a medically approved substance will automatically invalidate it for Schedule I. States also have their own controlled substance systems, though, and while about half of them automatically follow the DEA's lead, the others have their own ways of doing things. New York and Colorado, for example, require specific legislation to reschedule a drug—a burdensome political and bureaucratic undertaking.

MAPS has already started working with states that don't automatically reschedule to try to get bills introduced and passed to ensure a smooth transition post-FDA approval. Coming full circle, Doblin also reached out to Frank Sapienza, the former DEA agent who participated in the 1985 scheduling hearings, for help shifting MDMA to the appropriate schedule at the federal level. "I give Rick Doblin a lot of credit," said Sapienza, who is now a partner with the Drug and Chemical Advisory Group. "I didn't think he would have been able to accomplish what he has accomplished. But he took the bull by the horns and he's come a long way."

Developments abroad are also underway. Starting in July 2023, authorized psychiatrists in Australia will be able to legally prescribe MDMA for PTSD. In Europe, MAPS is training researchers so they can conduct a MAPS-sponsored Phase 3 study with an additional seventy participants. Once that is done, the European Medicines Agency (Europe's FDA equivalent) will evaluate those data alongside the U.S. findings. In Brazil, pilot studies have already been completed, and an additional fifty Brazilian clinicians are being trained to administer MDMA-assisted therapy in trials with 140 participants over the next few years. "In Brazil, we don't have the same big issue of war veterans, but we have a huge issue with violence, gangs, robberies, sexual abuse, and shootings," said Eduardo Schenberg, director of Instituto Phaneros, a nonprofit psychedelic research and therapy group in São Paolo. Study preparations are likewise being finalized in Armenia, and other efforts are beginning to be explored in Iraq, Rwanda, South Africa, Bosnia, and Somaliland.

Back in the United States, the VA has finally come around, too. On October 12, 2021—more than twenty-five years after Doblin and David Presti first tried to get the VA to take an interest—a veteran with PTSD received MDMA-assisted therapy at the Loma Linda VA in California. Yehuda, who has been working within the VA system since 1987, has also started trials of MDMA-assisted therapy with sixty combat veterans at the VA in the Bronx, where she and her colleagues treated their first PTSD patient in February 2022. Another study to test MDMA-assisted therapy in a group setting is making its way through the approval process at the VA in Portland, Oregon. "We're really at a tipping point where this would not have even been a feasible conversation two or three years ago," said Chris Stauffer, a psychiatrist and researcher at the VA Portland Health Care System, in a Horizons panel discussion in 2021.

Most scientists see the uptick in interest in MDMA-assisted therapy in the United States and beyond as only the beginning, not the end, of research. Studies can help refine the treatment itself—from the ideal number of sessions a patient undergoes for preparation, integration, and MDMA-assisted therapy to what kind of physical setting and music would be most effective and for whom. British psychiatrist Ben Sessa, for example, thinks that the psychedelic community's stereotypical emphasis on Eastern mysticism will not connect with the majority of people. "Pictures of the Buddha and Indian sitar music and incense? Most people are not hippies," Sessa said. "Why not put up a picture of Beyoncé or Manchester United, if these are our patients' power objects? We have to meet patients where they are rather than expect them to adapt to us."

Yehuda also emphasized that, like any medical treatment, MDMA-assisted therapy will not work for everyone, so identifying who it *won't* work for is just as important as homing in on who it most likely will benefit. Xenakis agreed: "We need to drill down a whole lot more to identify who responds to what, and what it is about not just the drug, but also the therapy they get while on the drug, that produces the response."

Another way to ensure that MDMA-assisted therapy is optimized for healing—and minimized for risk of causing inadvertent harm—is to untangle exactly how the drug produces its therapeutic effects in the brain. Fortunately, groundbreaking new research is beginning to elucidate this formerly inscrutable biological process. If these findings hold up, the implications not only for mental health, but also potentially for all classes of disorders that originate in the brain, are huge.

# A CRITICAL PERIOD

ALEXANDER FLEMING HAD just returned to work after a two-week holiday in Suffolk when he noticed something strange in one of his petri dishes. While the Scottish bacteriologist had been vacationing, a fungus had apparently taken up residence in a staphylococci colony he was growing in his lab at St. Mary's Hospital in London. Normally, this would warrant a trip to the rubbish bin. But Fleming stopped short of tossing the colony when he noticed that the bands of agar gel immediately surrounding the fuzzy fungal blobs were intriguingly clear of bacterial growth.

A year later, in 1929, Fleming published a journal article showing that "mould juice" from *Penicillium notatum*, the fungus in question, inhibited bacterial growth in vitro. He hypothesized that penicillin, as he called his discovery, could be used as an antiseptic. Scientists at the University of Oxford took it from there. After isolating the molecule that gave penicillin its antibacterial properties, the Oxford team conducted clinical trials with 170 patients in 1941 and 1942. Their findings demonstrated penicillin's remarkable effectiveness in fighting bacterial infections.

The discovery of this "miracle drug" saved thousands of Allied soldier and civilian lives in the final years of World War II. As one triumphant 1944 poster declared, THANKS TO PENICILLIN . . . HE WILL COME HOME! Clearly, penicillin worked—and yet no one knew exactly *how* it worked. It wasn't until 1965, nearly four decades after Fleming's initial revelation, that a pair of pharmacologists at the University of Wisconsin, Madison, finally teased apart the exact mechanism: the lifesaving drug dashed infections by inhibiting bacterial cell wall synthesis. While this discovery wasn't pertinent for saving lives in the immediate term, it did enable researchers to start designing even more effective antibiotics, and eventually to better understand and combat antibiotic resistance.

MDMA seems to be following a similar timeline of mechanistic discovery. Therapists in the late 1970s clearly saw that the drug produced positive benefits for many of their patients, but they had no idea how it worked. Researchers conducting the clinical trials over the past two decades have likewise remained in the dark about why, exactly, MDMA seems to be such a potent therapeutic catalyst. In terms of gaining clinical approval, this glaring unknown doesn't actually matter, because the FDA does not require applicants to prove how a new drug works—only that it is safe and efficacious. Regardless, many scientists still want to know what exactly is going on.

MDMA's acute effects—the flurry of serotonin and other brain chemicals that it triggers—are not context-dependent. They happen regardless of whether a person takes MDMA at a rave, at home with a lover, or in a therapist's office. But given that most people are not spontaneously recovering from trauma after attending all-night dance parties, experts surmise that there must be something more going on—something specific to the context of taking the drug while primed to address trauma and healing. In such settings, MDMA seems to culminate in "a softening and opening up," said psychiatrist Eric Vermetten. The solutions patients arrive at are often found "in metaphorical terms, beyond the cognitive domain."

The ineffableness of MDMA-assisted healing does not preclude scientists from taking a closer look under the neurological hood, though, to find out "why this short experience is having such a transformational effect," as neuroscientist Rachel Yehuda put it. The answer to this question could help clinicians maximize healing and minimize harm. And it would also provide new insight into one of the greatest biological mysteries of all, the human brain.

*

GÜL DÖLEN, A neuroscientist at Johns Hopkins School of Medicine—whose first name rhymes with "cool"—did not set out to solve the mystery of how MDMA produces its therapeutic effects. For years, Dölen's scientific investigations focused on topics ranging from schizophrenia to theory of mind and social behaviors, not psychedelic drugs. Her interest in MDMA began simply because its unique prosocial effects made it a means to an end for trying to answer other questions.

Dölen grew up in San Antonio, the first-generation daughter of two Turkish doctors. Her parents immigrated to the United States to do their residencies but then got stuck when a coup broke out back home. By the time things had settled down in Turkey, the kids were in school, so the family decided to stay.

Dölen had always excelled at math and science, but her interest in becoming a scientist was solidified in elementary school on a visit to see her grandmother in Antalya, a Turkish resort town on the Aegean Sea. Prior to the trip, the only bodies of water Dölen had experienced were the sterile swimming pools of Texas. She was at first horrified by the strange sea creatures she saw washed up on the beach and lurking beneath the Aegean's clear water. Her grandmother, a biology teacher, quickly intervened to show Dölen that there was nothing to be afraid of. She dissected a sea urchin and explained the animal's radically different anatomy: a stomach equipped with teeth, spines that enabled sensing and locomotion, and gonads that were the brilliant orange shade of a pumpkin. Under her grandmother's guidance, Dölen realized that nature in all of its mind-boggling variation was something to be celebrated and scientifically pursued, not feared. "That's how I've been lured into science, through that childlike wonder and amazement over all the weird, crazy stuff out there," Dölen said. "There's a sort of magic to the unknown."

Dölen considered becoming a marine biologist, but in college she shifted her focus to what seemed to her to be nature's ultimate unknown: consciousness and the human brain. She also discovered firsthand that psychedelic drugs could be powerful tools for better understanding the workings of her new favorite organ—and for exploring "the strangeness of the world, the magic of the weird," as she put it.

But Dölen wasn't particularly interested in undertaking studies of psyche-delic drugs herself, and she also thought other scientists were on the cusp of getting these compounds to spill their mechanistic secrets, which struck her as probably being pretty straightforward. She remembers seeing side-by-side drawings of the chemical structures of LSD and serotonin in an undergrad-uate textbook and thinking, "Ah-ha! That's how we're gonna understand consciousness and how these things work." Like many other scientists, she assumed the answers would boil down to the specific receptors that psyche-delics activate. As Dölen recently pointed out, though, "biology is unfortu-nately more complicated than we'd like it to be."

For several years after graduating with a PhD and MD from Brown University and MIT, Dölen worked as a postdoc in a lab at Stanford Univer-sity that focused on the neural circuits underlying social reward learning—the intrinsic reward that humans and most mammals derive from social inter-actions. Meanwhile, other labs began publishing studies purporting to eluci-date the mechanisms behind psychedelic drugs by highlighting how they affected activity in various human brain regions. Most of these papers were authored by psychiatrists and psychologists rather than neuroscientists, and most relied on functional magnetic resonance imaging (fMRI), a technique that infers neuronal activity by measuring changes in blood flow in the brain. Dölen was not impressed. Given that the human brain consists of several hundred billion cells linked by hundreds of trillions of connections, relying on fMRI to answer basic questions "is like trying to solve a traffic problem in New York City by taking pictures of cloud cover from Saturn," she said. "There may be a correlation between a cloudy day and traffic, but where I'd put my money is looking closer and at a better time scale."

Neuroscientists like Dölen prefer to use much more detailed techniques such as whole-cell patch-clamp electrophysiology, in which scientists use elec-trodes inserted into a neuron extracted from a mouse brain. This allows them to measure activity down to the level of a single cell. "It's like the French kiss of communicating with a neuron—we're creating a direct inside-the-cell to inside-the-electrode relationship," Dölen said. The data produced from experiments of that sort, she added, are "just orders of magnitude more mechanistic, informative, and useful for developing new therapies and under-standing how the brain works."

Dölen watched the advances in psychedelic science from afar with increasing interest, feeling more and more that she could contribute to the field by providing more granular insight. Yet early in her career, she didn't think psychedelics would be something "considered legitimate for me to study." It wasn't until she got hired at Johns Hopkins—specifically, in the Solomon H. Snyder Department of Neuroscience—that she realized, in fact, psychedelics could be a possibility for her. Snyder, the namesake of Dölen's new department, was of course a close friend of Sasha Shulgin's, who had also dabbled in some psychedelic research himself. As Snyder recounted to me of the early 1970s, "the rules and regulations were much more lax in those days, so I was able to get Hopkins undergraduates to spend a day doing new Shulgin drugs." Snyder was winding down his lab by the time Dölen arrived, but the open-minded culture he helped to instill in the department lived on.

*

IN SOME WAYS, the story of Dölen finding her way to MDMA begins not with neurons, molecules, or her new position at Johns Hopkins, but with geese. In 1935 an Austrian zoologist named Konrad Lorenz hatched a greylag gosling he named Martina. Lorenz was the first thing Martina saw after she pecked her way out of her eggshell, and she latched on to him as though he were her mother. In work that later earned him a Nobel Prize, Lorenz performed similar experiments with many more baby geese and ducks. He postulated that the birds were imprinting on him because he was there at a key moment in their development—a critical period.

Lorenz's discovery provided the mechanistic basis for an observation that the psychologist William James made back in 1890. While "most performances of other animals are automatic," James wrote, humans come into the world with the blank slate of their minds primed to become fluent in any language, to adapt to any culture, and to learn any skill. But given that the number of things we could potentially learn far outstrips our brain's finite capacities, most of the skills we develop "must be the fruit of painful study," James reasoned.

The younger we are, the less painful that study is. Adages like "You can't teach an old dog new tricks" contain a core, intuitive truth about the brain and learning: the older we get, the more set we become in our ways. "This goes way back to Aristotle, this very old concept that the young brain is more malleable or sensitive to the environment," said Takao Hensch, a neurologist and molecular and cellular biologist at Harvard Medical School and Harvard University, who specializes in critical periods. "For centuries, we've known earlier is better for learning, but why is that?"

Scientists now believe critical periods are a key part of the answer. Starting in infancy and lasting into early adulthood, the memories and skills we learn during these finite windows of malleability solidify into automated habits that will serve us for the rest of our lives. We lose behavioral flexibility as we grow older and some neuronal networks are pruned, but as part of that trade-off other networks are strengthened, and we become adept at the skills we most often use in daily life.

Neuroscientists have sought to elucidate the mechanistic underpinnings of critical periods since the 1940s. Their research to date has primarily focused on critical periods related to sensory processing systems such as sight and hearing, simply because those are the easiest to study in lab animals. But as Hensch noted, "there are probably as many critical periods as there are brain functions."

This includes learned social behaviors, such as the rules of connection, interaction, and cultural appropriateness—things that are "hugely important for human beings, and really central to who we are," Dölen said. Teenagers, in particular, are exquisitely sensitive to the rewards and punishments of having behaved correctly or incorrectly according to the social standards of whatever group they're trying to fit into. Fortunately, this phase passes. As we get older, social habits, skills, and preferences established in youth harden into tried-and-true behaviors. "This is why adults aren't as susceptible to peer pressure, or why it's hard for us to fit into a new culture," Dölen said. "Every time I go to Japan, for example, I fear I'm going to make some horrible faux pas and act like a bear in a china closet."

Critical periods close for a reason, and normally that's a good thing. It simply wouldn't be efficient to go through life in a state of constant impressionability and openness. Learned behaviors and skills from childhood become second nature in adulthood, from the ability to differentiate between reality and fantasy to being able to skillfully navigate the physical and social environment. "When you're older, it's something of a relief to have your habits and preferred styles and social groups," Dölen said. "You become less playful, but also more stable."

In some cases, though, it would be desirable to reopen certain critical periods after they close. Children with a lazy eye, for example, can have their vision relatively easily corrected up until about eight years old, after which the corresponding vision-related critical period closes and interventions become much more difficult. Cochlear implants likewise work best if given to deaf or hearing-impaired children before the age of three, while children born with bilateral cataracts must have corrective surgery before the age of five or they will be blind forever. As Dölen said, "We're oftentimes not able to fix things not because we've got the mechanisms wrong, but because by the time we get around to fixing them, the relevant critical period has already closed and the brain is no longer responsive."

If doctors could reopen critical periods that correspond to these and other conditions, they could potentially correct those problems anytime over a person's lifespan. For decades, neuroscientists have been searching for ways to safely, efficiently, and selectively do this. It's tricky, though, because in tampering with critical periods, scientists do not want to destabilize the entire infrastructure of the brain that supports learned habits and behaviors, and possibly induce seizures in the process. Opening critical periods willy-nilly could potentially make a person's entire suite of memories "vulnerable to erasure," Hensch warned. "It would really impact who you are."

*

IT WAS THE quest to find a way to safely reopen critical periods that ultimately led Dölen to MDMA. In 2015 she unexpectedly discovered an unknown critical period—or, to put it more accurately, her postdoc, Romain Nardou, did. Rather than relate to sensory processing, this critical period dealt with social reward learning, one of Dölen's specialties.

Nardou spent two years conducting experiments with hundreds of mice across fourteen age groups using a common assay for learned associations called "conditioned place preference." Researchers originally developed this experimental model to test how animals come to associate drugs of abuse with reward. They would give mice the choice to hang out on two types of bedding, one of which would be paired with access to heroin or cocaine, and one that would have no drugs available. Afterward, even when the drug wasn't around, mice of all ages showed a preference for the bedding they had come to associate with getting their fix. As Dölen noted, "There's not a critical period for cocaine reward learning. Adults love cocaine as much as kids."

Nardou wanted to test the learned reward value not of addictive drugs, but of social interactions. His mice took turns spending twenty-four hours in an enclosure they shared with several other mice, and then in another one in which they were alone. Like the drug studies, both enclosures had different types of bedding. When Nardou later gave the mice a choice between these two beddings, the younger mice—especially those that were the equivalent of teenagers—showed a clear preference for hanging out on the bedding they associated with their friends. The older mice, on the other hand, neither preferred nor avoided the social bedding. "After two years of Romain doing a ton of really painstaking and repetitive experiments, he convinced me, yup, there's a big change across development, and we can define this as a critical period," Dölen said. The equivalent of these findings in humans, she added, would be "like why people of a certain age have warm fuzzy feelings about mid-century modern furniture that reminds us of our grandmothers. It feels homey and cozy."

Dölen and Nardou validated the behavioral observations in mice on a cellular level by extracting live neurons from the animals' nucleus accumbens, a node-like structure that plays a central role in the brain's reward circuit. During her postdoc, Dölen had pinpointed the nucleus accumbens as being especially important for social reward learning. Using whole-cell patch-clamp electrophysiology, she and Nardou computed the frequencies of the neurons' firing to see if the cells behaved differently when they were bathed in oxytocin. They chose to apply oxytocin to the neurons because of previous findings Dölen and her colleagues had reported in *Nature* in 2013, showing that the hormone is a necessary component for social reward learning in the nucleus accumbens.

They found that the cells from juvenile mice responded to the oxytocin bath with a sudden and significant change in electrical activity, as measured by a hair-thin electrode connecting the inside of the cell to a computer. The cells of older mice, on the other hand, did not respond to the oxytocin at all. The difference indicated that the younger mice's neurons were still in a state of openness and malleability that permitted them to receive oxytocin's prosocial signal, whereas the older mice's cells were not. "That oxytocin-induced synaptic plasticity is how we think that social bonds are formed," Dölen said.

Dölen and Nardou coined their discovery the "social reward learning critical period." While Dölen thought the findings represented a "cool mechanism," at first it didn't occur to her that there would be any chance of figuring out any practical application for humans. She suspected that oxytocin could be key for such a reopening, but she also knew that that hormone does not cross the blood-brain barrier. "When people try to give oxytocin through the nose or in injections, it targets a lot of other receptors all over the body, but it just doesn't get into your brain," Dölen pointed out.

In chewing over her hunch about oxytocin, though, an image came to Dölen's mind: the sixty-person-strong cuddle puddles of blissed-out Burning Man attendees rolling on MDMA. As Dölen noted, "People in the recreational drug scene have known about the extremely prosocial effect of MDMA for a long time."

Dölen checked the existing scientific literature and confirmed that there was indeed evidence that MDMA causes "massive oxytocin dumps" in the brain, as she put it. Compared to other, more high-tech options, giving mice MDMA seemed like a much simpler solution for testing whether oxytocin could reopen the social reward learning critical period. And if her hunch was correct, she knew this could also have important implications for humans.

To run the experiment, Dölen needed money. But this was around 2016—before the mainstream media and scientific establishment had started to get on board with the so-called psychedelic renaissance. "I'd go to conferences and bring this up, and clinicians would just look at me like I was crazy," Dölen recalled. The National Institutes of Health (NIH) likewise didn't get it, and rejected her application seventeen times. Inevitably, the grant reviewers would tell her something along the lines of, "Even if this is theoretically true, it'll never be practical because we'll never get approval to give humans a dangerous psychedelic drug."

Dölen finally gave up on trying to get funding from the NIH for any application containing the words "psychedelics" or "MDMA," and instead just submitted an application for research on the social reward learning critical period without any mention of drugs. This time it worked, and she also managed to secure some private foundation money to cover the MDMA expenses. With funding now in hand, she and Nardou repeated the original experiment, but with the addition of various injections for the mice. Some of the rodents received MDMA (sourced from David Nichols's original master stash), while others received cocaine or a saline placebo.

The adult mice that received coke or saline showed no behavioral or neuronal changes with regard to social reward learning. The behaviors and brains of adults that received MDMA, however, transformed to resemble younger mice. Importantly, though, MDMA only produced these changes if the adult mice hung out with their friends on the social bedding while they were on the drug, or in the two weeks immediately after. If they were left alone, they showed no increased preference for the social bedding, and their neurons also did not respond to oxytocin. The presence of their friends, in other words, was important for unlocking MDMA's ability to help them acquire new, rewarding memories of social encounters.

Seeing this important distinction, Dölen immediately thought of the Phase 2 clinical trial results of MDMA-assisted therapy for PTSD. She realized that her lab's findings could represent a biomarker for what clinicians were observing in their offices. Severe PTSD, after all, tends to be triggered by social interactions gone awry, from childhood abuse and sexual assault to the horror of killing or of witnessing others killed. The maladaptive habits that result from these traumas and become symptoms of PTSD also largely pertain to the social environment, including distrust, guilt, paranoia, fear, and disconnection from the self and others. If MDMA reopens the social reward learning critical period, then that could explain why the drug combined with therapy is so much more effective than therapy alone. People are literally given the ability to rewire the neural memory circuits they've built around the personal narrative of their trauma. The memories are not erased, but they can be recontextualized.

MDMA, moreover, seems to do this with surgical precision: it only opens the brain up to a cognitive reappraisal when the right memory circuits are primed to be activated. Just as Dölen's rodent subjects required interactions with other mice for MDMA to produce a lasting change, human participants also have to go into the experience with preset intentions to engage with traumatic memories in order for the drug to permit the possibility for healing. Psychotherapy also likely plays an important role in guiding this process. While many Indigenous cultures have long recognized the importance of proper context for psychedelic experiences, Dölen and Nardou's findings represent the first time this millennia-old knowledge has been confirmed in an animal model.

*

DÖLEN, NARDOU, AND their colleagues published their findings about MDMA and the social reward learning critical period in *Nature* in 2019. The story could have ended there, but just for due diligence, Dölen decided to repeat the same experiment in mice given LSD rather than MDMA. She had no reason to think that LSD would reopen the social reward learning critical period. The subjective effects of that classic psychedelic are significantly different from MDMA, including with regard to social behavior. If anything, people tend to become antisocial on LSD, seeking alone time rather than hugs.

To Dölen's incredulity, though, the results indicated that LSD also reopened the social reward learning critical period in mice. "Well, you fucked it up," she told herself. "Do it again." Yet again and again, her lab got the very same results. "It just kept happening," Dölen said.

Pondering this, she wondered if the social reward learning critical period wasn't being opened up by the biological mechanism that encourages cuddle puddles after all. Maybe it was being opened instead by whatever mechanism it is in MDMA—and also in LSD—that makes people feel connected to themselves, to others, and to the universe. To put this idea to the test, Dölen and her colleagues repeated the experiment this time using ketamine, a drug that usually does not make people feel connected to anything at all (including their own bodies). But lo and behold, they found that ketamine produced the same results. And tests with psilocybin and ibogaine did, too.

Dölen was stunned. But in puzzling out these findings, it dawned on her that the subjective sensation of being in an altered state of consciousness could just be what it feels like to be in a neurochemical state of critical period openness. The thing that might unite psychedelics, then, is that they all open critical periods. Once Dölen had this eureka-moment realization, she said, "we were off to the races."

Dölen set her sights on pinpointing the shared biological mechanism across psychedelics that is responsible for reopening the critical period. After ruling out a couple of commonly hypothesized culprits behind how psychedelics work, the team turned their attention to genes. They identified sixty-five genes whose expression seems to be unique to the open critical period state. These findings provide a road map for future investigations into how psychedelics function at the most fundamental level of DNA transcription—a question that Dölen guesses will keep her lab occupied for the next decade.

Already, though, scientists are beginning to regard Dölen and her colleagues' research as paradigm-shifting. Not only do their latest findings—due to be published in the scientific literature in 2023—seem to uncover the long-searched-for biological commonality behind psychedelics' therapeutic effects but they also imply that mind-altering substances could be the master key that neuroscientists have been searching for to safely and precisely reopen critical periods. As Dölen said, "Not to be too arrogant, but to me, this is like, holy shit! It's pretty amazing."

Nearly a dozen outside experts I spoke to about Dölen's findings were complimentary of the work. According to David Nutt, director of the Neuropsychopharmacology Unit at Imperial College London, Dölen's research so far is "very, very exciting. Opening up these critical periods and allowing the brain to relearn—I think that's an extremely credible theory."

Rachel Yehuda agreed, and added that the findings are in line with what we know about the subjective experience of taking psychedelic drugs. "When people use the metaphoric shorthand of 'the reset button,' what they mean is we're searching for a mechanism exactly like this that will explain how something that is so short in duration can have lasting and transformative effects that go well beyond the time period that the drug is in there," she said. "Here, we have something that can be modeled in an animal that really explains why this works. Dölen has opened up a field of inquiry—this is beautiful work."

Frederick Barrett, a cognitive neuroscientist at Johns Hopkins Center for Psychedelic and Consciousness Research, added that Dölen's meticulously investigated research provides "one of the cleanest stories in psychedelic neuroscience right now in terms of what she predicted, what she found, and the relevance of the mechanism across different compounds. More research is always needed, but so far, this is really great work."

Now that the work on critical periods is gaining traction, however, a number of outside researchers—primarily chemists and psychologists—are "trying to fuzzy the border," Dölen said, between their findings and hers. This has especially shown up in papers that talk about psychedelics creating "plasticity" in the brain, which is different from what Dölen found. Plasticity—the capacity of neural connections to change and reorganize—is something a host of drugs induce. It's one of the properties thought to underlie the addictiveness of cocaine and certain other substances, and in the case of cocaine, it indiscriminately occurs all over the brain rather than in one particular area.

The reopening of critical periods, on the other hand, represents the plasticity of plasticity itself. Put another way, it's the ability of plasticity to change over time. As Dölen's experiments confirm, psychedelics do not induce cocaine's addiction-driving hyperplasticity, and cocaine, in turn, does not reopen the critical period. "I know that seems like nuances, but we need to understand nuance if we're going to understand what makes psychedelics different than SSRIs or cocaine," Dölen said. "We have to get sophisticated, and this is where the neuroscientists have a lot to say."

Dölen's findings also raise questions about various research efforts, primarily being undertaken by psychedelic pharmaceutical start-ups that aim to engineer out the "messy" elements of mind-altering drug trips and shorten their duration—in theory, eliminating the journey and leaving only the therapeutic properties behind. Most of these companies are focused on developing products that induce plasticity, however, and some are even aiming to make drugs that people could take at home, without any professional oversight. "That's misguided, because it misunderstands how these drugs are working," Dölen said. "They could end up just turning a psychedelic into an addictive drug like cocaine."

The jury is still out about whether the psychedelic experience itself is indeed necessary for realizing the therapeutic benefits of MDMA and related substances. Dölen's guess, though, is that the psychedelic effects are playing an important role in activating specific memory circuits that need to be available for modification in order to enable healing. "The more we understand how psychedelics are working, the more we can build versions that minimize things we don't want and maximize things we do want," Dölen said. "But we will never know how to do that until we understand how they're working."

Dölen's findings themselves are too new for another lab to have reproduced yet—the gold standard in science for ensuring that results actually hold up. "The work is cutting edge enough that some people are unsure what to think until another lab replicates it," said neuroscientist Jennifer Mitchell. "The biggest problem is there isn't money to really suss these things out and get at these answers quickly." Even so, she added, Dölen's work thus far "is *very* intriguing."

One recent study, though, strongly hints that Dölen's findings will hold up. In 2021 Sandra Siegert, a neurobiologist at the Institute of Science and Technology in Austria, was giving mice ketamine to test the drug's effect on brain immune cells with relation to vision processing. Siegert and her colleagues weren't trying to reopen a critical period—"We came from a completely different angle to this story," she says—but to the researchers' surprise, after several doses of ketamine, the extracellular environment of the adult rodents' brains returned to a state resembling juveniles', and their vision-related critical period reopened. As in Dölen's study, though, this only happened when the mice also underwent a vision-related exercise while on ketamine—a nice way of describing an experiment in which a mouse's eyelid is temporarily sutured shut and scientists use an electrode implanted in the animal's brain to measure how the loss of that eye affects cellular activity. In adult mice with closed critical periods, nothing changed, whereas in juveniles or adults with open critical periods, the cells from the still-open eye got stronger while the cells from the closed one got weaker.

The findings suggest the tantalizing possibility that psychedelics could indeed be the master key for reopening other critical periods, not just the one for social reward learning. "What if someone blind for the last thirty years has the opportunity to see again? What if someone with auditory impairment could hear again?" Mitchell said. "Those are the questions that will keep some of us busy for the next fifty years, and will definitely benefit different populations of people if the critical period work holds up."

*

DÖLEN'S FINDINGS ALSO shed light on one other important question: the window of time the critical period stays open. In mice, she and her colleagues found that the social reward learning critical period stays open even after the various psychedelics' acute effects have worn off, and that the length of time that window stays open parallels the duration of human trips on the corresponding drugs. Ketamine trips, for example, only last half an hour or so in humans, and in mice, ketamine keeps the critical period open for forty-eight hours. MDMA and psilocybin's four- to five-hour trips in humans translated into two weeks of critical period openness in mice; LSD's eight- to ten-hour trips resulted in three weeks of openness; and ibogaine's monster up to seventy-two-hour human trips translated into at least four weeks of critical period openness in mice (at which point Dölen and her colleagues stopped taking measurements).

These findings also seem to line up with the durability of therapeutic gains made under the influence of different psychedelics. For example, people who undergo an initial series of ketamine infusions for depression usually have to come back for boosters every two to three months. Based on the clinical trial results of MDMA-assisted therapy, the positive effects of that treatment seem to last at least a year. And people who take one- to three-day trips with ibogaine to address their addiction to opioids regularly report being cured for life.

Given the physiological differences between mice and humans, the findings don't necessarily support a one-to-one comparison between the length of the open state in rodents and how long it might be for us. People who undergo MDMA-assisted therapy could have their social reward learning critical period open for a couple of months or more, Dölen guessed, which could help to explain why a majority of the Phase 2 participants continued to get better in the weeks and months after their last session concluded.

This possibility also warns of problems that could arise if people who undergo psychedelic-assisted therapy are not treated with care while they remain in this impressionable state. As Dölen noted, "It's really important that people are not taking these medications and then just returning to the chaos of their normal lives." In the worst case, people who return to an abusive environment while their critical period is still open could be retraumatized and have those negative memories become even more entrenched than they were prior to therapy. This emphasizes the necessity of careful, attentive, and ongoing integration and support after psychedelic-assisted therapy. As Dölen said, "We really need to be designing clinical trials with more emphasis on that postdrug period so people won't be further injured by reentry, and we can maximize the therapeutic effect."

Three months after Dölen made these comments to me, a *New York* magazine and Psymposia podcast called *Cover Story: Power Trip* aired an episode that seemed to confirm some of Dölen's concerns about the vulnerable state people could be left in even after the acute effects of MDMA have worn off. Leah and Mel, two of the women who were interviewed for the podcast, were participants in the Phase 3 MDMA-assisted therapy trial for PTSD. Both women felt strongly that the integration sessions they received were not sufficient, and that they were harmed as a result.

"As I was coming down off the medicine there was just this deep knowledge that something had been left wide open and completely unresolved," Leah described on the podcast. "I got stuck, I felt like I got stuck. I don't think they assessed the dangerousness of the territory that they were leading me in."

Mel made similar comments: "I've equated it to like someone did open heart surgery, you know, and they tore open my chest and they repaired the little damage in the heart there, but then everyone just walked away from the table and my chest was still wide open."

As it happens, that word, *open*, is the same one Dölen and her colleagues used in their 2019 *Nature* paper to describe what is happening on a cellular level. "The critical period stays open," Dölen explained, "and patients need to be supported after the acute effects have worn off because they will continue to exhibit heightened sensitivity, malleability and vulnerability during the open state."

Inadvertent harm is only one example of what can go wrong if people in an open critical period state are not treated with care. There's also the possibility of intentional harm. Perhaps the most horrific example of this is the

Manson Family. Charles Manson repeatedly gave his followers LSD and then took advantage of their impressionability to indoctrinate them into his ideology—brainwashing them to the point of committing unspeakable murders. While the Manson Family is the most well-known example of what can go wrong when psychedelic drugs are abused, Manson was far from the only "mind vamp" who has preyed on hapless trippers. According to Martin Lee and Bruce Shlain in *Acid Dreams*, in 1960s psychedelic hubs like San Francisco's Haight-Ashbury and New York City's East Village, "there was a certain type of character who got off on attacking people while they were high and trespassing on their brains."

Dölen worries about something similar happening today, should MDMA and other psychedelics become more widely available and get into the hands of nefarious actors ranging from exploitative religious organizations to sexual predators. "These are very powerful drugs, and if we don't take the time to think through these ethical dilemmas, it could end badly," Dölen said.

However, if these ethical dilemmas are acknowledged and carefully controlled for—and if scientists are thoughtful and thorough in how they go about studying psychedelics—then the potential positive applications of the critical period findings could be huge. In theory, tremendous gains could be made not just for mental health, but in applications involving critical periods related to vision, hearing, motor function, and more. The specific critical period a therapeutic or medical team targets for reopening would come down to the context in which they gave a patient a psychedelic—an idea Dölen is already preparing to test.

In 2021 Dölen teamed up with a group of Johns Hopkins doctors, scientists, and engineers called Kata Design Studio to collaborate on a project using MDMA-assisted motor learning to help stroke patients recover movement. "There are four hundred thousand Americans every year who have a stroke and will have enough loss of function that it has moderate to severe impact on their lives," Dölen said. "It's a big patient population."

Rather than pair MDMA with talk therapy, stroke patients will take the drug and then play a therapeutic video game called *I Am Dolphin*. The game, developed by Kata, immerses patients in the underwater world of a dolphin named Bandit. A powerful 3D tracking camera allows patients to control Bandit through their own hand and arm movements, helping them to regain function by keeping them engaged in the game. The Kata team's results sans MDMA already indicate that *I Am Dolphin* is more effective than traditional occupational therapy. But the gains stroke patients achieve through *I Am Dolphin* tend only to compensate for lost movement, rather than provide full recovery. The idea, now, is to see if MDMA in combination with the *I Am Dolphin* technology can bring patients closer to true recovery by reopening their motor learning critical period—"an unbelievably powerful idea," said Kata member Steven Zeiler, a stroke physician and neurologist at Johns Hopkins Medicine.

Dölen hopes to see these trials underway in 2023. If the findings are encouraging, then a similar approach could be tested for a range of other conditions, from restoring sight, smell, or hearing to addressing obsessive-compulsive disorders or various substance- and behavior-based addictions. There's even anecdotal evidence that psychedelics could help banish allergies: celebrity doctor Andrew Weil famously lost his cat allergy after interacting with a friendly feline while on LSD. There could also be room for more personal-improvement-oriented applications, such as giving adults the ability to learn a foreign language or new skill with childlike ease.

As Michael Silver, the director of the UC Berkeley Center for the Science of Psychedelics, noted, "It's fascinating to think of set and setting as variables we can manipulate and study—and there's an infinite number of dimensions one could vary."

# THE ADDICT'S NEED

DAVE POUNDS WAS on the overnight ferry from Dover, England, to Amsterdam with twenty-odd lads from his football team when he met a girl. She was from Denmark, and "we got on like a house on fire," Dave recalled. Rather than join the guys getting plastered at the bar, he spent the entire evening just sitting and talking with the Danish girl.

When the boat docked at Amsterdam at ten A.M., the two reluctantly said their goodbyes. "It would be great to stay in touch," the girl told Dave.

"Yeah, but when would we see each other?" he said. He lived in Leicestershire, she in Denmark. "There's no point, given the geographical distance between us."

They left it at that, and Dave headed to a hotel to get some sleep.

When he woke up, the afternoon sun was streaming through the window. It was a beautiful day, and he had the entire weekend partying with his mates to look forward to. His first thought, though, was of the Danish girl. He knew a relationship was a nonstarter, but still, he could have at least gotten her number so they could stay in touch, as she had suggested. Why hadn't he done that? Now he had no way of even reaching her.

"If I want to see her, I can't see her—I can't see her," Dave realized. "It's completely out of my control."

Dave suddenly felt a crushing sense of claustrophobia, as if the walls of the hotel room were closing in on him. His heart began to race, his hands started to shake, and his breath quickened. He had no idea what was happening. "It was like being buried alive—it was pure terror," he said.

The panic eventually subsided, leaving Dave with an acute sense of dread. He didn't tell his mates what had happened, but he struggled that day to focus, and he couldn't manage to eat until around midnight—after copious drinking had numbed the fear.

Nearly forty years later, Dave's bright blue eyes still tear up when he recalls that first panic attack in Amsterdam. It would be the first of many, and it marked the beginning of a decades-long mental health struggle. Panic attacks would overtake him in seemingly innocuous situations: in elevators, at work, while driving, or at home watching TV. Dave knew his fear was irrational, but it was also completely impervious to logic. He tried seeking professional help, and when the National Health Service failed to provide any solution, he turned to the private sector. Over the years, he spent tens of thousands of pounds traveling all over the country to see around sixty doctors, therapists, and counselors of different sorts. None had an answer, and frequently they dismissed his concerns. "There's nothing wrong with you," one doctor told him. "Pull yourself together." Others tried various treatments that had no effect.

The one thing that did bring relief, Dave learned, was alcohol. When trapped in the vise grip of adrenaline, drinking was the only surefire way to soothe his nerves. At times, it took eight pints for him to calm down enough just to eat a meal.

Years passed like this. Dave moved in with a partner, had three kids, and held a steady job. An avid athlete, he'd always been health-conscious—at fifty-eight, when I met him, he looked no older than forty-five—but he started drinking more and more just to manage. "I found that grabbing a bottle of vodka and having three or four chugs took the edge off," he said. Dave knew that it wasn't the alcohol per se that was his problem, but the panic attacks—and whatever it was that was causing them.

Eventually, Dave and his partner split up. Living alone, he found the panic attacks increased in frequency and intensity—as did the drinking. "It became lunchtime, then mornings," Dave said. "There were weeks-long binges where, if I was awake, I was drinking." In 2014 Dave woke up in the hospital after consuming three 750-milliliter bottles of vodka in a single day. "The paramedics said I should have been in a coma," he said. He was committed to a rehab center in London, where his children and his father visited him and held a moving intervention, and where he bonded with other patients. "We bared our souls," he said. "It was quite powerful."

Dave gave up alcohol completely for a couple of years. But the drinking began again after he decided it would be okay for him to have a beer at a mate's stag party in Edinburgh. It wasn't as bad as before, but he could feel himself backsliding.

Hours sitting in front of his computer scouring the scientific literature for possible answers brought him to an article about MAPS's MDMA-assisted therapy trials for PTSD. Dave respected the law and had never tried an illegal drug of any kind, and he was especially wary of psychedelics after reading about a bad acid trip in one of Sam Harris's books. But he was desperate and willing to try anything.

Some googling led Dave to Bristol-based psychiatrist Ben Sessa, who had published extensively about psychedelics in the scientific literature. He reached out to Sessa to inquire about psychedelic-assisted therapy, and they set up a call. "I've spent three decades searching for things that could help me," Dave told Sessa. "Where can I try this, is it legalized in other countries in Europe?"

Sessa explained that, unfortunately, psychedelic therapy is not legalized anywhere nearby. But Sessa was wrapping up recruitment for a study he planned to conduct on MDMA-assisted therapy for alcohol use disorder, and he might just be able to squeeze Dave in.

*

THE IDEA OF using psychedelics to treat addiction is not new. As Michael Pollan reported in *This Is Your Mind on Plants*, for decades Native Americans have held peyote ceremonies to address the drivers of alcoholism in their communities, including multigenerational trauma caused by genocide and colonialism. Western medicine in the 1950s likewise discovered that LSD seemed to be effective for this purpose. In 1951 Alfred M. Hubbard, known by some as the "Johnny Appleseed of LSD" for turning thousands of people on to the drug, and Humphry Osmond, the psychiatrist who coined the word *psychedelic*, set up an LSD and mescaline center at a hospital in Saskatch-ewan to treat patients with alcohol use disorder, among other things; similar psychedelic treatment centers soon spread to other locations in the province and in British Columbia. Bill Wilson, the founder of Alcoholics Anonymous, also endorsed LSD's effectiveness as a tool to treat alcoholism after Osmond gave him tabs to try. (Wilson's board of trustees forbade him from publicly acknowledging this, however.)

More recently, in 2014, scientists at Johns Hopkins University conducted a study using psilocybin to help longtime smokers break their habit. After six months, 80 percent of the fifteen participants were still abstaining from cigarettes. In comparison, varenicline, a pharmaceutical drug considered to be the most effective treatment for helping people quit smoking, typically has a 35 percent success rate at the six-month mark. In a 2017 paper, the Johns Hopkins researchers followed up on their psilocybin subjects and found that 67 percent were still abstaining from smoking at the twelve-month mark.

Sessa's interest in MDMA and other psychedelic drugs was sparked in 1990, when he was a long-haired, soulful-eyed, eighteen-year-old DJ immersed in London's rave scene. When he started medical school, he brought his interest in psychedelic culture to his studies and read all the decades-old liter-ature about the medical use of these substances. He asked his psychiatric tutors about LSD-assisted therapy in the 1950s and 1960s and its former promise of becoming the next big tool for healing. Inevitably, though, the senior psychiatrists would look at Sessa like he was crazy. "That never happened," he remembers more than one of them telling him. "LSD is a dangerous, addictive drug. If a patient takes LSD, the correct treatment is to tie them to a table and sedate them."

In 2004 Sessa wrote what is likely the first paper in the British scientific literature since the 1960s on psychedelics' use for psychiatry. "That got published, and I quickly found myself a part of what was then a very small international group interested in psychedelics," Sessa said. He met Rick Doblin and the Mithoefers, and in 2006, when David Nutt at Imperial College London injected him with psilocybin, he became the first person to be legally administered a psychedelic in the United Kingdom in forty years. Of all the psychedelic drugs Sessa had read up on and tried himself, though, MDMA struck him as most suitable for treating trauma-based conditions. "If you were going to invent a drug for psychotherapy, it would be MDMA," Sessa said. "It ticks every single box that you would want as a psychotherapist."

Sessa was interested in conducting studies on MDMA-assisted therapy with the aim of legalizing the treatment in the United Kingdom, but he didn't want to just repeat what MAPS was doing with PTSD. "I'm interested in novel research no one else is doing, and in things with a large public health benefit," he said. He chose alcoholism because it's such a huge problem, and because the current treatments are so poor.

An estimated 237 million men and 46 million women around the world have alcohol use disorder, according to the WHO. In 2016 alcohol was to blame for three million deaths worldwide, representing 5.3 percent of total lives lost that year and making the condition among the top five causes of years of life lost for people aged fifteen to forty-four. According to a 2021 study in *Addiction*, only one in six people with alcohol use disorder ever receives treatment, and of those who do, up to 75 percent relapse within a year. "In some ways, this is a low-hanging fruit to choose to study because you can't really do any worse than the current situation," Sessa said.

According to addiction and trauma expert Gabor Maté, addiction entails any behavior a person engages in to find short-term relief or pleasure, but that inflicts long-term suffering on them or others and that they are unable to stop. In the short term these behaviors, whether substance-based or not, can be a highly effective strategy for banishing pain. In the long term, though, they are maladaptive.

Substance- and behavior-based addictions in general represent one of the world's largest unmet medical needs, affecting some 1.3 billion people. But despite addiction's ubiquity, gross misconceptions about the condition prevail. One common one is that addiction is a choice. Another is that it is a "disease." While the disease label can capture various aspects of addiction, it does not come close to explaining the phenomenon itself, let alone provide solutions for freeing people from it, Maté said. Contrary to popular lore, evidence increasingly indicates that addiction also is not primarily caused by genetics. As Maté pointed out in *The Myth of Normal*, there has never been a single addiction gene found, and while there might be a set of genes that predisposes some people to susceptibility to substance abuse, studies in both humans and animals show that this risk can be offset by a positive environment.

Another major misconception is that taking any drug by itself will produce an addiction—that certain drugs, in other words, are so powerful that the brain cannot help but yield to their addictive force. In fact, 70 percent or more of regular drug users—including of alcohol, cocaine, prescription medications, methamphetamine, and even heroin—do not meet the criteria for addiction, reported Carl Hart, a psychologist at Columbia University, in *Drug Use for Grown-Ups*.

The Vietnam War provided real-world evidence of this. While stationed in Southeast Asia, many soldiers began regularly taking heroin, barbiturates, and amphetamines. According to research published in the *Archives of General Psychiatry*, a whopping 20 percent of those serving in Vietnam met the diagnostic criteria for addiction. When the soldiers returned home, however, 95 percent of them stopped using drugs. This is because their addictions were being driven not by something inherent to the drugs themselves but by the need to mentally escape the circumstances of war. "Under certain conditions of stress many people can be made susceptible to addiction, but if circumstances change for the better, the addictive drive will abate," Maté explained in *In the Realm of Hungry Ghosts*. "Drugs, in short, do not make anyone into an addict, any more than food makes a person into a compulsive eater."

That said, all addictions do have a biological dimension, and this applies regardless of whether the addiction is behavioral- or substance-based. Addiction causes neurological changes tied to either dopamine, a key neurotransmitter in the brain's motivation system, or to the brain's natural opiate systems, which deal with pleasure and reward—or to both. "In effect, people become addicted to their own brain chemicals," Maté wrote. Repeatedly engaging in behaviors that tamper with dopamine and other brain features produces, over time, chemical, physical, and epigenetic alterations that contribute to the cravings and long-term risk of relapse that are associated with addiction.

Importantly, though, while it is possible for anyone to become physically addicted to alcohol or other habit-forming drugs, it's those who have suffered trauma who usually wind up developing the most harmful addictions—and who have the most difficulty breaking them. Sessa recalled, for example, a patient of his who began drinking every night with her rugby team while they were on tour. By the end of the month, she was having ten pints a night. When she got back to medical school and stopped drinking, a day or so later she started sweating profusely, her hands shook, and she had a seizure. She had become addicted to alcohol. Just as quickly as she'd formed the addiction, though, she sought help and was able to break it. "So anybody can become addicted," Sessa said. "But the point is, you usually don't become addicted if you have that bedrock of underlying positive narratives, and if you have that positive attachment style and do become addicted, you usually respond very well to treatment."

Usually addictions arise to generate feelings that a healthy brain would normally experience, but that trauma and stress interfere with. Maté has treated and spoken with thousands of addicts over his career, from those hooked on substances like alcohol, pills, or inhalants, to others who engage in compulsive online shopping, pornography viewing, or binge eating and purging. He has never met anyone whose long-term addiction did not at the outset serve to satisfy some essential unmet need. Common reasons Maté encounters that drive people's addictions include achieving a sense of social connection; finding inner peace and respite from the self; feeling empowered; and being graced by a fleeting sensation of love and belonging. Emotional pain, stress, and social disconnection are the central drivers behind all of these reasons, he emphasized.

Not surprisingly, PTSD and addictions frequently go hand in hand. Up to 63 percent of veterans with PTSD, for example, also suffer from alcoholism. Research likewise shows that adolescents with histories of abuse are three times more likely to binge-drink and two to four times as likely to use drugs than those who were not abused. In Maté's twelve years working in Vancouver's Downtown Eastside neighborhood with some of the city's most severely addicted residents, literally every female patient he saw had been sexually abused as a child or adolescent. Addiction also frequently accompanies other psychiatric diagnoses. An estimated one third of people with major depression, for example, also have a problem with alcohol. According to the U.S.

Department of Health and Human Services, 9.2 million Americans have a co-occurring substance dependency and a mental health condition such as anxiety, ADHD, or bipolar disorder.

Just as no gene exists for addiction, none has been found, either, that definitively causes the mental illnesses that tend to accompany substance use disorders. This may sound confusing because it runs counter to what years of media headlines, popular culture, and even medical professionals have led most of us to believe, so it's probably worth repeating, Maté said: no one has ever found a gene or set of genes that decisively determine whether someone will develop a particular mental health condition.

As radical as this may sound to some, it's not a new revelation. Alexander Shulgin, for example, made this argument back in 1987 to his students: "There is tremendous drive to find some biochemical marker, some biological marker, some test, that will say this person is insane, this person is not insane, this person is mentally ill, that person is not mentally ill, so we can classify easily by an objective test and put these in the hospital and treat them, and leave these out running around doing their thing outside the hospital. But this has been almost a total disaster because I really don't believe there is that kind of a conspicuous biological abnormality going on up there, any more than you can give a chemical test to determine intelligence, happiness, sadness. You've got to communicate with a person."

Evidence has continued to build in support of this argument, with more scientists and doctors reconsidering earlier assumptions about the role of genes as primary drivers of mental health problems. "In terms of genetics, I have a strong inclination to agree with Gabor Maté," said Bay Area addiction expert Howard Kornfeld. For example, although medical textbooks still point to the significant role genes play in the likelihood that someone develops alcoholism or schizophrenia, many of the conclusions are based on studies comparing twins reared together and apart. "However," Kornfeld said, "if you dig deeper into these studies, there are legitimate, fundamental questions being raised about their assumptions and validity."

That said, what Maté and some others who agree with him *do* believe is inherited is a person's baseline level of sensitivity—how deeply they feel, and how easily stress can overwhelm them. Extremely sensitive individuals are more vulnerable to developing a mental health condition in response to the stress they face in their lives—but that does not mean they have inherited a genetic sensitivity for a specific illness. As the geneticist Richard C. Lewontin has written, "Genes affect how sensitive one is to the environment, and environment affects how relevant one's genetic differences may be."

These observations are reflected in the scientific literature. In a 2022 *Molecular Psychiatry* study, for example, researchers examined blood samples from 489 children aged nine to thirteen, some of whom had experienced trauma and others not. They followed up on the participants around seventeen years later and found that those whose childhood blood samples revealed trauma-related epigenetic changes—how genes are turned on or off by environmental factors—were significantly more likely to suffer in adulthood from depression, addiction, serious medical problems, social problems, or poverty. The epigenetic changes related to trauma did not occur in all of the children who had experienced a traumatic event, however, and they also did not correlate to any demographic variables. This points to the fact that trauma does not impact every person in the same way; some individuals seem to be inherently more sensitive to it. As Maté said, "Trauma is not what happens *to* people, but what happens inside them"—and sensitivity is one important variable in how that process plays out.

Under positive, supportive circumstances, sensitive people are often more aware, empathetic, inventive, and artistic compared to individuals with hardier dispositions. Pediatrician and psychiatrist Tom Boyce at UCSF has likened the deeply feeling children he regularly works with to orchids: "Exquisitely sensitive to their environment, making them especially vulnerable under conditions of adversity but unusually vital, creative and successful with supportive, nurturing environments." Maté has also seen evidence of this dichotomy in many of the adult patients he has encountered over the years. "When you go to jail and work with some of the most hardened criminals— I'm talking about killers—they become the sweetest and most loving people," he said. "Why? Because they're so sensitive. They've become hardened because when they were hurt, their hearts closed down more."

Pointing to a robust body of scientific evidence for conditions as diverse as psychosis, depression, ADHD, and disordered relationships with food, Maté argues that virtually every mental health condition we know can trace its origins to trauma, stress, or childhood adversity. He is not alone in this thinking. "The evidence of a link between childhood misfortune and future psychiatric disorder is about as strong statistically as the link between smoking and lung cancer," writes Richard Bentall, a clinical psychologist at the University of Sheffield and fellow of the British Academy.

Childhood misfortune can mean overt abuse, neglect, or maltreatment, but it can also entail subtler but just as damaging forms of emotional injury, especially a lack of quality relationships. "Our major finding is your history of relational health—your connectedness to family, community and culture—is more predictive of your mental health than your history of adversity," write Oprah Winfrey and psychiatrist Bruce Perry in *What Happened to You?* "Connectedness has the power to counterbalance adversity."

Indeed, scientists now know that emotional nurturing is on par with nutrition and physical security in terms of importance for a child's developing brain. For this requirement to be satisfied, a child needs at least one reliable, protective, psychologically present, and relatively unstressed adult in their life. "Kids need some kind of anchor, some kind of caregiver during their childhood to teach them the rules of attachment," Sessa said. "They need to be taught that love is a thing, that care is a thing, and that people can be good. When they don't have anything like that, then their version of the world is very skewed."

Without a healthy attachment relationship, abnormalities can form in the developing brain, impacting learning and behavior. Because human children cannot survive without adults, evolution has also programmed them to love their caretakers above all else. So when children are abused, molested, or simply do not get the attention, support, and connection they need, rather than turn on their caretaker, they assume they did something to deserve it and internalize that they are bad. This causes traumatized children to frequently grow into adults with "this very pervasive, core sense of being damaged goods, disgusting and defective," according to psychiatrist and author Bessel van der Kolk. They will be more reactive to stress throughout their lives, and as a result more likely to develop mental health conditions and to form addictions in an attempt to self-soothe.

If trauma's role in driving addiction and other problems is still not the mainstream perspective, that's not for lack of scientific evidence, Maté argues: literally thousands of published research papers elucidate the link between stress and health, including trauma's role in increasing the risk of developing mental illness or a substance use disorder, or of dying from cancer, stroke, or heart disease. Rather than a lack of evidence, he continued, it's our cultural ideology that informs the mainstream perspective that addiction is a choice or a disease, and that mental health conditions are primarily dictated by genes rather than life experience. "Genetic determinism has been drummed into people's heads for decades, despite poor evidence and despite the scientific evidence disproving it," Maté said. "But the mainstream perspective does not look at the science of trauma and brain development."

Slowly, though—as evidence continues to build and people's general awareness about trauma grows—things are beginning to change. Rather than viewing addictions and other forms of mental distress as "illnesses" caused by some outside force, Maté and others continue to urge their medical and scientific colleagues, and society at large, to consider what these conditions might be expressing about the lives in which they arise. Only by opening our eyes to the true drivers behind our afflictions, Maté said, can we take effective steps toward addressing and healing them.

*

AFTER SEVERAL PREPARATORY sessions with Sessa and his colleagues, Dave arrived at the research clinic in Bristol nervous but eager. This was an open label pilot study, meaning every participant would be receiving two sessions of MDMA-assisted therapy, and everyone knew they would be taking the drug. Forty-five minutes after swallowing his MDMA capsule, Dave still wasn't feeling anything. He was becoming anxious that "it wasn't going to kick in at all," he recalled. But then "this amazing, wonderful, warm calmness flooded my body."

"Ben, I think it's happening!" Dave gleefully announced.

"Okay, just put the headphones and eye mask on," Sessa advised. "Just close your eyes and see what comes up."

Trauma, Dave's subconscious decided, was exactly what needed to come up. Dave never talked about it and tried not to think about it, but when he was twelve years old, his mother had been murdered in their home—and Dave had been present for the whole thing.

A co-worker had given Dave's mom a ride home from the restaurant they both worked at, and she apparently invited him in for a cup of tea after dismissing the babysitter. Dave was awake in bed, and he could hear the two of them downstairs, talking. With a growing sense of discomfort, Dave heard the man make a pass at his mom, and she politely turned him down. Suddenly the talking stopped, and Dave heard thudding noises. Then there was silence.

Dave could sense something was terribly wrong, and when he heard unfamiliar footsteps coming up the stairs, his instincts told him to pretend to be asleep. His door slowly swung open, and he closed his eyes. All he could hear was fast, panicky male breathing. The panting sounds went on for what seemed like ages before the man turned away from Dave's bedroom. Dave could hear him opening all the other upstairs rooms and then, finally, receding footsteps as he left the house.

Dave lay there for at least an hour, frozen, until he heard banging on a window. He flew down the stairs and threw open the curtain to see his dad standing outside. The key was in the kitchen door, and his dad was locked out.

"Dave, what's wrong?" his dad asked when he saw his stricken son.

Dave could only gesture toward the lounge. He and his dad went in together, and "it was just a disaster," Dave recalled. "Mom stabbed so many times—God knows. My only hope is she was knocked out before the knife came out and before she was raped."

The murderer was quickly arrested, convicted, and sentenced to life in prison, and Dave and his father tried to move on. Dave never spoke to his family or friends about what happened, and he only brought the incident up once with his father, when he was thirty-one and felt compelled to tell his dad that he hadn't actually been asleep that night. "I was a bloke's bloke," he explained. "It was chest out, get on with it."

But his mother's loss—along with the horror of what happened to her—was always with him. He was also haunted by the guilt of wondering whether he could have done something to stop her murder from happening. What if he had gone downstairs after hearing the man hitting on his mom? Would this have prevented her death—or would the outcome have been even worse?

Over the years, Dave had realized that his panic attacks must be connected to this early trauma, and a host of therapists had also reached that conclusion. But as Dave learned firsthand, "most therapies for trauma-related issues are ineffective."

The MDMA cut through his mental defenses, however, and brought him straight back to that night. As though having an out-of-body experience, he saw his childhood bedroom and his twelve-year-old self in bed. But the room was warmly lit, not dark and terrifying. When his mother's murderer opened the door, the young Dave sat up in his pajamas, looked the man straight in the eye, and calmly spoke. "I'm pretty sure I know what you've done downstairs, and I'm pretty sure you could kill me," he said. "But I just wanted you to know that I'm not frightened of you."

Dave's mom—lovely and whole—then came into the room and addressed the man, too. "You're probably going to go to prison for a long time," she said. "You need to understand what's caused you to do this and get some help for that."

His younger self and his mother then gave the man a hug.

*

IN ALL THE many visits Dave had made to various mental health professionals over the years, of those who *had* made the connection between his childhood trauma and his drinking, only a few could make any positive difference, and none could provide him with any genuine, lasting relief. "Most of them simply lack tools that are of any use, to me, anyway," Dave said.

This is not surprising, given that doctors do not receive adequate training, if any, in trauma. "The average medical student in most medical schools never so much as hears a single lecture on emotional trauma, its impacts and health consequences, let alone how to treat it—that's just how it is," Maté said. "When was the last time you went to a physician with an inflamed gut or joint or skin or nervous system and they asked you about the trauma in your life?"

Doctors also tend to be swayed by society's preference to blame addiction on a person's weak or hedonistic disposition, or to point the finger solely at genetics. "There's a fundamental failure to see addiction as rooted in human suffering," Maté said. For those on the receiving end of this oversight, the results can be catastrophic.

Fortunately, Dave had the unwavering support of his father, children, and close friends, and he also had the resources to keep himself housed, clothed, and fed even through his worst moments. Others are not so fortunate. Addicts are frequently ostracized by their families and by society and, in the case of those who seek relief through banned substances, put behind bars.

This is a particular problem in the United States, the world's leader in incarceration, where each year about 1.5 million people are arrested on drug charges, and about half of the federal prison population is there because of lower-level drug offenses. Minority communities in the United States as well as other countries bear the brunt of this burden. Despite making up just 6 percent of the U.S. population, Black men compose 40 percent of the prison population; in the United Kingdom, Black men are ten times more likely to be imprisoned for drug offenses than white men. Similarly, in Canada, Indigenous people make up no more than 5 percent of the general population, yet they amount to nearly 30 percent of those behind bars.

An estimated 65 percent of the U.S. prison population has an active substance use disorder, and by criminalizing and locking up drug users, countries like the United States, United Kingdom, and Canada perpetuate a vicious cycle of suffering that further traumatizes these individuals. At a fundamental level, Maté suspects that our continued failure to see addiction for what it is, and our tendency to treat addicts with disdain instead of compassion, is because people are conditioned to resist critical self-examination. We also do not like to take responsibility for our own failings. Acknowledging the outsize role that trauma plays in driving addiction would require taking an honest, difficult look at how the society we've built generates suffering, including through racism, poverty, and inequity.

Rather than face an uncomfortable confrontation with that reality, we favor simple explanations and quick fixes—another preference of modern society. For harried doctors, this means prescribing a pill (or several pills) to "treat" a patient's addiction, depression, or other mental health conditions. This proves to be much easier than asking patients about their lives. As Maté told me, "It takes me two minutes to give you a prescription for Prozac. For

THE ADDICT'S NEED  199

me to ask you, 'When did you learn to push down your emotions?'—that's a much longer conversation."

*

FOR DAYS AFTER Dave's first MDMA-assisted therapy session, he felt enveloped in a warm glow. He came to call this his "MDMA mindset."

"I'd go running down by the canal outside my village, and I could smell the earth like never before," he said. "I could see the colors and hear the birds with a new acuity."

Dave felt anxious, however, going into his second session, and as the MDMA started to kick in, he sensed a panic attack coming on. "It took everything I had not to race out of the room and just find the nearest pub," he said. "I was just incredibly scared."

Sessa and his colleague managed to calm Dave down a bit and encouraged him to interrogate his feelings. Dave's panicked reaction, he realized, was because his amygdala, his brain's fear center, had been calling the shots—not just that afternoon, but ever since Dave's mother died. Dave began to reprimand his amygdala out loud, as though it was sitting in front of him on the floor.

"I've had fucking enough of you!" he declared. "Clear off."

After a couple of hours of this, Dave felt his amygdala back down, as it were, and in its place his heart emerged. He began talking out loud to his heart, just as he had his amygdala. "We're thankful for the amygdala—it's been trying to keep us safe—but its job is done now," Dave told his heart. "It's just me and you, big guy."

Recalling this unusual experience, he told me, "it sounds like I was off my head, but I wasn't—I was absolutely lucid."

Despite the day's rough start, Dave found himself in a good place after his second session. His MDMA mindset returned, and even several years later, he's now able to summon that outlook when he needs to. "I don't consider myself 'cured,' whatever that means," Dave said. "But do I feel stronger and more resilient than I ever have? Yes, I do. Am I looking forward to the future now more than I ever have? Yes, I am."

Dave was one of fourteen people who took part in Sessa and his colleagues' small Phase 2a safety and tolerability pilot study, which was the first ever to test MDMA-assisted therapy for alcohol use disorder. All of the participants suffered from trauma that was ultimately underpinning their drinking, and all enjoyed some relief from unhealthy levels of alcohol consumption immediately following the trial. At the nine-month mark, three participants (21 percent) had relapsed to their original levels of drinking. Nine of them (64 percent) were still abstaining from alcohol completely.

These findings "blow out of the water" those typically seen for treating alcohol use disorder, Sessa said. For comparison, prior to conducting the MDMA study, he and his colleagues carried out an observational study with a similar group of twelve patients to see how they fared after completing a fourteen-day detox program for alcoholism. All of the patients left the program alcohol-free. But just three months later, 66 percent had relapsed to pre-detox levels of drinking, and by nine months, 75 percent had. "And that is the best treatment you can get," Sessa pointed out.

Sessa's MDMA study was just a preliminary pilot, so larger randomized, controlled trials will be needed before researchers can establish for sure whether the treatment really is efficacious for addressing alcohol use disorder. "But in terms of a starting point to ask if there's a role for MDMA for treating alcoholism," Sessa said, "the answer seems to be yes indeed, there is a very strong role."

He and his colleagues are now organizing a Phase 2b efficacy study involving 120 participants to test this hypothesis—but they're already betting that the results will be favorable. In October 2021 Sessa and a cofounder opened Awakn, Europe's first psychedelic medical clinic, in Bristol. The ribbon-cutting ceremony had taken place the night before I toured the bright, airy space, and champagne flutes and empty bottles of Moët were still scattered around the small lobby, which featured a mix of modern and Georgian elements. For now, Awakn patients can only receive ketamine-assisted therapy for a range of disorders, but the plan is to add MDMA- and psilocybin-based therapy once those substances become legally available. The company has opened additional locations in London and Oslo and has plans for another twenty clinics across the United Kingdom and Europe in the coming years.

Sessa is betting, too, that MDMA-assisted therapy will have a range of applications for psychiatry, because, like Maté, he believes that unaddressed trauma is at the heart of almost all chronic, unremitting mental disorders. For many if not all of these conditions, there is a desperate need for better treatments. "Forty years of top-down biological psychiatry has created this learned helplessness within the field in that we don't believe we can cure people," Sessa said. "Psychiatrists these days are more like palliative care doctors, looking after patients for life and giving them drugs like SSRIs to manage their symptoms so they can ride it out for the next sixty years. No other branch of medicine would accept the kind of poor outcomes we do in psychiatry."

While Sessa and others conduct more research on the possibility of using psychedelic-assisted therapy to address various conditions, Maté is not waiting. When he first heard about psychedelic healing around 2009, he felt a knee-jerk skepticism about taking one substance to address addiction to another. But after trying ayahuasca, "I got it immediately," he told me. He has since developed a "reverence" for the synergistic power of psychedelics and therapy, he said, because he has seen firsthand what can be accomplished by treating patients using this model. "I talk about it very publicly, I don't care," he said of his underground work.

Maté has helped patients enroll in ayahuasca ceremonies and has administered MDMA- and psilocybin-assisted therapy himself to people with various diagnoses, including addiction, depression, PTSD, anxiety, chronic fatigue, degenerative neurological illness, multiple sclerosis, rheumatic diseases, and terminal cancer. "The potential goes way beyond PTSD, because PTSD is only a small sliver on the trauma spectrum," he told me. Some of Maté's patients, but not all, have recovered from addictions and mental and physical health conditions following psychedelic-assisted therapy. "I can't say that everyone found everything they were seeking," Maté wrote in *The Myth of Normal*. "What I can say is that most people took major steps forward on their way to authenticity and found significant liberation from their limiting or even deadening mind patterns and behaviors."

Sessa, like Maté and many others, emphasized that MDMA and other psychedelics are not a panacea. The drug-therapy combination might give traumatized, addicted patients the opportunity to feel love for the first time, or to tackle the rigid self-narratives that they've told themselves all their lives. But in order to achieve lasting benefits, they must translate these revelations into meaningful behavioral changes. "MDMA is just the beginning of the journey," Sessa said. "It's the platform on which to move forward."

Dave agreed with that assessment. He's encountered a few bumps since taking part in the MDMA trial in 2019, but his drinking is now under control, and he doesn't have full-fledged panic attacks anymore. When he does feel emotionally triggered, he is usually able to calm down more quickly and with less hurt than before. He's come to see himself as having central agency in his own healing process and said that, overall, the benefits from his participation in the trial have been "profound."

Dave's experience with MDMA-assisted therapy also gave him a new purpose in life: helping others. He spent his pandemic lockdown planning ways to share his story through volunteerism, workshops, coaching, and motivational talks. "If there's any silver lining or good to come out of this disaster, it's me doing whatever I can to help as many people as I can," he said.

In getting his story out, he also hopes to encourage legalization of MDMA-assisted therapy. "Where would I get to if I had another one, two or three sessions?" he said. "I want that for myself and for other people."

# 10
# GROWING PAINS

RICK DOBLIN'S BABY-BLUE attic is part hobbit hole, part psychedelic hoarder's paradise. On plywood shelves covering a back wall, books about consciousness, mysticism, healing, and drugs vie for space with a lifetime's worth of knickknacks: framed photos of Doblin with Leo Zeff and with his wife, Lynne; a copy of NIDA's infamous "Brain after Ecstasy" postcard; Harvard student IDs; a commemorative 2010 Shulgin Tribute Dinner mug; wolf statues; cannabis floss; a ceramic chalice made by an ex-girlfriend; MAPS stickers, buttons, pendants, and soap; and a certificate of completion for the New York City marathon. Yet more newspapers, magazines, books, scientific journals, and old MAPS bulletins cover most of the floor. Cutting through this cluttered landscape of paper plateaus and magazine mesas, a narrow valley of dusty carpet—just wide enough for a person to pass—leads to an L-shaped desk enshrouded in folders, letters, pencil holders, photographs, obsolete electronics, and one very large, very bright green bong.

On an October morning in 2021, Doblin was stationed, as usual, in this unlikely command center for the push to gain federal approval for MDMA-assisted therapy, watching his screen as a MAPS Zoom room filled up with employees signing in for their weekly all-hands meeting. In the more than three decades since Doblin founded MAPS, the organization has grown from a tribe to a corporation. Within a few minutes, 134 people had joined the meeting. "The team just keeps getting bigger!" said Kris Lotlikar, MAPS's deputy director, kicking things off. "And that's good, because we've got so much work to do."

One of the main items on the agenda that day was the monetary fuel that MAPS will need to secure in order to scale MDMA-assisted therapy up for hundreds of thousands, or even millions, of people. Traditional revenue streams are off the table, and purposefully so. For one, Doblin made sure early on that MDMA cannot be patented for profit. Although Merck's patent on the molecule, which ran out years ago, precludes a second patent being issued for the same thing, Doblin knew it was still possible to obtain patents for novel uses of a substance. If he had wanted to, for example, he could have at some point sought a patent for MDMA to treat PTSD.

In the early 1990s, however, he witnessed firsthand "the destructive nature of the use of patents," as he put it. Specifically, he watched from the sidelines as complications that arose from patent fights on ibogaine and noribogaine for treating opioid dependence blocked research from moving forward. Likewise, in the years since *Psilocybe* mushrooms came to broader public attention following the publication of a 1957 article in *Life* magazine, there have been dozens of attempted and successful patents filed for the mushrooms' active compounds, raising ethical questions about Indigenous rights, cultural heritage, and ownership over nature.

Doblin decided to get ahead of this problem for MDMA, so he went to the same attorney who had secured the ibogaine patent and hired him to instead develop an *anti*patent strategy. The easiest way to keep MDMA from being patented, the attorney advised Doblin, was to publicize as much evidence as he could about all of the different uses for the drug, so that no one else could claim to be discovering something novel. So far, this black diamond legal maneuvering has worked. As neuroscientist Gül Dölen appreciatively noted of Doblin's strategizing, "Rick can come across as a wide-eyed hippie who's done a ton of drugs and is super enthusiastic, but despite the cuddly teddy bear appearance, Rick is hardcore, he's dead serious. He's been very shrewd about avoiding some of the pitfalls that have fucked over psychedelic research in the past."

This has also allowed MAPS to avoid conflicts of interest that come from primarily profit-seeking development of a drug, as pharmaceutical companies currently practice for the vast majority of new products. As Michael

Mithoefer told me, "The nonprofit public benefit model of drug development is one of the most exciting parts of this whole thing. It's only about doing the best science as possible. If there's ever anything we feel needs to be done to make the science better, Rick's said, 'Okay, I'll find the money for it.' "

Finding that money has been a challenge for Doblin and his colleagues from the beginning, though. Federal agencies typically do not support clinical research on Schedule I compounds, eliminating a huge pool of potential support. MAPS has also missed out on the billion-plus dollars that for-profit psychedelics companies have raised from venture capitalists in just the past few years alone. Doblin instead chose to pursue a philanthropy-based model not because he hates capitalism or doesn't know how to run a company but because he bet that in the long run, this would best serve the MDMA cause.

Absent government, VC, and Big Pharma money, Doblin tapped into one of his greatest assets, his personality, and put it to use fundraising. I saw this firsthand in December 2021, when I got to be a fly on the wall of what's probably the most stunning private home I've ever been inside, whose owners were sponsoring the annual MAPS New York City benefit dinner. Masked servers passed out truffle tater tots and pinkie-sized fish tacos—a bold move, I thought, given the home's immaculate white carpet and white cloth furniture—and elegantly dressed guests compared notes on their second homes in Aspen. When I asked one West Coast attendee what time he was flying out the following day, he shrugged and nonchalantly replied, "I just call the plane and they pick me up." I laughed, unsure if this was a joke or not.

Despite the vast economic gulf between me and the other guests, though, there was one shared interest that we could all talk about: drugs. As a woman was telling me about the underground MDMA trips she and her partner took throughout the pandemic with a facilitator on Zoom, Doblin stood up to give a speech. Starting with the story of his family's dinner table conversations about the Holocaust, he swiftly got attendees up to speed on his life and mission. "I'm so privileged and I could be so oppressed, but I'm not," he said. "So I should use the privilege and use the freedom to work towards something." That something, he continued, is ensuring that consciousness prevails over catastrophe—and psychedelics are one key for doing that. Nods and murmurs of approval filled the room.

MAPS has managed to raise an impressive $140 million–plus in donations and grants over its thirty-six-year history, and the diversity of individuals who have contributed gives insight into the breadth of interest across various sectors of society. Major donors have included the late Ashawna Hailey, a trans computer scientist; Richard Rockefeller, the great-grandson of John D. Rockefeller; Peter and Jennifer Buffett, Warren Buffett's son and daughter-in-law; and David Bronner of Dr. Bronner's natural soaps. Support has also come from more unexpected ideological spheres. Doblin caught flak, for example, when he accepted a $1 million donation from Rebekah Mercer, daughter of Robert Mercer, a right-wing hedge fund billionaire who helped Donald Trump win the 2016 presidential election. "That was a controversy, but I'd totally do it again," Doblin noted.

Similarly, when I heard that Elizabeth Koch is another major MAPS donor, I was skeptical but intrigued. Elizabeth's father, Charles, is regularly ranked on lists of the world's wealthiest individuals, as was Elizabeth's uncle, David, until his death in 2019. I first became acquainted with the Koch name in 2012, when I wrote a story for the *New York Times* about an ad campaign sponsored by the Heartland Institute—a libertarian organization supported by Charles Koch's charitable foundation—that compared people who believed in global warming to "Unabomber" Ted Kaczynski and other "notorious killers." Since then, thanks to reporting by the *New Yorker*'s Jane Mayer and others, the Koch brothers have come to be widely known for their hugely influential role in pushing conservative agendas— waging a disinformation campaign against climate change, opposing efforts aimed at reducing greenhouse gas emissions, fighting to repeal the Affordable Care Act and block a major election reform bill, and working to quash labor unions. Empathy, healing, connection, and consciousness expansion do not immediately come to mind as attributes of the Koch brand.

I was curious what would motivate a Koch family member to become a major philanthropic supporter of psychedelic therapy, so I visited Elizabeth at her Santa Monica office on one exceptionally rainy afternoon in December 2021. The moment I walked through the door of the loftlike space, the slender forty-five-year-old greeted me with a hug, a blanket, and not one but two very L.A.-appropriate canned drinks ("energy booster" and "prebiotic popping soda") from the office's meticulously organized fridge.

Elizabeth's bubbly enthusiasm and disarming warmth immediately put me at ease, and within minutes I felt as though I were chatting with an old friend.

Elizabeth's uncanny ability to endear herself to others is a skill she has been cultivating nearly her entire life, and it's actually a symptom of her trauma. In hearing her story, I would learn that MAPS's fundraising success doesn't just boil down to Doblin's prowess as a salesman, or to wealthy people simply loving MDMA, but to the fact that trauma and suffering are universal. Not even the most privileged individuals in the world are immune to mental anguish, and they can face the same limitations as the rest of us in finding relief for that pain.

Elizabeth's "fall from Eden," as she described her index trauma, occurred when she was five years old. After a close friend of her parents severed his spine by diving into a shallow pond, the family went over to pay their respects to the now wheelchair-bound man. The atmosphere in the house was oppressively somber, so to lighten the mood for her little brother, Elizabeth began singing the Humpty Dumpty song. In one refrain, though, she absentmindedly replaced "Humpty Dumpty" with the name of the paralyzed man. Suddenly, all the tension in the room was directed at her. "I see my dad looking over his shoulder and giving me this death stare," she recalled.

When the family got home, Elizabeth's father sat her down. "You kids don't get it," she recalled him saying. "You have everything that everyone wants, and you'll be hated for it your entire life. Your job, always, is to be the nicest person in the room, and the hardest worker in the room—the one who picks up garbage that everyone leaves behind. You have to be aboveboard because if you aren't, you'll not only be hated by everyone else but also by yourself."

Looking back on this incident with an adult's perspective, Elizabeth now understands that her father was trying to protect her. "He was absolutely terrified that my brother and I would grow up to be spoiled, piece-of-shit monsters," she said. As a five-year-old, however, she interpreted his lecture to mean that she could only be loved if she were good. That pivotal message came to hold sway over nearly every facet of her personality and life.

In *The Myth of Normal*, Gabor Maté wrote, "A child who does not experience himself as consistently and unconditionally lovable may well grow to be preternaturally likable or charming"—which was exactly the path

Elizabeth followed. It started with a nightly ritual: before bed, she would review everything she had said and done that day to make sure she had been the nicest person and the hardest worker, and that she hadn't accidentally hurt anyone's feelings. If something bad happened to her—say, she tripped and skinned her knee—she would tell herself that it was because the universe was punishing her for not being good enough. In classrooms, during extracurricular activities, or on sports teams, she would always beeline for whichever kid she thought would hate her the most—usually the one who appeared to have the least money, or the one who looked the least like her—and try to win them over by telling them funny stories about her family's dysfunction.

Over the years Elizabeth rose to the top of her class, won competitions for her writing, and made many friends, but she lacked joy. "I have to do this to prove that I deserve to be alive," she would tell herself each time she accomplished something. "I have to earn my existence." Her paranoia about what others thought of her intensified, as did her unhappiness. She realized she needed help and began trying various mental health solutions, including yoga, silent meditation retreats, and, briefly, medications. She read books about Buddhism and neuroscience and gained glimpses of insight. But no amount of knowledge, learning, or practice brought genuine relief.

When a friend suggested in 2016 that she try psychedelic-assisted therapy with a "consciousness cowboy" he knew—an ex-military man who called himself Doug the Lovebunny—she agreed. Doug filled a silver balloon full with "some kind of vapor smoke," Elizabeth recalled, and instructed her to breathe in and hold it. She had no idea what she was in for: he had given her 5-MeO-DMT, a short-acting but incredibly potent tryptamine. The ego-abolishing drug dissolved Elizabeth in totality. It was terrifying.

Doug the Lovebunny hadn't prepared Elizabeth for this harrowing and destabilizing experience, and he did not provide any support or integration for her afterward. For weeks, she would wake up in the middle of the night, she said, "scrambling to try to grab hold of my body." She wanted to know more about what she was going through, and research led her to MAPS. She attended a psychedelics conference in Los Angeles, where she was moved and inspired by the firsthand accounts shared by war veterans who had taken part in the MDMA-assisted clinical trials for PTSD.

MDMA sounded a lot more user friendly than 5-MeO-DMT—and perhaps, Elizabeth thought, it could help her, too. So in spring 2018 she found "someone off grid" who agreed to give her MDMA-assisted therapy following the MAPS protocol. Elizabeth wound up doing three sessions, and through that process she saw the vast amount of pain she had been harboring throughout her life. "I had been terrified of joy," she said. "The medicine showed me the degree to which all this buried stuff that I hadn't even been able to see was causing me to be reactive and feel constantly trapped, overwhelmed, and miserable."

The MDMA sessions (one of which she also paired with psilocybin) helped Elizabeth let go of the "intense self-hatred" she had been burdened with since she was five years old, she said, and to feel sympathy and love for herself. She's since become one of MAPS's top five donors. "MDMA is not going to save the world," Elizabeth said. "But together with conversations and experiences of going inward and self-investigating, I think it can help."

Following that thread, in 2018, Elizabeth founded a company, Unlikely Collaborators, that aims to bring people together who seem like they're on opposite sides of an issue, and then work with them to reveal their shared humanity and commonalities. If and when MDMA-assisted therapy gains FDA approval, Elizabeth also envisions Unlikely Collaborators providing community-oriented group integration services. "We each have our own relative hell realms that we have to learn to crawl out of," she said. "The only way to bridge divides out there are to bridge the divides within."

*

FOR ALL THE help that Elizabeth and other MAPS donors have provided, bringing MDMA to market and globalizing access will require, at a minimum, an additional $150 million. That's much more than philanthropy alone can realistically generate, especially over just a few years. "There's a big sadness for me of not making it all the way with philanthropy," Doblin noted. "But we vastly increased our costs and are now struggling to keep up with the core research in different areas."

The beginning of a solution to MAPS's economic challenges unexpectedly arrived in 2013, when Doblin—stoned and wandering around the buffet table at a fundraiser for a foundation his wife was leading—ran into a patent attorney he knew. The attorney told him about something called "new drug product exclusivity," an obscure 1984 Reagan law that grants a five-year period of exclusive data use for companies that bring new drugs to market for which patents are not available. Within those five years, no other company can market a cheaper generic version of whatever drug the founding company brought to market, even though the drug is not patented. All that matters is that the product has never been approved by the FDA before. A similar law also exists in Europe and grants exclusivity for ten years.

Despite being super high and off the clock, Doblin realized he'd just been handed a legal revelation of utmost importance. If MAPS could get MDMA approved for PTSD, then the five-year exclusivity period the group would be granted would allow MAPS to sidestep the patent issue yet still bring MDMA to market, with the goal of earning enough revenue through sales of the drug to be able to sustainably pay employee salaries and to support ongoing research, education, and outreach.

Data exclusivity is not a patent, though, so other pharmaceutical companies could get involved with the production and sale of MDMA if they generated their own FDA-approved uses for the drug. Companies could also develop new, MDMA-like drugs that they could patent and that could potentially offer some advantages over MDMA itself. Already, however, some of these groups are taking "a very traditional, very aggressive grab kind of approach," said Nicole Howell, cofounder of Clark Howell LLP, a law firm based in Santa Monica. At the same time other companies are challenging the notion that psychedelic compounds that have been used historically should be subject to private ownership at all.

To try to lay the groundwork for a psychedelic medicine industry that values more than just revenue, in 2020 Howell and cofounder Ismail Ali created the Psychedelic Bar Association, a group for attorneys from all practice areas who are interested in solving the novel legal and policy issues surrounding this emerging sector. "As lawyers, we play a very pivotal role in what the market winds up looking like," Howell said. "We need to ask ourselves if we're simply trying to bring psychedelics to the mainstream, or if we want to make the mainstream more psychedelic. If the answer is more psychedelic, then there are many, many things that need to be different, including how we practice law."

As of early 2022, the Psychedelic Bar Association's members numbered around one hundred, and another five hundred attorneys had applied to get in. One big issue the group has been working on is the feasibility of inserting public benefit requirements into state laws for any group seeking a license to produce and sell psychedelics. Howell and her colleagues have also been collaborating closely with the North Star project, an effort that has brought around one hundred psychedelic stakeholders together to establish a set of principles to help guide the movement into commercialization. "The industry saying 'This is how we want to be regulated' is where the most powerful message will come from," Howell said.

MAPS is also playing a role in shaping that industry. To better manage the economic and commercial side of things, in 2014 MAPS split into two organizations: the nonprofit arm that Doblin started in 1986, and the MAPS Public Benefit Corporation (PBC). The latter is essentially a pharmaceutical company that conducts R&D and will oversee the commercialization of MDMA post-FDA approval. MAPS PBC is wholly owned by MAPS the nonprofit, and both share the same core mission of maximizing access to psychedelics.

The easiest way for MAPS PBC to have earned the requisite funds to get MDMA-assisted therapy over the finish line would have been to sell stock. But from the outset, Doblin and his colleagues purposefully steered clear of this path, to avoid being beholden to shareholders who expect profit. This is something that already happened in the cannabis industry, which developed under "a very traditional, extractive capitalist framework," Howell said. "It was largely considered to be necessary then, but it isn't here, and it shouldn't be how we do it for psychedelics."

They settled instead on a model called revenue financing, in which a company sells a future proportion of revenues to generate immediate capital. In 2021 MAPS entered into an agreement with a lead funder, Vine Ventures, a venture capital firm focused on novel approaches to health and wellness, to raise seventy million dollars in exchange for 6.1 percent of earnings from MDMA sales in North America. The agreement will expire eight years after the first quarter that MAPS earns at least five million dollars in revenue from the sale of MDMA, and the percentage of revenue that funders get will decrease if the return on their investment hits certain levels. In summer 2022 Elizabeth Koch also became a significant participant in this new funding model (she declined to name the exact amount she invested).

"This revenue financing allows for sharing of some economics without sharing governance," said Andrew "Mo" Septimus, the chief financial officer and cohead of business development at MAPS and MAPS PBC. "They can't tell us what to do, there are no board seats given to our revenue financing funders as part of this arrangement."

MAPS is looking at "a bouquet of options" to raise the additional runway needed to get to commercialization, added Federico Menapace, MAPS's chief strategy officer. These options include possible partnerships with other companies to conduct research on MDMA-assisted therapy for different indications—for example, eating disorders, alcohol use disorder, or traumatic brain injury—or help bring the treatment to different countries. Crowdfunding is another idea for generating support, as is having charitable foundations invest and then put their returns back into their own philanthropic efforts or into patient assistance funds. Selling equity, if absolutely necessary, could also be a possibility down the line. The exact recipe of funding components MAPS and MAPS PBC will settle on is still a work in progress, but whatever the eventual solution, "it's going to be a creative approach," Menapace said. If MAPS does manage to pull this unique business model off, then the group could provide a blueprint for other companies interested in a different way of financing and pursuing social change.

Another primary focus of MAPS PBC in the lead-up to FDA approval is securing market access to the product—pharmaceutical-speak for getting insurance companies and government payers to agree to cover MDMA-assisted therapy. "While maintaining complete control over the drug development, commercialization, and potential cash flow is a core focus while considering fundraising options, patient access is the most important goal, and we will do whatever is necessary to get an approved commercialized drug in the hands of patients who need the treatment," Septimus said.

Because of the treatment's novelty as a combination of both medication and therapy, this presents some challenges for payers, which are used to dealing with those things as separate line items. There's also some concern about payers trying to lower costs by watering the treatment down, for example, by cutting the number of sessions or shortening them. So far, though, MAPS has gotten "really strong positive responses" from payers, said Joy Sun Cooper, chief of patient access and head of commercialization at MAPS PBC. "Payers indicated that PTSD is an area of very high unmet need, and they saw our evidence of safety and efficacy as very compelling."

Not everyone has insurance, though, and some of those with insurance may have plans that choose not to cover MDMA-assisted therapy or have high deductibles that may make the treatment unaffordable. MAPS PBC is working on a patient assistance program that will help uninsured or underinsured people access care through subsidized or even free MDMA-assisted therapy. As Doblin and his colleagues are well aware, in many cases people who otherwise cannot afford the treatment may be the most in need of it. This especially pertains to people impacted or traumatized by racism, intergenerational trauma, inequity, discrimination, and other societal-level forces that put them at greater risk of developing a suite of physical and mental health conditions. These problems are only exacerbated by the fact that minority communities have also traditionally been overlooked in terms of access to care.

According to some experts, the newness and uniqueness of the MDMA-assisted therapy model presents the medical community with a chance to correct for some of these long-standing disparities from the ground up. "Essentially, this could be an opportunity for a new wave of engagement with mental health support for people of color who have not accessed it in the past," said Joseph McCowan, a clinical psychologist and psychotherapist in Los Angeles, and a cotherapist in the MAPS Phase 3 trials.

Ensuring that MDMA-assisted therapy reaches minority communities will most likely require a concerted effort that goes beyond just providing the treatment for free or at a subsidized cost, though. Participation in the clinical trials for MDMA-assisted therapy was free, for example, yet in the first Phase 3 trial, 77 percent of participants were white. The lopsided demographics "raises deeper seated questions about equity and access to treatment," said Albert Garcia-Romeu, a research psychologist at Johns Hopkins University School of Medicine.

There are a number of factors that might explain the low enrollment of minority participants in clinical trials of MDMA-assisted therapy. For one, not everyone who has PTSD can afford to take days off work to undergo therapy, or has the means to travel to the closest city where the therapy is being offered. In some communities of color, there's also a cultural condemnation of illegal drugs of almost any sort, because of those substances' association with the destruction of families and neighborhoods, said Nicholas Powers, an author, poet, and associate professor of literature at SUNY Old Westbury in New York. "The drug war has left people very reticent about anything except weed, which kind of got a pass because it was cool."

In some marginalized communities, the traumatized experience has also been normalized through generations of oppression. Strength and self-sufficiency are valorized while vulnerability and surrender—key components of not just psychedelic experiences but therapy in general—are associated with potential harm. "Often, the therapy space isn't considered a safe space," McCowan said. In part, this is because therapy was designed by white people for white people, and the vast majority of therapists today are white. While effective therapy does not require that the therapist come from the same background as their patient, it can be a problem if the therapist isn't aware of their own biases, fragility, and blind spots. "If anger by someone who's Black in a therapy session is pathologized by a white therapist, then that's not a good fit," McCowan said. "It really comes back to therapists doing their own work so they're prepared to work with diverse populations."

MAPS has taken some steps to try to recruit a more diverse group of therapists and participants for their trials, yet its efforts have sometimes revealed just how stubborn issues of equity can be. In 2015 the organization reached out to clinical psychologist Monnica Williams to see if she would be willing to lead a Phase 3 study site that focused on treating participants of color. "I was like, 'Wow, if white people are getting this, I want to make sure the Black people get it, too,'" recalled Williams. "I thought about the wonderful potential to use this for people suffering from racial trauma."

Williams was enthusiastic about the trial, but after three years of setbacks, her study site at the University of Connecticut ultimately had to shut down due to what she described as "a perfect storm" of racism, sexism, and stigmatization around psychedelics. In the end, she and her colleagues only completed treatment of one participant. On top of that major disappointment, she and two other Black female colleagues on the MDMA study ran into difficulties during an optional MAPS training session in Colorado, where study therapists had the opportunity to take MDMA in a onetime clinical setting. Challenges they ran into during the training revealed larger issues surrounding the need for culturally sensitive interventions.

Sara Reed, a licensed marriage and family therapist based in Louisville, Kentucky, who was a member of Williams's team, remembers going into her MDMA-assisted therapy session in Colorado feeling "a little nervous" but "ultimately trusting the process." As the 120-milligram dose took hold, Reed's late grandmother appeared to her and brought her to a space of intense love, divinity, and freedom. "For the first time in my adult life, I felt free as a young Black woman," Reed recalled. "Words don't do justice to what that sense of freedom was like."

This level of liberation was short-lived. As Reed came back into her body, she reconnected with the weight of the trauma she had been carrying her entire life. But as she began to process her experience out loud with her white MAPS therapists, there were moments where she struggled and started to become dysregulated, she said—largely due to a lack of culturally sensitive care. "Some of the moments of feedback are making me more confused, angry, and frustrated," Reed reflected back to the therapists. "You all don't understand what I'm really trying to say."

"Maybe there is a part of you that doesn't want to be understood," one therapist replied.

Reed couldn't believe what she'd just heard. In processing her trauma, there was nothing *more* she wanted than to be understood. "When you're under the influence of psychedelics, you are emotionally more raw and vulnerable, and the risk of harm increases," she told me. "Telling someone that there's a part of them that doesn't want to be understood misses the mark. On the contrary, it showed that this therapist didn't understand that part of me."

There were other gaffes, too. Williams, for example, was thrown off by the new-agey music played during her session. "MAPS is like, 'This is a neutral playlist because there's no words.' For us, it's like, 'Okay, that's very white person music,' " she said. "They made a lot of missteps that did unfortunately cause some harm."

Reed's experience in particular left her strongly concerned for future MDMA-assisted therapy participants whose therapists are not prepared to best serve them. "To me, it's a more systemic issue: most therapists are trained to track symptoms, not trained to track and intervene in culturally sensitive ways," she said. While training more therapists of color should be a priority, her experience also highlights "the importance of incorporating culturally responsible care in training programs and teaching white therapists how to not do harm, especially when working with people from BIPOC communities," she said.

Regardless of how culturally competent a white therapist may be, McCowan emphasized that representation is still very important. If a person of color goes onto a care provider's website and sees that everyone on the team is white, that can be an immediate turnoff. This isn't something that's unique to psychedelic therapy. Garcia-Romeu remembers a presentation by Gregory Vidal, a Black oncologist from Memphis, for example, who talked about how much of a struggle it was to convince Black women to come to the hospital, despite the fact that they suffered from higher rates of breast cancer than white women. The one thing that did bring them in, Vidal said, was having a Black doctor in charge. "There's still wariness of going into a biomedical setting that looks like it's run by and for some people," Garcia-Romeu said. "Walking around Hopkins, most people you see that look like me are going to be taking out the trash and cleaning the floors—that's just the way it is. But it makes it harder for Black folks and other people of color to really feel like they have a vested ownership or any sort of ability to steer the ship in some of these settings."

There are some signs that the field is moving in the right direction. Through concerted effort, for example, only 48 percent of the subjects in MAPS's second Phase 3 study were white. Independent of MAPS, Williams has also launched a training program for psychedelic-assisted therapists who want more guidance on navigating cultural issues and racial trauma. Garcia-Romeu also recently met with representatives from Howard University, a historically Black college in Washington, D.C., who expressed interest in starting their own psychedelic research program. Positive change "is percolating right now," Garcia-Romeu said. "But these are things that can take generations."

While equitable health care is only part of the solution to endemic social exclusions, Williams does wholeheartedly believe that MDMA-assisted therapy will be beneficial for some marginalized people, and preliminary findings seem to support this. In 2021, she and her colleagues surveyed more than three hundred BIPOC respondents who had taken MDMA or a classic psychedelic in a nonclinical setting. The participants reported various ways that psychedelics ameliorated their symptoms of racial trauma, including a reduction in depression, anxiety, and stress. In particular, Williams thinks MDMA-assisted therapy could help certain individuals see their suffering as something originating outside themselves. This is important, she said, because "people of color are socialized to think that we're the problem."

MDMA-assisted group therapy, McCowan added, could be an especially beneficial tool for promoting connection and collective healing from racial and intergenerational trauma in underserved and minority communities. First, though, psychedelic therapists need to develop relationships with communities and listen to people's concerns and hesitations regarding this new form of treatment. "This isn't missionary work, and it's important that we don't fall into the savior role when working with underserved communities," McCowan said. "Rather than bringing these medicines and treatments to communities, we need to focus on developing relationships with them and learning from them."

\*

ON A CHILLY December morning in 2021, psychiatrist Julie Holland took to the podium at Horizons, an annual psychedelics conference in New York City. Holland—whose 2001 book *Ecstasy: The Complete Guide* was one of the first comprehensive works on MDMA—wasn't here to talk about the promise of psychedelic healing, or the exciting prospect of impending FDA approval for MDMA-assisted therapy. She was here to issue a warning to the psychedelic community.

"The bad news is, there's some weeding that needs to be done and some pruning that needs to be done," she said, her voice brimming with emotion. "It's unfortunate, and uncomfortable, but in the long run, it'll be better."

Horizons is the world's largest, longest-running annual psychedelics gathering, and the event's growth alone is a bellwether of the broader change rocking the formerly close-knit community. Kevin Balktick—an articulate event producer with a passion for vintage books and obscure Shulgin molecules—launched the conference in 2007 after discovering a dearth of public forums to bring people together to discuss psychedelics. "At the time, it was mostly private salons and secret meetings, it felt closed," Balktick said.

Just a handful of researchers and activists (including Doblin) showed up for Balktick's inaugural conference, held over the course of a single afternoon at Judson Memorial Church opposite Washington Square Park. For the first few years Balktick regularly fielded emails from paranoid attendees asking him if their name would wind up in an FBI file if they bought a ticket to Horizons, or what safety measures he was taking to prevent undercover cops from infiltrating the conference. "People have forgotten about this, but the belief, for a very long time, was that users of psychedelics were a priority for law enforcement and if you got anywhere near them, the government was going to come after you," Balktick said. "Very few people would openly host any events about psychedelics, and people were often very closeted."

Things began to drastically change after the FDA designated MDMA-assisted therapy a breakthrough treatment in 2017, and then Michael Pollan's *How to Change Your Mind* came out the following year, triggering a surge of public interest. As of 2021, Horizons spanned five days of forums, workshops, classes, and talks with 2,800 attendees, including corporate PR representatives, Silicon Valley microdosers, and investors in Patagonia vests. "Now you're also dealing with venture capital bros at psychedelic meetings," said Matthew Johnson, a professor of psychedelics and consciousness research at Johns Hopkins University School of Medicine. "I've actually met some really nice ones, but that's been a total change in landscape."

While many of the developments around research, destigmatization, and education are welcome, Holland, Johnson, and others who have been at the forefront of the psychedelics field for years have expressed concern at the speed at which things are growing—and the way in which some of the changes are transpiring. "There's a sense we need to make up for lost time, but on the other hand, we need to take it one step at a time and not get too far ahead of ourselves," said Charles Grob at Harbor-UCLA Medical Center. "What will blow this field out of the water is if there's a spate of adverse outcomes."

Laura Mae Northrup, a ketamine psychotherapist from Oakland with curly purple-and-blue hair, spoke at Horizons 2021 about one of the most serious of these potential adverse outcomes: sexual abuse of patients by psychedelic therapists. Northrup knows of no research that's been conducted on the prevalence of abuse in psychedelic-assisted therapy. But according to a 2017 analysis of data derived from a national pool of mental health professionals across the United States, an alarming 7 to 12 percent admitted to having had erotic contact with a patient or patients. Given that these data are based on self-reporting, this is likely an underestimate. As Northrup told the Horizons audience, "Clinicians can and do abuse their clients. Psychedelic therapy is only as safe as the therapist providing it."

In general, predatory therapists are more likely to abuse people who have experienced sexual trauma as children, representing 32 percent of victims, according to one study. Adding psychedelics to the mix could make the likelihood of abuse even higher—and the potential negative outcomes worse. As we know, MDMA and other psychedelic drugs cause the brain to revert to a childlike state of openness and suggestibility, and MDMA, especially, also deepens feelings of connection and trust, including with a therapist. It's precisely these attributes that seem to make MDMA such a boon for facilitating effective therapy—yet these features of the drug also render people more vulnerable to verbal or physical transgressions committed by the person entrusted to care for them. "It's unfortunately very common that there's weird sexual dynamics that come up in non-drug-assisted psychotherapy, not just male-female, but male-male and female-female," Holland told me. "Psychedelic therapy is just going to catalyze and amplify the problem. It's not going to go away."

Whether psychedelics are involved or not, sexual abuse at the hands of a therapist can lead to feelings of suicidality and symptoms of trauma similar to those experienced by incest survivors, including self-blame. In certain cases, a patient might think that being sexual or partnered with their therapist is going to heal them, so they will consent to or even pursue a relationship.

Given the lopsided power dynamic between therapists and patients, however, any relationship—even one that is purportedly consensual—is still "clearly abuse," Northrup said. This is even more so the case when altered states of consciousness are involved, because a therapist has an even higher level of power over their patient than usual. "Similar to date rape, the victim is drugged," Northrup said.

There is ample evidence of sexual abuse occurring in the realm of psychedelic therapy over the years, including with MDMA. In 1989, for example, Richard Ingrasci, a psychiatrist in Massachusetts who had testified at the DEA hearings about MDMA-assisted therapy's medical value, surrendered his license after former patients accused him of sexual abuse. According to a story published in the *Boston Globe*, Ingrasci told a patient with cancer that having sex with him was an integral part of her healing process, and at least two of his alleged victims said that MDMA was involved in their abuse. Another prominent member of the early psychedelic therapy community, Francesco DiLeo, was sued by a patient in 1990 who alleged to have developed PTSD after DiLeo began giving her MDMA and having sex with her. According to court documents, DiLeo—who also lost his license—told her that sexual contact was a "way of partial fulfillment of [her] oedipal wishes."

A more recent case of abuse involved therapist Richard Yensen and psychiatrist Donna Dryer, a husband-and-wife team who were providing treatment for a MAPS Phase 2 trial site in Vancouver. Yensen had been friends with both Ingrasci and DiLeo, and he was considered to be a "prominent leader in psychedelics research for many decades," reported the webzine *Mad in America*. In a 2016 lecture at the California Institute of Integral Studies, Yensen addressed the issue of sexual abuse by therapists, recalling that in the early 1980s, when many therapists were legally using MDMA, "I ran across unfortunately large numbers of people where there was sexual acting out and difficulties, where therapists would be involved with multiple patients sexually." Sharing the stage with his wife, he added that this is why cotherapist teams are "really, really important for being able to deal with that . . . and to temper the tendencies to act things out."

What Yensen did not share with the audience was that he was actively engaging in sexual activity with one of his own patients, a MAPS trial participant named Meaghan Buisson who had undergone MDMA-assisted therapy with Yensen and Dryer in 2015. Buisson, a competitive inline speed skater in her thirties, suffered from PTSD caused by multiple traumas, including from childhood abuse and a violent rape that occurred in her twenties. Buisson declined an interview request for this book, but her story is extensively detailed in *New York* magazine and Psymposia's 2022 *Cover Story: Power Trip* podcast.

On paper, Buisson was an MDMA-assisted therapy success story. In 2016 she published an essay on MAPS's website about what she saw then as a complicated but overall positive experience in the clinical trial, and she also spoke at a conference about the powerful healing she underwent. "I learnt how much I craved as much as I feared touch," she told the audience. "And in the MDMA sessions, I was hugged. . . . And I am grateful every single day now for those hugs."

Buisson later said she was putting up a facade. Her actual experience following her MDMA-assisted therapy, according to the account she shared on *Power Trip*, was more akin to "a frog being boiled alive." After Buisson's MDMA sessions concluded in October 2015, she continued to receive conventional therapy from Yensen and Dryer. She also began working for them as a sort of assistant, and growing closer to the couple on a personal level. "It's hard to say it, but there were a lot of positives in my relationship with my therapists," Buisson said on *Power Trip*. "There were moments of laughter and there were moments of support and there were moments of healing, and that is part of the mind fuck."

According to Buisson's account, in December 2015 Yensen started touching her. A few months later, Buisson said, he digitally penetrated her, and Buisson had a panic attack. Yensen, she said, reassured her by framing this violation as "exposure therapy." Soon after, he progressed to having intercourse with her. When Buisson later began to rebuff Yensen, she said, he called her "selfish," "seductive," and "a manipulative bitch." In spring 2017, she escaped.

In 2018 Buisson filed a civil court claim in British Columbia alleging that Yensen sexually assaulted her, and she also named Dryer as a defendant, reported Olivia Goldhill for *Quartz*. Buisson additionally filed ethics complaints against Yensen and Dryer to the College of Psychologists of British Columbia and the BC College of Physicians and Surgeons, and she alerted Michael Mithoefer at MAPS about what happened. (Buisson has repeatedly said that she called Brad Burge, MAPS's former director of communications, and alerted him months before she reached out to Mithoefer, but that Burge did not act; in Goldhill's story, Burge denied that this happened.)

"Once we heard about it, we acted immediately," Doblin told me. "We contacted Richard, and he admitted it happened. His wife, Donna, also said she knew it was happening and tried to block it, but didn't know what to do."

MAPS barred both Yensen and Dryer from all MAPS-related activities or affiliations in the future, and submitted a report about what happened to the FDA, Health Canada, and the clinical trial's review committee. (MAPS had already terminated Yensen and Dryer's involvement in the trial a year earlier, in part because of their failure to provide study records in a timely and organized fashion.) MAPS also agreed to pay Buisson fifteen thousand Canadian dollars on a compassionate basis so she could obtain additional therapy while her lawsuit against Yensen and Dryer was in process. MAPS did not make Buisson sign an NDA in exchange for the money, but they did make her agree to waive her right to sue. In 2019 Yensen, Dryer, and Buisson settled their case outside of court, according to Goldhill's reporting, and MAPS released a public statement summarizing the violations.

In early 2018, prior to learning of Buisson's abuse, MAPS had already begun work on a stronger code of ethics for the MDMA therapy training program, as well as the creation of a patient bill of rights that would outline a clear, official process that participants could use to file grievances. "In retrospect, what more could we have done to prevent this? I don't know," Doblin said. "This never should have happened, but it does happen in that profession. It's human weakness."

On Twitter, Buisson characterized these types of statements as "misogynistic" and dismissing of sexual assault as "an 'inevitable' part of psychedelic therapy." In other tweets, she described MAPS's response to her case as "horrific" and accused the organization of fostering, enabling, and covering up abuse. An expert who spoke to me on the condition of anonymity agreed that MAPS's response to Buisson's case was not ideal. "I think they needed to be a lot more courageous and take responsibility at every level of their organization," the expert said. "I'm not saying they needed to punish themselves for this, but rather to really consider, 'How the hell did this fucking happen?' "

Lily Kay Ross, the cocreator of *Power Trip*, told me in an email in April 2022 that multiple people every week reach out to her to share stories about their negative experiences with psychedelic-assisted therapy, sexual in nature or otherwise. "The problem is much larger in scale than many realize, and there's evidence of serial abuse over decades," she wrote. " 'Power Trip' was the tip of the iceberg as far as what evidence we have, and how many abusers and unethical therapists we are aware of in different organizations and institutions, underground and above."

More research is needed before Ross will be able to share any numbers to try to quantify the problem, she said, but the bottom line is that she does not think MDMA- and other psychedelic-assisted therapy can safely move forward without first creating a more robust ethical framework that better protects patients. "The field has actively avoided (and, at times, covered up) these issues for decades," Ross wrote to me. "It will take many years and consultation with many experts to make up for what has been lost due to the decisions that people made to prevent rigorous discussion of these topics."

Doblin pointed out that in MAPS's case, at least, more than 360 patients have been through the trials, and so far sexual violations have occurred just once that the organization is aware of. "That doesn't excuse what happened," he said. "But it's pretty rare, and we're trying to learn from it and make it even rarer." It also doesn't seem balanced, he added, to call for a halt to MAPS's research or approval of MDMA-assisted therapy because of a single patient's experience with sexual misconduct. "What about the people with PTSD in MAPS's studies who have benefited from MDMA-assisted therapy, and the more than 10 million people in the U.S. alone who still suffer from PTSD?"

While sexual violence is not unique to psychedelic therapy, Northrup thinks the field in general could benefit by incorporating more education about the problem into therapist training sessions. Those doing the training should also be attuned to trainees who do not strike them as safe or ready for this kind of work. "It's the trainer's responsibility not to train them, or to tell them to get more healing themselves," Northrup said. Normalizing conversations among therapists about power—and what it means to take advantage of it—is also important, she added.

Legalizing MDMA-assisted therapy will not prevent sexual abuse from happening, but it will at least ensure that victims have a professional body to appeal to and that practitioners who commit violations can be held account-able, said Franklin King, a psychiatrist and instructor at Massachusetts General Hospital and Harvard Medical School. "Not that regulation fixes everything, but when things are secret and underground, there's shady shit and bad things that happen."

Acknowledging the need for more oversight, in 2020 a handful of doctors and therapists founded the American Psychedelic Practitioners Association, a self-governing body for the rapidly growing field. Another group, the Board of Psychedelic Medicine and Therapies, will certify psychedelic-assisted psychotherapists in an attempt to ensure competent, safe, and ethical care. "This is one of those situations where you're putting down the tracks and the train is right behind you," Holland said. She hopes, though, that these types of groups will provide a mechanism for reporting abuse and for holding psychedelic practitioners accountable for their actions.

Whatever precautions are taken in developing MDMA- and other psychedelic-assisted medicine, Northrup warned, there's still "going to be people who are harmed." And harm can take more forms than just sexual infractions. There is a chance, for example, that eventually someone who receives MDMA-assisted therapy will commit suicide in the days after treat-ment, or that someone will have a fatal physical reaction during their session. "There will be casualties," Johnson said. This isn't something specific to MDMA-assisted therapy, though. "Blood draws, endoscopies—they all have risks," Johnson said. "One out of so many thousands, something happens."

"A person committing suicide after MDMA therapy is possible and seems more of a realistic risk than a fatal physical reaction," Doblin said. "Yet there should be a risk-benefit balance."

As far as MAPS is aware, no one who has received MDMA-assisted therapy as part of the clinical trials has ever tried to commit suicide following treat-ment, but a number of people have experienced suicidal ideation immedi-ately after. In a way, this is not surprising: people who have severe PTSD already suffer from higher rates of suicide, and 90 percent of the first Phase 3 trial participants reported a history of suicidal ideation. "It can stir things up, which is why careful attention and support afterwards is needed," said Michael Mithoefer. "While some people do just fine with little or no support, some people will die if they don't have adequate support."

This only emphasizes the need to ensure that care providers and payers do not try to cut back on the amount of integration that patients receive after their psychedelic-assisted sessions. "The industry is going to expand, and that's good for getting these treatments into patients' hands," Johnson said. "But are people going to start cutting corners, and will safety standards be held up? This is not plug and chug, there are real risks."

While some negative experiences are inevitable as MDMA-assisted therapy is scaled up, what will probably be a much more common outcome, Northrup predicted, are lukewarm, disappointing results. "You might go in thinking, 'I'll be completely healed, I won't be depressed or suicidal anymore,'" Northrup said. "But you might come out and just be more capable of asking for help. That's huge, but it's not the same as your PTSD being gone."

Doblin concurred: "It's not like MDMA is a miracle cure and works for everyone and makes all of their problems all of a sudden go away."

The next few years will begin to reveal the community's effectiveness at addressing some of these challenges—which will only intensify as psychedelics become more mainstream. As those involved with bringing MDMA-assisted therapy to market contend with medical and equity issues, others, however, are grappling with another equally serious challenge: how to reduce risks and increase safety for the largest MDMA participant pool of all—recreational users.

# THE PROBLEM WITH PROHIBITION

JULY 20, 2013, WAS a glorious Saturday in Oxford, England, and Martha Fernback was going to take full advantage of the rare blue skies by spending the day outside with her friends. The fifteen-year-old laced up her white Converse All Star High-Tops and headed to Hinksey Park, a favorite hangout a few minutes' walk from her house. The plan was to kayak on the lake, soak up the sun, and do some MDMA.

It wasn't Martha's first time trying the drug, and she'd had good experiences before. Within twenty minutes of swallowing her powdered MDMA this time, however, she started showing signs of distress. Her friends helped her over to a tree where she was shielded from public view. At first they hesitated to call for help, because they were worried about Martha getting into trouble for taking an illegal drug. But after she collapsed, they realized the situation was serious.

Anne-Marie Cockburn, Martha's single mum, was at home that morning when an unknown number appeared on her mobile phone. The stranger on the other end said something that at first Anne-Marie did not understand: "Your daughter is gravely ill and we're trying to save her life."

Martha was rushed to John Radcliffe Hospital, where ER doctors pumped her chest. But from the moment Anne-Marie saw her daughter's half-open blue-gray eyes, she knew she was already gone. "I was calling to her in the same tone I last heard when I gave birth to her. A tone so unearthly and raw that it haunted the entire corridor of medical staff," Anne-Marie recounted in her diary, which she later published as a book about Martha's loss, *5,742 Days*. "I couldn't breathe once they announced what I already knew."

I visited Anne-Marie at her home a couple of weeks shy of what would have been Martha's twenty-fourth birthday, and when I arrived, the Converse sneakers she'd been wearing when she died were waiting for me. Anne-Marie had also set up a poster displaying a chillingly prescient tweet that Martha had sent out less than a month before her death: "its kinda scary how your whole life depends on how well you do as a teenager."

In the weeks after Martha's death, Anne-Marie pieced together the circumstances that had culminated in tragedy. She came to see that, more than just a series of unfortunate decisions Martha made, larger political and societal forces had been at work, playing a significant role in increasing the risk of harm befalling her daughter and other children like her. The more she learned, the more convinced she became that Martha's tragic loss had been entirely preventable—and the more determined she grew to campaign for policy changes that would prevent other parents from going through the same suffering.

*

FOR MILLENNIA, HUMANITY has recognized that all drugs have a two-faceted nature. As Michael Pollan pointed out in *This Is Your Mind on Plants*, the Greek word *pharmakon* means both "poison" and "medicine." For almost anything we put into our bodies, the difference between healing or harm, pleasure or pain, depends solely upon context, including dose and setting.

The chance of a drug leading to an adverse outcome increases significantly, though, under the constraints of prohibition. When drugs are illegal, provision of the substance falls to an unregulated criminal market, and consumers are left to piece together safety for themselves. Due to the illegal nature of drugs, as in Martha's case, users or their friends may also be less likely to promptly seek help should something go wrong.

"So many of the drug harms we deal with are artifacts of prohibition and the war on drugs rather than the pharmacology of drugs," said Steve Rolles of the Transform Drug Policy Foundation in the United Kingdom.

"The risks associated with MDMA, for example, are almost all dosage, adulteration, or environment-slash-behavioral, such as polydrug use, overheating, or hydration issues."

Even under prohibition, though, the risks of MDMA remain relatively low. In a 2000 analysis, for example, drug researcher Russell Newcombe in Liverpool found that the risk of death associated with Ecstasy use at dance parties—about one in a hundred thousand—is on par with the risk of a British citizen being killed while engaging in soccer, rugby, or snow sports; of choking to death or succumbing to food poisoning; of fatally falling down a flight of stairs; of dying in a fire or drowning; or of being victim of a deadly train or airplane accident.

According to Wim van den Brink, a professor of psychiatry and addiction at the University of Amsterdam, such findings highlight the fact that life, in general, "is a riskful thing." We manage risks, though, by weighing the chance of something bad happening against the likely rewards. From drinking alcohol or eating sugary foods to having sex or playing sports, risk assessments are a part of daily life. Yet society places certain drugs into a special category deemed somehow outside the bounds of normal decision-making, van den Brink said. "I think that's just not rational."

Even more irrational is the fact that risk assessments have no bearing on a drug's legal status, with many legal drugs—notably, alcohol and tobacco—being significantly riskier than many illegal ones. In 2010 David Nutt, the current chair of neuropsychopharmacology at Imperial College London, and the former chair of the British government's Advisory Council on the Misuse of Drugs, analyzed a suite of twenty legal and illegal drugs based on criteria related to the harms each substance produces in individuals and to others and society. Each drug received a score, with 100 being the most harmful possible. As Nutt and his colleagues reported in *The Lancet*, alcohol, with a score of 72, far surpassed all the other drugs in terms of its total harm. It was followed by heroin at 55 and crack at 54 (tobacco, with a score of 26, ranked the sixth most harmful). MDMA scored 9, making it the fourth *least* harmful drug in the analysis—just behind LSD (7), buprenorphine (7), and magic mushrooms (6).

Fed up with the lack of rational discussion around drug policy, in 2009 Nutt authored another article on the same topic, this one published in the

*Journal of Psychopharmacology* and titled "Equasy—An Overlooked Addiction with Implications for the Current Debate on Drug Harms." Nutt had learned of this "harmful addiction," he wrote, after treating a woman in her thirties who had suffered permanent "equasy-induced brain damage" that had resulted in severe personality change, behavioral disinhibition, and an inability to work. About one in every 350 people who are exposed to equasy in the United Kingdom suffer serious adverse events, he reported, including permanent neurological damage and around ten fatalities a year. What is this dangerous activity? "Equine Addiction Syndrome," aka horseback riding. The fact that horseback riding is legal but Ecstasy—something nearly thirty times less likely to cause acute harm—is illegal, Nutt wrote, "reflects a societal approach which does not adequately balance the relative risks of drugs against their harms."

Nutt's paper was not well received by his colleagues in government or the media (not to mention the horse-riding community). "The right-wing press went absolutely ape," he told me. "Some people believed it was a new drug at first!" Several months after the equasy paper's publication, UK home secretary Alan Johnson fired Nutt from his position as chair on the government's drug advisory group. As the Conservative party's shadow home secretary, Chris Grayling, told *Nature* at the time, "Professor Nutt's comments earlier this year, comparing the risks of ecstasy with those of horse riding, were particularly ill judged." Given the sensitive nature of the drug debate, Grayling added, Nutt had failed in his "responsibility to act cautiously and be mindful of the fact that messages given by official advisors can and will influence the behavior of the public."

Clearly, however, the public wasn't waiting around for some bureaucrat's approval to take Ecstasy. While no reliable data exist quantifying just how many people around the world use MDMA, the drug's popularity over the years has proven to be "really resilient," Rolles said, "because it provides effects that people want and like."

According to a 2021 United Nations Office on Drugs and Crime (UNODC) report, in 2019 alone, somewhere between nine and thirty-five million people worldwide aged fifteen to sixty-four used Ecstasy. National surveys estimating drug use based on weighted data indicate that, as of 2019, 7.3 percent of Americans over twelve years old have tried Ecstasy at least once, while 9.6 percent of people aged sixteen to fifty-nine in England and Wales have done the same as of 2020. Experts point out that these data are likely an underestimate of true use, given that some people lie on surveys and because certain groups, such as the homeless or prison inmates, are typically excluded.

Various papers and reports provide different indications of trends in Ecstasy's popularity over time—and most indicate that the drug is not going away any time soon. According to the UNODC's 2021 report, Ecstasy use in North America and Europe is stable, whereas in Australia and New Zealand, it's increasing. But based on what he's seen, Mitchell Gomez, executive director of DanceSafe, a nonprofit group that provides drug testing and education services in the United States and Canada, thinks that Ecstasy is undergoing "not just an increase, but a *large* increase in use."

For one, Ecstasy seizures around the world are on the rise, jumping 38 percent from 2018 to 2019, to sixteen tons—and quadrupling since 2011. Van den Brink pointed out, however, that the price for Ecstasy has stayed stable and low throughout this time. "Thus it seems that seizures represent only a very small fraction of the total amount that is produced and trafficked," he said. Thanks to the dark web, MDMA is also easier to access than ever before. In 2019, 67 percent of MDMA users around the world said they obtained their drugs this way, according to the Global Drug Survey. "It used to be that you'd have to know somebody and have a certain risk tolerance," Gomez said. "Now it just requires a certain level of technological expertise."

Another proxy Gomez pointed to for MDMA's increasing use is the electronic dance music (EDM) scene, which has transformed since 2000 into a multibillion-dollar global industry that, in some ways, purposefully sought to divorce itself from early rave culture. Following the passage of the Illicit Drug Anti-Proliferation Act in 2003, American party promoters felt they needed to distance themselves from any association with drug taking, so they stopped calling their events "raves" and instead began referring to them as "dance music festivals." Formerly subversive house music was also commodified by the mainstream and rebranded as EDM, which was pumped out at megafestivals such as Tomorrowland, Electric Daisy Carnival, and Ultra that now draw hundreds of thousands of attendees.

Most dance culture purists saw EDM as a violation of all they stood for, but by the mid-2000s, it had seemingly won the day. " 'Rave' had become a bad word and the festival scene was the biggest thing around," said Joseph Palamar, a drug researcher at New York University Langone Medical Center. Ecstasy also started being referred to as "Molly," a cutesy shorthand for "molecule," which was supposed to indicate pure MDMA. Many youngsters mistakenly thought Molly was a new drug, when in fact it was just Ecstasy rebranded and sold in powder or crystal form. While not everyone who goes to EDM clubs or attends music festivals is on Molly, many are. "Molly is a big part of it," Palamar said. "You cannot remove Molly."

The risks of taking Ecstasy or Molly can be enhanced by the festival or club environment, where temperatures can be high and water scarce, and attendees often mix MDMA with alcohol or other drugs. These factors are not required, though, for the drug to be dangerous. Martha, for example, was not a typical party kid. In the evenings, she was more likely to be at home having dinner with her mom or in her room listening to David Bowie than out on the town with friends. But Martha did have "some demons," as Anne-Marie put it, especially stemming from the fact that her parents had split when she was ten months old, and she seldom saw her father. "That clouded her a bit, her relationship with her dad not being fully formed," Anne-Marie said. A typical teenager, Martha also had some insecurities about what others thought of her. "She was a very sensitive child," Anne-Marie said. "She definitely was reaching out to Ecstasy to numb certain things, and to fit in as well."

Martha's friend bought the Ecstasy that wound up killing her from a seventeen-year-old boy in Oxford. As Anne-Marie pointed out, "a teenager can get any kind of drug they want from their mobile phone, easier than they can get a pizza." Almost certainly, though, the drugs ultimately traced back to a lab in the Netherlands, which over the last thirty years has risen to become the world's top MDMA producer. In 2017 alone, Dutch underground labs produced an estimated 972 million Ecstasy pills that, along with methamphetamine, generated at least €18.9 billion in revenue, according to a report issued by the Dutch Police Academy. (Some experts have questioned the numbers cited in this report, however.) An estimated 99 percent of MDMA made in the Netherlands is destined for foreign markets, not just in Europe and the United Kingdom but as far as Australia, Brazil, and Japan. The United States, however, is not a major destination for direct shipments of MDMA from the Netherlands, because of the risk of extradition for dealers. Instead, most MDMA that winds up there seems to come from Canada and Asia.

The Netherlands has become a hub for MDMA production for a number of reasons. Decades before the drug hit the scene, that country had already become a center of illegal amphetamine synthesis. Speed gangs built up well-established distribution networks and had strong ties to the Dutch chemical industry, so for many of those groups, pivoting to Ecstasy in the late 1980s and early 1990s was "a logical evolution," said journalist Philippus Zandstra, based in Haarlem. "They see this new drug in town, MDMA, the recipe for which could be found in the university library. That was how they made the change to Ecstasy."

The Dutch labs tend to be run by networks of criminals who may or may not have ties to other larger illicit enterprises. The people producing the MDMA itself usually do not know who they're working for, and tend to lack any sophisticated chemistry knowledge. "Mostly, they will be directed to a fully-equipped lab where they will find a note from the 'master chef' with instructions on how to operate everything," Zandstra said. Because the master chef never has any direct contact with the cooks, he's insulated from any legal repercussions in the event that the lab is busted.

"When the police enter a lab, they may find just two guys who have no clue what they're doing there," said Tim Surmont, a scientific analyst at the European Monitoring Center for Drugs and Drug Addiction. "The main guy almost never comes into the picture."

Over the years, the perks for MDMA producers of working in the Netherlands have only increased. There are liberal drug laws and fast Wi-Fi, plus a massive flow of cargo in and out of Rotterdam—the largest seaport outside of East Asia. To top it off, the Netherlands has also set its sights on becoming one of Europe's financial centers, a convenience for anyone trying to conceal illegal earnings. As Zandstra wryly noted, "We're very good at money laundering."

Although the Netherlands is renowned for producing the world's best MDMA—the Ecstasy version of what Colombia is for cocaine, or Scotland is for whisky—given the criminal nature of the trade, there's still no telling what a given pill or baggie of crystals actually contains. "Within a single club, you can have pills that are completely fake to ones that are really, really strong,"

Newcombe said. "If it's weak, it means there could be lots of nasty toxic adulterants, and if it's really strong, it means the person can overheat."

One way to approximate just how many people are unknowingly taking adulterated drugs is to ask them what they think they've recently taken, and then test their hair to see what they've actually taken. On a frigid November evening, I joined two of Palamar's undergraduate researchers in front of 3 Dollar Bill, a club in Brooklyn that was hosting a popular dance party called I Feel. Alexis Wasserman, one of the students, enthusiastically implored the glittery, sequined patrons shivering in line to take part: "We're with NYU Langone—do you want to take a fun little survey about drug use? It's completely anonymous and we'll give you ten dollars, cash!"

Most people said no, but about fifteen minutes in, a couple of gay guys said sure, they'd help out. Working their way through a lengthy iPad questionnaire that asked about everything from poppers and 2-CB to NBOMe (pronounced "N-bomb") and "purple drank," they finally got to the MDMA part: Have you ever knowingly used Ecstasy/Molly/MDMA?

"No, I've not done Molly, but I want to," one of the guys said after reading the question out loud and agreeing to chat with me.

"I've done Molly once, and it was not great," the other chimed in. "I did, like, the smallest amount you could possibly imagine. And I was like, 'No.'"

"Are you sure it was real Molly?" I asked.

"Dang—okay! You're really hitting the real question!" the guy replied with feigned incredulity. "I mean, it was about seven years ago, so I don't know for sure. But probably not? Oh my god, the sass outta you!"

Sassy or not, it's a legitimate question. Palamar and his colleagues have found clear indicators that people are being unintentionally exposed to other drugs. "Molly is supposed to mean pure MDMA, but we've found that at least here in New York City, Molly is often the furthest thing from pure," said Palamar. "It's often just a mystery powder."

The composition of that mystery powder has shifted over time, according to a 2021 study Palamar's team published. In 2016 they analyzed ninety hair samples collected from people who said they had taken MDMA over the past months and found that among those *not* reporting use of the following drugs, 31 percent tested positive for new psychoactive substances; 28 percent tested positive for synthetic cathinones ("bath salts"); 22 percent tested positive for methamphetamine; and 19 percent tested positive for ketamine. When Palamar did the same analysis in 2019 using seventy-two new samples from self-declared MDMA users, the prevalence of unknown exposure to adulterants had dropped significantly, to 6 percent for meth and 3 percent each for new psychoactive substances and bath salts. Ketamine was the exception, increasing to 35 percent. While ketamine isn't more dangerous than MDMA, the others are, and even with the changing trends, "that's a substantial portion of people—assuming they were honest on the survey—who have been unknowingly exposed to potentially more dangerous drugs," Palamar noted.

There's also a powerful lesson here about the unintended consequences of drug-war policies: the shifting patterns of MDMA adulteration are partly explained by the cat-and-mouse game between law enforcement and underground drug producers at a global scale. In 2008, authorities in Cambodia raided a series of woodland processing plants and confiscated more than thirty-three U.S. tons of safrole oil, the main precursor at the time for making MDMA. Another raid the following year resulted in an additional 5.7 tons intercepted. According to the nonprofit environmental group Fauna and Flora International, the oil had been extracted from the roots of illegally felled *mreah prew phnom* trees, and the second, smaller seizure alone represented enough precursor to make forty-four million tabs of Ecstasy, with a street value of $1.2 billion.

The safrole oil seizures triggered a global drought in MDMA availability, and on the prohibition side of things, "everyone was like, 'Yay, success, enforcement works!' " Rolles said. But the celebrations were short-lived. To fill the gap in the market, dealers began subbing in other products passed off as Ecstasy, including more dangerous drugs such as synthetic cathinones like mephedrone. Some pills were even laced with PMA and PMMA, chemicals that are significantly more toxic than MDMA. PMA and PMMA have a slower biological uptake than MDMA; users still waiting to experience any effects an hour after taking the first pill would often conclude they'd swallowed a dud and consume additional doses. Eventually, though, the pills would all kick in and produce a tsunami release of serotonin. In some people this would cause a potentially lethal condition called serotonin syndrome, in which abnormally high levels of that neurotransmitter can trigger dangerously elevated blood pressure and hyperthermia. In England and Wales alone, deaths attributed to PMA and PMMA shot up from just one in 2011 to twenty in 2012; twenty-nine in 2013; and twenty-four in 2014. As Nutt said, "We'd created a new monster in this failed attempt to stop people from accessing MDMA."

After several years of increasing adulteration, criminal entrepreneurs realized that rather than make MDMA from safrole oil, they could simply order other chemical precursors—namely, PMK—directly from China. Authorities caught on pretty quickly, though, and responded with new controls on PMK—to which the labs in China responded just as quickly by tweaking their formulas slightly to escape regulation. "Basically, each time a new chemical appears, legislation comes in to control it, and they make another new chemical," Surmont said. "This has led to a business on its own, with Polish and Romanian gangs buying these chemicals, converting them to PMK and selling them to the Dutch. What you actually wind up getting by trying to control illegal labs are more labs."

By 2010 producers had also figured out a way to create a different precursor, PMK-methyl-glycidate, that bypassed entirely the need to order controlled chemicals from abroad. "If those chemists had kept that recipe a secret they probably could have made a billion dollars," Gomez said. "But they put that information online. I think the decision was philosophical: they didn't like the fact that there were all these misrepresentations being sold as MDMA."

Even if PMK-methyl-glycidate was somehow stamped out, manufacturers, Gomez added, will always find a way to meet demand. Someone recently published a proof-of-concept formula online for making MDMA using Styrofoam as a precursor. Other groups are working on creating genetically modified yeast to generate banned drugs or key ingredients needed to make them. In 2020, for example, researchers from Stanford University reported in *Nature* that they'd succeeded in engineering baker's yeast to biosynthesize propane alkaloids—a group of chemicals that includes cocaine. "We're entering an age that's a technological kill shot to the drug war," Gomez said. "If you can home brew safrole oil and manufacture MDMA from that, then prohibition has collapsed."

For now, though, the glut of new precursors has permitted cheap, topnotch Ecstasy to come surging back onto the scene. But this has created yet another unexpected and harmful side effect: pills that contain dangerously high doses of MDMA. These pills are often scored and meant to be broken in halves or even quarters, but users may or may not realize that.

In the 1990s and 2000s, average MDMA tablets ranged around 50 to 80 milligrams, whereas in 2019 the average tablet in Europe was 180 milligrams. "Super pills" are now regularly found in the 250-to-350-milligram range. In November 2021 a new record for the world's most potent Ecstasy pill was set by a "Blue Punisher" tablet seized at a club in Manchester that contained 477 milligrams of MDMA—up to five times the normal oral dose. That amount of MDMA "is enough to kill a small, susceptible person, and to make a more regular user feel very unpleasant," Newcombe said. Ecstasy-related deaths in the United Kingdom have been creeping up in the past years, reaching a height of 131 in 2020, the last year the government provided data for. Experts suspect this is because of the increasing potency of pills. As Nutt pointed out, "People are now dying of Ecstasy poisoning, which hardly ever happened before."

Unlike the United Kingdom, in the United States, solid data on the number of deaths even associated with MDMA (or what users think is MDMA) do not exist. Coroners in the States frequently have no medical training, let alone toxicology expertise, so information surrounding cause of death when drugs are involved is often highly questionable or incomplete. A 2018 study in *Science* found, for example, that a quarter of the nearly six hundred thousand officially reported U.S. drug-related deaths between 1979 and 2016 didn't even list the drug in question on the death certificate. Even if MDMA is listed on a death certificate, though, the federal government does not track the number of deaths attributed to that drug. Instead, it classes MDMA-related deaths within a catch-all bucket of "psychostimulants," which includes methamphetamine, among other things.

Whatever the exact number, people do die every year around the world from taking adulterated Ecstasy or Molly, or by unknowingly taking too much pure MDMA. Drug testing is one way to help prevent this, and a number of countries already provide such services, including Austria, Colombia, Luxembourg, Portugal, Spain, and Switzerland. The Netherlands, in particular, is "harm reduction heaven," Zandstra said. Two dozen stations exist throughout the small country where people can bring their drugs for free testing, plus get tips while they're there about how to safely use them.

MDMA producers make signature pills based on unique artwork and color—from blue Volkswagens to orange Donald Trump heads—so the staff at testing facilities first examines a pill that someone's brought in to see if it's already in their existing database. "If they don't have it in the system—which I had one time, I felt quite special—they'll take the entire pill for testing," Zandstra said. "It's a bit of solidarity with other ravers." Because of the ease of these services, most MDMA users Zandstra knows and has interviewed are "really fanatical" about testing, he said, and it's just become a natural part of planning a night out.

In some countries with governments that are less proactive or supportive of drug testing, grassroots initiatives are stepping up to fill the gap. New Zealand provides a particularly inspiring example. Drug-checking initiatives, as Kiwis call these services, began in 2014, when a risk management consultant named Wendy Allison was working at an EDM festival and witnessed a spate of serious medical problems when a few attendees took what came to be known as "the black pills." (No one ever found out what these pills were, but Allison suspects they were some sort of synthetic cathinone.) "The medics came to us and said, 'Look, if you don't do something about this, someone is going to die,' " Allison recalled.

Allison had just gotten a degree in criminology, and she knew that in places where festivals take a zero-tolerance approach to drugs—for example, by bringing in sniffer dogs and performing strip searches—the death rate among attendees is actually higher. "It makes sense, because people see the cops and do things like swallow their entire stash," Allison said. Drug checking seemed like a more prudent approach, but it occupied a legal gray area at festivals and clubs in New Zealand because the law criminalizes anyone who knowingly permits a venue to be used for drug consumption. Allowing drug checking on-site would mean implicitly acknowledging that people do drugs there.

Despite this, Allison managed to convince one festival sponsor to allow her to discreetly set up a tent. Of the forty-eight samples she and her colleagues tested, most were presumed to be MDMA, but only 20 percent turned out to actually be what people thought they were. Half the people whose drugs turned out to be something else told Allison they did not intend to take them as a result. This seems to be a standard reaction. A 2017 paper analyzing data tied to 529 presumed MDMA samples tested by DanceSafe at events across the United States revealed that people were significantly less likely to say they still intended to use their drugs if their sample turned out to not actually contain MDMA.

Since 2015, KnowYourStuff New Zealand, as Allison's group came to be called, has quietly carried out more than 6,200 tests at festivals across the country. Depending on the year, up to 90 percent of samples were presumed to be MDMA. While the organization cannot prove that its drug checking has saved any lives, up to 75 percent of people whose samples turned out *not* to be what they expected said they wouldn't be taking the drug. Additionally, 86 percent of people who have used KnowYourStuffNZ's services said that they have changed their drug-taking behavior as a result, including no longer taking anything that isn't tested first and refraining from taking more than one substance at a time. "One of the important things in terms of our trajectory is we didn't ask permission from the government," Allison said. "We knew if we asked permission, we'd be denied out of hand. We waited until we had the data to show it's effective."

That strategy seemed to work. When KnowYourStuffNZ went public, rather than condemn the group, the country's police minister, Stuart Nash—who had a teenage daughter of his own—publicly voiced his support. "That created quite a stir and got the conversation going," Allison said. In 2021 New Zealand set a historic first by passing the Drug and Substance Checking Legislation Act, which permits drug checkers to become licensed and to operate at festivals and in communities, with the support of government funding. While drug checking has been happening in other places for over twenty years, no other country has permanently legalized these services. "Every other country operates clandestinely or in some legal gray area with tacit support but no legal backing," Allison said. "There was a bit of quiet smugness going on, like 'Yeah, we did it, we changed the world!'"

New Zealand's practical, forward-looking approach to drug testing stands in stark contrast to the United States, United Kingdom, and most other countries, where these services are still illegal in many contexts. Users can order kits online to do their own tests at home, but there's often nowhere they can go to get more precise analyses done by professionals. And while there are groups that try to get around this, they usually run into problems similar to those Allison did prior to government endorsement of KnowYourStuffNZ.

To test at festivals or clubs in the United States, for example, DanceSafe has to get permission from party promoters, who risk running afoul of the 2003 Illicit Drug Anti-Proliferation Act, which holds event organizers and venue owners liable for acknowledging drug use on site. While no one has ever been charged for allowing harm reduction, "the fear of the law is real," Gomez said.

In the United Kingdom, a group called The Loop provides on-site testing services at some festivals, but for the last few years they have usually been limited to examining drug samples seized by security or surrendered in anonymous "amnesty bins." So rather than being able to provide personalized results, the organization can only put out general alerts on social media and flyers, should something dangerous be found. As Newcombe said of the British government's approach, "Harm reduction isn't really on a back burner at all, it's been thrown off the stove. And death is the worst harm of all."

*

BEFORE SHE DIED, Martha sometimes used her mom's computer to log in to Facebook, and Anne-Marie wound up getting hold of her daughter's password this way. Periodically, she would check Martha's private messages to keep an eye on things. One day, about six months before she lost Martha, she saw a series of telling texts in a group chat: "I'll have a half," someone said. "I'll have a quarter," someone else said.

"Shit," Anne-Marie thought.

She sat Martha and her best friend down and asked them if they were doing drugs. Neither of the girls denied it, and their honesty and almost blasé attitude threw Anne-Marie off. She considered herself to be a confident parent, but she had never done drugs herself and had no knowledge base to draw from. So she did what years of war-on-drugs conditioning had taught parents in her position to do: she started shouting at her daughter about danger and poor decisions. "No parent wants a child to do anything dangerous, so you say the most extreme thing possible to stop it," she told me.

Looking back, Anne-Marie now sees that she'd punished her daughter for telling the truth. "That's the problem with prohibition," she said. "I didn't have the tools to be able to be open-minded enough to listen to what she was saying, or to know the reality of what she was doing to herself."

By the time Martha took the MDMA that killed her, she had done the drug on at least three prior occasions with her friends. "I think she had really good experiences taking it, and I think they thought they knew what they were doing," Anne-Marie said.

Martha, in fact, had done her own research. When Anne-Marie checked the search history on her daughter's computer in the days after her death, she found scientific articles about MDMA from the *Lancet*, one of the world's most esteemed medical journals. "She was trying to find good harm reduction information," Anne-Marie said.

Martha would have had no idea of the content of what she took on that Saturday morning, but a sample from the same batch that authorities later tested revealed that it contained 91 percent pure MDMA. Martha had consumed 500 milligrams of that substance, a dose four to five times higher than the normal amount an average person at a rave would take, or a therapist would give a client. Anne-Marie has no idea whether Martha took this high a dose on purpose—"maybe she thought that taking more could get you extra high," she speculated—or if this was just a measurement error that wound up having fatal consequences.

After Martha died, Anne-Marie's only escape from the pain was in sleep. Her life had become a living nightmare, and at times she despaired. As she wrote about a month and a half after losing her daughter, "Give me what Martha took then I can join her—half a gram of white powder and I'd die deliriously happy too, as high as a kite and full of love and rainbows."

Yet even in her darkest moments, Anne-Marie knew that following her daughter in death was not an option. "I could have just gone to bed and given up and said my life ended with hers, but it didn't," she told me. "I have a future and I have a life—that came into my head really loudly in the very moment Martha died."

Anne-Marie's life had irrevocably changed, though. Whereas before her purpose had been to raise her daughter, now she had to find new meaning.

Within a few weeks after Martha died, that meaning, she realized, could be helping to prevent other families from needlessly losing loved ones to drugs.

Anne-Marie was certainly not the first parent who had been inspired to take action after losing a child to MDMA. The United Kingdom's most well-known case of parent activism occurred in 1995, surrounding the death of eighteen-year-old Leah Betts, a middle-class girl from Essex. It was Leah's birthday, and as she was preparing her house for a party that evening, she and a friend took around 80 milligrams of Ecstasy. Leah's dad was a former police officer and her stepmom was a volunteer antidrug worker, and she had heard about the importance of staying hydrated while on MDMA by drinking plenty of water. Leah wasn't dancing or sweating, but she seemed to have gotten paranoid that she was becoming dehydrated, and she consumed seven liters of water within a two-hour period. This resulted in hyponatremia, a condition that occurs when excess water dilutes the blood and causes plasma sodium levels to drop. This can lead to potentially deadly cerebral edema, in which brain cells swell with water. Especially in young women, MDMA also causes the release of an antidiuretic hormone that helps the body retain water, heightening the chances of water poisoning even if a person doesn't drink as much as Leah did.

Leah fell into a coma and died several days later. Her family met with Prime Minister Tony Blair, who promised them he would never ease restrictions on MDMA, and they released photos of Leah to the media, including one of her intubated in the hospital. Another image of the smiling teenager wound up on antidrug billboards published at fifteen hundred locations across the country with the caption "Sorted. Just one ecstasy tablet took Leah Betts." According to Nutt, links were eventually found suggesting that the multimillion-pound advertising campaign had been paid for by the alcohol industry, which had been experiencing drops in sales for the first time in decades due to Ecstasy's popularity.

Whatever the case, publicity surrounding Leah's death "really turbocharged the imperiled child narrative and the criminal justice pushback against MDMA and raves," Rolles said. Over the years the media played an essential role in propagating that narrative, never failing to publish hysterical headlines each time an Ecstasy-related death occurred. In 2008, for example, MDMA was linked to 44 deaths in the United Kingdom that generated forty-seven media stories (106 percent coverage), whereas the 685 deaths caused by alcohol that year generated just fourteen stories (2 percent coverage). "There's been a whole series of tragic MDMA-related deaths where parents have often been, to a certain extent, exploited by politicians or the media to condemn drug taking and call for harsher sentencing," Rolles said.

By the time Martha overdosed on MDMA, though, nearly two decades had passed since Leah Betts's death. Years of tough laws and heavy-handed messaging about abstinence had not stopped kids from taking MDMA. Neither had it stopped some of them from dying every year. There had to be a more effective approach, Anne-Marie thought.

The day before Martha's funeral, Anne-Marie found the website for Transform, the group Rolles works for. She called them and asked how she could help. Rolles and his colleagues linked her up with experts like Nutt, who got her up to speed on drug policy, the problems caused by prohibition, and the arguments in favor of more sensible and compassionate laws pertaining to the use of all drugs, not just MDMA.

As she learned more, Anne-Marie came to see the ideal approach to drugs as a legalized, strictly regulated system that would "give people the right to choose," she said, and empower them with information to support those choices. In other words, a system similar to what is already applied to other legal drugs, including alcohol and tobacco. "We know that tobacco is dangerous and bad for health, but we don't say, 'You're not having it,'" Anne-Marie said. "You give people a choice, you give them the truth."

Ethan Nadelmann, the founder and former executive director of the Drug Policy Alliance, a New York City–based nonprofit group dedicated to ending the war on drugs, agreed with this assessment. "The core principle, to my mind, of drug policy reform is that nobody deserves to be punished or discriminated against based on what we put in our bodies, so long as we don't hurt anyone," he said. "That applies across the board, both to those substances we see as more elevated and those we see as less elevated." An analogy, he continued, would be the First Amendment of the U.S. Constitution: it equally protects all forms of speech, regardless of whether they are judged by others to be lofty or despicable. "You recognize that protecting those other forms of speech is essential to protecting broader freedom," Nadelmann said.

Columbia University neuroscientist Carl Hart also makes this argument but takes it a step further. By banning Americans' ability to decide what to put into their own bodies, he asserts, the U.S. government is actually violating the fundamental rights of its citizens. As the Declaration of Independence states, the government's purpose is to secure "certain unalienable rights," among them, "life, liberty and the pursuit of happiness"—not to restrict these rights, as it currently does with drugs. "Our right to make decisions based on the outcome of [risk-to-benefit] calculations is not outlawed by the government, except when it comes to certain recreational drugs," Hart wrote.

There are also less philosophical, more practical arguments in favor of ending prohibition. Considering that American taxpayers spent approximately thirty-five billion dollars fighting the war on drugs in 2019 alone, regulated legalization of drugs would save money. Manufacturing of illegal drugs, including MDMA, is also behind environmental destruction and pollution. Authorities in the Netherlands estimate that more than 560,000 pounds of waste from MDMA and other illicit drug production is generated in their country each year, and most of it winds up dumped in the countryside. There's also, of course, the criminal justice argument, and the case for dismantling organized crime by eliminating the need for consumers to buy illegal products.

The strongest argument in favor of ending prohibition, though, is simply to reduce harm and save lives. Legalization would not only guarantee that lawfully purchased drugs are what they purport to be, it would also ensure that people know the exact amount they are given and have access to reliable safety information. "If something regulated had landed in Martha's hands that day, she would have read on the package that it's 91 percent pure, and she would have had the recommended dose," Anne-Marie said. "She could have made a more informed decision."

In the span of just two years, Anne-Marie gave approximately two hundred media interviews. Martha's story—and Anne-Marie's message about the importance of more sensible drug policies—rocked the country. She participated in a historic debate on drug policy at Westminster, and Parliament discussed what happened to Martha on at least seven separate occasions. "When I do my political stuff, I say, 'Martha wanted to get high, she didn't want to die,'" Anne-Marie said.

All the publicity created a snowball effect, with more and more families who had lost loved ones speaking up in favor of sensible policies. With Rolles, Anne-Marie helped launch Anyone's Child, a campaign that brings together families whose lives have been impacted by current drug laws and who want to change them. On those families' behalf, she helped to deliver a petition in favor of drug law reform to Prime Minister David Cameron. "It's one of these things where you cannot argue with what the families are saying," Anne-Marie said. "This is what happened to us, and it could happen to you."

If and when MDMA and other currently banned drugs are regulated for legal sale, experts imagine a three-tiered system of control, depending on the drug's abuse potential. As is already happening in many U.S. states, the least potentially harmful drugs, like cannabis, would be subject to the most lenient controls, while drugs on the opposite end of the spectrum, like heroin, would be administered in clinical settings, as already happens in places like Switzerland, the Netherlands, and Canada. "People are like, 'What, legalize even heroin!?' " Anne-Marie said. "But that's like saying we're going to legalize beer but not vodka. Then vodka would be sold on the black market. If something is 'dangerous,' it means it should be regulated."

Under this model, club drugs like MDMA would occupy a middle ground, available for purchase in limited amounts from specialized pharmacies. "What would legal MDMA look like? You'd go to a pharmacist during the day, independent of the club, who would give you advice that is relevant to you," Rolles said. "They'd ask you questions like whether you've done MDMA before and what environment you'll be using it in, and they'd tell you things like not to mix it with alcohol. The whole thing would be geared towards not just safer products but encouraging more responsible use."

Requiring people to obtain a license ahead of purchasing MDMA could be an additional option for enhancing safety, added Rick Doblin at MAPS. As with getting a license to drive, an MDMA license would require first passing a test about how to safely and responsibly use the drug. If the license holder wound up causing harm through abuse of MDMA, then their license could be suspended.

In the Netherlands, van den Brink imagines a system for legally selling MDMA similar to what's already in place for marijuana at the country's coffee shops—in this case, X-Shops. This was the conclusion reached in 2021, when he and seventeen interdisciplinary colleagues sought to quantify the best approach for reducing harms and risks associated with MDMA. Rather than start with a foregone conclusion, they analyzed a spectrum of strategies that the Dutch government could take with regard to MDMA, from more enforcement to legalization, and then predicted what outcomes each of these strategies would most likely result in, including for health, law enforcement, criminality, and financial issues. Based on the measured differences between those predicted outcomes, they concluded that the optimal policy outcome would indeed be regulated MDMA sales. Politicians in the Netherlands have expressed a willingness to engage on the issue of Ecstasy, so there is a chance that something like this could be adopted in the coming years. As van den Brink pointed out, "There's so many people using Ecstasy now, it's not only youngsters but also the middle-aged. Ecstasy's use is more and more normalized, it's mainstream."

The United Kingdom has been more hesitant. In 2009 the Advisory Council on the Misuse of Drugs recommended that MDMA be reclassified from a class A drug—those that carry the highest legal penalties—to a class B drug, but the government rejected this advice. And although more and more members of Parliament from all parties now say they agree that drug policy reform is warranted, nothing has changed since Martha's death. In fact, things have only gotten worse. In 2016 the British government passed the Psychoactive Substances Act, a new law banning the production and sale of any substance that "affects the person's mental functioning or emotional state," with the exceptions of alcohol, tobacco, caffeine, and "any substance which is ordinarily consumed as food." One of the law's primary aims was to legally control any new psychoactive substance "before they appeared or had even been imagined," Newcombe said. "I was very surprised when the act was passed, as I expected it to fail as a bill or get radically toned down, at least on human rights grounds. Instead, most British organizations and people made very little noise about it."

Given the approach at home, realistically, Anne-Marie thinks it will take some other country—namely, the United States—leading the charge before policymakers in the United Kingdom feel comfortable taking steps of their own. "It'll be 'OK, America's done it, let's go along with it,'" Anne-Marie predicted. "It'll get to the point where our hand will be forced."

This is more than a pipe dream. Doblin and others are hoping that medical use of MDMA in the United States will pave the way for legalization of recreational use, as has been the case for marijuana in a growing number of states. This has happened despite the fact that cannabis has not been approved by the FDA to treat any disease or condition, and that federally, it remains a strictly banned Schedule I substance. Doblin thinks this is because, whether for cannabis or MDMA, research and medicalization "changes peoples' understanding of the risk-benefit," he said. "They start thinking more carefully and start to wonder, 'Why are we putting people in jail for this?' "

While marijuana's increasingly mainstream status seems natural and is even taken for granted in certain places now, just a few years ago, van den Brink pointed out, it seemed like an impossibility. "Nobody could have predicted the legalization of cannabis not only for medical use, but recreational use," he said. "We had all the international drug treaties and laws, we didn't think it could change, but it's very clear now that quick changes can occur. So I'm more positive now that we can have an open, rational discussion about Ecstasy."

Indeed, more and more people are coming around to this. Even Duke University professor emeritus Allen Frances—the most critical outside expert I consulted with regarding MDMA's use for treating PTSD—told me that he is pro-legalization. "[MDMA's] risks in pure form, while not negligible, pale in comparison to the risk of street 'Ecstasy' with its unknown dosage and potential adulteration with lethal fentanyl," he wrote in an email. "I personally would legalize all drugs (despite the considerable harms of doing so), because the 'war on drugs' is such a dismal failure, and the cause of much greater individual and societal harm."

In *Chasing the Scream*, journalist Johann Hari likened the current state of the battle to end the war on drugs to the situation gay activists found themselves in during the 1969 Stonewall riots in New York City. At that time, change seemed like an impossibility: antigay positions were encoded into every major religious text and into the laws of every country, and gay people—like drug users today—"were representatives of one of the most despised minorities in the world," Hari wrote.

After nearly fifty years of untold numbers of activists risking their reputations, freedom, and even lives, in 2015 the U.S. federal government finally legalized gay marriage. Within a single lifetime, their efforts had transformed domestic culture and policy, and created a domino effect that spread to other countries, too. As in 1969, the final end to the war on drugs "is so distant we can't see it yet," Hari wrote, "but we can see the first steps on the road, and they are real, and they can be reached."

"We're getting there," Anne-Marie agreed. "But sadly, it won't be saving lives today, which is what I want."

# THE SOCIAL SPECIES

OCTOPUSES ARE ABOUT the closest we can come on Earth to encountering aliens. A five-hundred-million-year evolutionary gulf separates our two species, making the eight-armed invertebrates more distantly related to us than dinosaurs. Not surprisingly, then, octopuses' brains are vastly different from our own, lacking the major anatomical features of the vertebrate brain, including key regions neuroscientists typically associate with complex social behaviors. Octopuses, for example, do not have a cortex, basal ganglia, or nucleus accumbens, and most of their neurons are actually distributed across their arms rather than in their heads. Many species of octopus are also fiercely antisocial, going out of their way to avoid others of their kind save for brief trysts during mating season. Yet at the same time octopuses are highly intelligent, capable of what scientists describe as "high-order cognitive behaviors" such as tool use and problem-solving.

It's precisely this mix of extreme intelligence and extreme dissimilarity to humans that attracted Gül Dölen at Johns Hopkins to studying octopuses. Most neuroscience research is done on mice, mammals with a brain "remarkably similar to our own," Dölen explained to me in early 2021 for a *Scientific American* article. While mouse studies are helpful precisely because the rodents' brains are so closely related to ours, octopuses are useful for the opposite reason: because they're so dissimilar. Comparing and contrasting our brain to a complex yet very different brain like the octopus's "gives you that logical power of reduction," Dölen said. Ultimately, this allows scientists to find commonalities that reach far back into evolutionary history and point to the origins of things like consciousness, social behavior, and the fundamental roles of various brain chemicals.

In particular, Dölen wanted to compare and contrast what happens when octopuses are given MDMA. If the animals responded much as humans do, then it would point to an ancient, conserved role for the mediation of social behavior by serotonin, the key neurotransmitter MDMA mimics.

Dölen and marine biologist Eric Edsinger holed up for two days in Dölen's mouse lab turned temporary aquarium, tending to seven California two-spot octopuses (an extremely antisocial species) on loan from Woods Hole Marine Lab in Massachusetts. Dölen actually had her doubts that MDMA, a synthetic drug not found in nature, would do much for the octopuses. Whether the marine invertebrates even had the same serotonin binding sites as in the human and mouse brain, let alone would get a buzz, was anyone's guess.

It took Dölen a few tries to get the dosing right, but then, with just a few days left before she had to return the octopuses to Woods Hole, she found the sweet spot. She uses words like "astonishing," "extraordinary," and "remarkable" to describe what happened next. After she diluted MDMA into the creature's tank, a tightly wound octopus visibly loosened up and began to perform what might be described as water ballet. It gracefully floated across the tank, ran its arms through streams of air bubbles and even undertook aquatic somersaults. Basically, it looked "like he was really just having a good time," Dölen said.

Most striking, though, was what the normally hermitic creature did with its tank mate. The experimental set up featured a central "neutral" area with two side chambers: one contained a control, a plastic figurine placed under a pot with holes large enough for the octopus to see inside, while the other held an identical pot beneath which sat a second, fully sober octopus. In control trials without MDMA, the free-range octopus stringently avoided the other cephalopod under the pot. In contrast, under the influence of MDMA, the drugged animal not only approached its tank mate, but also wrapped its body around the pot in an eight-armed embrace. It wasn't just a fluke, either: all of the octopuses tested with the same dose spent significantly more time in the chamber with their potted friend than they did when sober.

Dölen also analyzed data produced by other researchers who had sequenced the octopus genome to confirm that the cephalopods do possess the serotonin transporter proteins that serve as MDMA's primary binding site in humans and rodents. She and Edsinger likewise found the same conserved sequence of protein-coding amino acids in almost all species they looked at, including fruit flies, *C. elegans* worms, and naked mole rats. The fact that the serotonin binding site is conserved across species indicated that the neurotransmitter *does* do something in the octopus brain, and the behavioral findings indicated that that "something" includes social behaviors. Taken together, this suggests that serotonin's role in mediating social behaviors "must not only be a function of serotonin, but one of the oldest functions of serotonin," Dölen said.

The media went wild for the octopus study, published in 2018 in *Current Biology*, transforming Dölen into something of a folk hero in the psychedelics community. But most people missed the study's deeper point. Humans have traditionally tended to think of complex social behaviors as being unique to our species, or perhaps to certain "higher" species we deem to be enough like us to also qualify; as Dölen pointed out, the octopus study suggests that the molecular origins of the complex social behaviors that govern our lives trace back more than half a billion years, to well before vertebrates even arrived on the scene. By powerfully manipulating serotonin and other brain chemicals, MDMA apparently taps into something almost unfathomably ancient. "Even though the octopus brain is totally different than ours, even though they're not normally social outside of windows of reproduction, this molecule that they're never seen before and didn't evolve with is able to create out of nowhere this social function," Dölen said.

Put another way, the findings suggest that the specifics of human brain anatomy—the features that countless researchers have spent whole careers obsessing over—are just historical accidents, red herrings distracting them from figuring out what's actually driving cognition, behavior, and consciousness. Instead, it's the molecular level that we should be looking to for essential insights into who we are, where we come from, and what makes us tick.

\*

PRESERVED THROUGH THE expanse of evolutionary time, serotonin's fundamental role in mediating social behavior helped us become the species we are today, and even significantly contributed to our eventual dominant role on Earth. While most people would probably credit our unfettered planetary proliferation to our use of language, our capacity for abstract reasoning, or our nifty opposable thumbs, research now suggests that the primary factor behind our species' spread was our ability to work effectively in groups.

Our social natures originally evolved out of necessity. Early hominins living alone would have been vulnerable to predators and struggled to feed and care for themselves, so over time selection pressures created a biological basis for sticking together. This behavioral adaptation unto itself didn't make our particular species special or more adept at survival compared to other relatives, though. When *Homo sapiens* diverged from our closest ancestors two to three hundred thousand years ago, we shared the planet with at least four other human species, some of which had brains just as big or even bigger than our own, and all of which also lived in small groups, write Duke University evolutionary anthropologist Brian Hare and journalist Vanessa Woods in *Survival of the Friendliest*.

For millennia *Homo sapiens* maintained only modest populations and could have easily been the ones to go extinct—until we reached a tipping point about fifty thousand years ago, and our numbers began to explode. As Hare and Woods pointed out, it wasn't diet, culture, brain size, or technology that allowed us to suddenly pull ahead and thrive when other human species began to fail. It was because we evolved to become friendlier through a richer repertoire of social cognitive skills, including an ability to communicate and work together toward common goals not just with family and friends but also with people we'd never met before. This behavioral adaptation permitted us to expand from limited bands of ten to fifteen individuals to groups of a hundred or more.

As our communities became denser, innovation accelerated and allowed us to outcompete our closest relatives and conquer new environments, creating a positive feedback loop of population growth. But the newfound social skills that enabled our proliferation also came with another survival-based hitch: the uncomfortable feeling of loneliness, which scientists now know often precedes depression and anxiety. In the same way physical pain evolved as a protection against physical danger—the unpleasant sensation of burning your hand prompts you to remove it from a hot stove, for example— loneliness evolved to protect the individual from the danger of remaining isolated, as a cue to return to the group, write University of Chicago social neuroscientist John Cacioppo and science writer William Patrick in *Loneliness*; "feelings of loneliness told them when those protective bonds were endangered or deficient."

The neurological wiring that contributes to our biological need to feel a sense of love and belonging likewise stems from necessity—specifically, from the fact that, as infants, we cannot survive without social support. Evolution's answer to this basic requirement isn't something we just outgrow and shed along with our diapers. "The price for our species' success at connecting to a caregiver is a lifelong need to be liked and loved, and all the social pains that we experience that go along with this need," writes UCLA social neuroscientist Matthew Lieberman in *Social*.

By social pains, Lieberman means literal pain. Recent research has shown that the same regions of the brain's dorsal anterior cingulate that register physical pain are also those that light up when we experience emotional pain such as rejection. Like many forms of physical pain, if left unaddressed, social pain also carries the risk of very real repercussions to our health, including accelerating the aging process, advancing the progression of Alzheimer's disease, and even contributing to the chances of early death. A 2010 *Plos Medicine* review of multiple studies representing more than three hundred thousand people found that those who experience subpar interpersonal relationships suffered an increased risk of death equivalent to smoking fifteen cigarettes per day. Other studies similarly found that loneliness and disconnection from others bring health risks equivalent to being obese or having dangerously high blood pressure. Still more studies show that social isolation inhibits the immune system, promoting inflammation and increasing the likelihood of strokes and heart disease. The despair of loneliness can lead to suicide, and in some cases sufferers direct that urge outward, against society. "Think of all those lonely people quietly radicalizing in isolation," writes psychiatrist Julie Holland in *Good Chemistry*. "It's not a coincidence that mass shooters are invariably described as loners."

Being socially connected, on the other hand, delivers tangible benefits, including lowering depression and slowing the physical decline associated with aging. One study found that having a friend who you frequently hang out with is worth the well-being equivalent of making an extra hundred thousand dollars a year, while simply seeing a friendly neighbor on a regular basis equates to a sixty-thousand-dollar bonus. Putting these benefits another way, a 2010 meta-analysis of 148 studies found that social connection is associated with a 50 percent reduced risk of early death. "Regardless of one's sex, country or culture of origin, age or economic background, social connection is crucial to human development, health *and* survival," wrote a team of researchers in a 2017 paper calling on social connections to be made a public health priority. "The evidence supporting this contention is unequivocal."

Social connections had been undergoing a precipitous and worrying decline well before the forced isolation of the Covid-19 pandemic. Some scholars argue that this gradual unraveling was kicked off during the dawn of the industrial revolution; others, that it dates all the way back to the late Renaissance, with the rise of the Protestant Church and its emphasis on individual responsibility. Most agree, though, that over the past few decades, this trend has been accelerating. As Instagram, TikTok, Facebook, Snapchat, and various streaming services supplant genuine connections, isolated living takes the place of multigenerational homes, and concrete replaces nature, we risk "disrupting biology that's older than our love of fire," Dölen warned. "We're really messing with fundamental animal biology."

Evidence of these disruptions is all around us. In 1985, for example, social scientists asked people to list all the individuals they'd discussed important life matters with over the past six months, and most provided the researchers with three or more names. When the same survey was given in 2004, just 37 percent of people listed three or more names, and 25 percent listed zero names—a dismal figure that just 10 percent of people reported in 1985. Likewise, compared to just a few decades ago, we sign fewer petitions; belong to fewer in-person clubs and organizations; know fewer neighbors; and meet up less with friends and family, reported political scientist Robert Putnam in his now-classic book *Bowling Alone*. By 2016 the percentage of Americans who said they are lonely had doubled from 20 to 40 percent compared to the 1980s, and as of 2014 one in five U.S. adults was taking at least one drug for a psychiatric problem. Social disconnection, Putnam argued more than two decades ago, has rapidly become a defining feature of contemporary American life—and it's only getting worse.

There are myriad reasons for this, ranging from increasing numbers of people living alone to changes in work structures and growing inequality. Materialism encouraged by a consumer society is also a contributing factor—a problem that is exacerbated by the fact that, since the 1980s, major companies dealing in everything from apparel to automobiles have been refining marketing strategies that exploit people's desire for connection by selling the promise of "meaning, identification and an almost religious sense of belonging through association with their brand," writes Gabor Maté in *The Myth of Normal*. By promoting self-interested goals like consumption, competition, and financial success, materialism breeds higher levels of depression, anxiety, and substance abuse in those who align with this value system, and lower levels of happiness, connection, and life satisfaction. While dozens of studies now support the association between materialism and negative mental health outcomes, this isn't a new revelation. As journalist Johann Hari points out in *Lost Connections*, philosophers have been warning for thousands of years that people who overvalue money, possessions, and how they come across to others will be unhappy.

Even as it virtually binds us, technology, ironically, is also playing an increasingly significant role in eroding genuine connections. In particular, the widespread use of smartphones has "diminished the quality of interpersonal exchanges, so much so that the problem of being *alone together* has emerged as a meaningful cultural reference," researchers warned in 2017. In the West, people check their phones an average of once every six and a half minutes, Hari reported, and 42 percent of smartphone owners never turn their devices off at all. Social media accounts for much of the time people spend scrolling on their phones, and while it does bring some real benefits, it does not create the deep, meaningful connections that people naturally crave and need, according to Lieberman: "Social media ends up serving as a very temporary distraction or placeholder for that, but it doesn't really work."

Put another way, Hari writes, "being online and being physically among people . . . is a bit like the difference between pornography and sex: it addresses a basic itch, but it's never satisfying."

*

ONE GROUP OF people who are particularly at risk of missing out on social benefits—and who serve as a sort of canary in the coal mine for the insidious effects of increasing disconnection—are autistic individuals. Autistic adults are more likely to experience high levels of loneliness than their neurotypical peers. While 7 percent of the general adult U.S. population meets the diagnostic criteria for social anxiety disorder, one in four autistic adults do. Autistic people are also four times more likely to suffer from depression and eleven times more likely to have suicidal thoughts—problems that frequently both stem from and exacerbate social isolation—and they are 2.5 times as likely to die early. As Cacioppo and Patrick write, "When our negative social expectations elicit behaviors from others that validate our fears, the experience makes us even more likely to behave in self-protective ways that spin the feedback loop further and faster toward even more social isolation."

Despite the serious setbacks that many people on the spectrum face due to living in a society that discriminates against those who are different, social anxiety, loneliness, and lack of connection are not inevitable parts of being autistic. According to a 2022 meta-analysis of thirty-four scientific papers, autistic adults are less likely to be lonely if—somewhat obviously—they have relationships, experience fewer difficulties with social skills, and have positive views and acceptance of themselves. While there are many different ways to achieve these things, some autistics have gravitated toward a certain particularly potent molecular tool.

Aaron Paul Orsini grew up in the suburbs of Chicago, and as a teenager he remembers oscillating between being on the periphery of social gatherings and being "overly performative and needing to take over a situation." At parties or at professional conferences as a young adult, he'd often feel overwhelmed by the bombardment of incoming sensory information. While this may not sound like "the end of the world," he said, for someone trying to fit in socially or to advance professionally, "that's an ill-suited challenge to have."

When he was twenty-three, Aaron started seeing a psychologist for depression, anxiety, and what he described as "feeling that I would never 'get it,' and not really having any answers about how or why that might be." During one session the psychologist handed him a questionnaire to fill out without really explaining what it was for. After evaluating Aaron's answers, the psychologist announced that Aaron was autistic.

In some ways, this news came as a relief. Knowing that he was autistic provided Aaron with a new way to conceive of his specific challenges and potential strengths. Yet even with this revelation—and to his distress—his lifelong habit of focusing on his deficits and limitations proved stubbornly resilient to change. "Even though I could tell myself, 'Oh, I have superpowers,' I was still feeling down and feeling a bit like, for the rest of my life, I wouldn't be able to do things," he said.

When Aaron was twenty-seven, he experienced something of a quarter-life crisis and wound up on a train from Chicago to the West Coast with only a backpack in hand. He befriended a group of free-spirited fellow travelers who gave him a tab of LSD—a chance encounter that changed his life. Sitting on a tree stump in a forest, Aaron felt his mind go still; his awareness widened, and his sensory issues suddenly seemed manageable. The LSD also bestowed him with an ability to better read between the lines of social interactions and emotions in ways "I quite literally could never have imagined," he writes in *Autism on Acid*, a book he published in 2019.

Aaron discovered MDMA shortly after LSD, when he was invited to a gathering of artists, musicians, and other creative types. By this time he was an old hand at classic psychedelics, but MDMA was unique, he found, in that the experience never strayed beyond the realm of his own narrative, "with my ego fully intact," he said. "It was like taking a crystallized form of intuition."

MDMA's use as a tool for reducing social anxiety was also made clear to Aaron that night, when he sat down next to a stranger and unhesitatingly struck up a conversation. He felt comfortable, he found, not only chatting but also just being silent with the other person and enjoying the shared moment. "In that instance, I struggled to feel like I had a problem, and I struggled to feel like, if a problem came up, it would be bad," Aaron recalled. "Everything seemed endurable, just because of how much love I felt for being alive. And for the other people with me as well."

Aaron has taken MDMA around seven times since then, adhering to a general rule of giving himself at least three months in between sessions. "I've intentionally kept myself at a distance from something that can be so great," he noted. But even the handful of times he's tried it, he said, it "feels like a lot of learning," especially with regard to social situations. As he explained, "I've been able to witness myself being social, rather than just contemplate why I am socially anxious."

Aaron isn't the only autistic person to have serendipitously discovered MDMA's usefulness for overcoming social anxiety. "We're a diverse bunch, but one of the traits that seems to be fairly universal for us is how curiosity-driven we are," said Nick Walker, a professor of psychology at the California Institute of Integral Studies. "A lot of autistic people do end up experimenting with psychedelics," she added. "I've certainly encountered people in the autistic community who have said they'd gone to a party, done MDMA, and felt much more comfortable than usual."

In 2012 Walker was presented with an opportunity to dig more deeply into these intriguing anecdotal accounts when Alicia Danforth—then a clinician at the Lundquist Institute at Harbor-UCLA Medical Center, and a colleague of Charles Grob—reached out to her about collaborating. Danforth was also in communication with MAPS, which had received some funds from a donor earmarked for research on MDMA and autism. Based on published data showing that MDMA could increase empathy in typically developing individuals, the MAPS team had originally thought about carrying out a study to test whether MDMA could also help autistic people feel more empathy. Both Danforth and Walker pointed out that for autistic people, however, this was misguided. As Walker said, "It's starting from false premises that the autistic community has been pushing back against for a couple decades now."

Indeed, since autism became a diagnosis in 1943, mainstream psychology and academia have pathologized autism and cast autistic individuals as being emotionally deficient, including lacking in empathy. Those flawed assumptions spring in part from neurological and behavioral differences that can exist between autistic and nonautistic people, creating communication difficulties. Because neurotypical people are in the majority, though, misunderstandings have traditionally been blamed entirely on autistic people, Walker said, and autistics have also been expected to shoulder the full burden of trying to fit into a world not built by or for them. While a rising tide of autistic academics such as Walker are working to change this—as is the autistic community at large—for now the dominant discourse still treats autism as a disorder in need of curing.

Danforth is not autistic, but her PhD research includes an analysis of data she collected from autistic individuals who had used MDMA. The hundred accounts shared with her revealed a wide array of benefits people perceived from taking MDMA, such as increasing their courage, communication skills, and feelings of connection. Many people also reported lasting healing with regard to trauma and social anxiety. Given Danforth's dissertation findings and Walker's real-world experience, they proposed that MAPS pursue a study trying to address something that autistic people themselves tend to identify as a problem, and that MDMA seemed to have a high likelihood of being able to help with: social anxiety. While social anxiety isn't an intrinsic aspect of autism, Walker emphasized, it is "something a lot of autistic people have because they have a lifelong history of social rejection."

The twelve autistic adults who wound up taking part in the MAPS-sponsored double-blind, placebo-controlled study all had very severe social anxiety, and most also had a history of trauma—a common occurrence for autistic people. Working in an autism-friendly space that Walker helped design, Danforth and Grob oversaw two eight-hour therapy sessions with participants who were given either a placebo or MDMA (75 to 125 milligrams, sourced from the original David Nichols batch). During the active sessions, Danforth and Grob guided participants through various methods for exploring and communicating their feelings, including art therapy and the use of a deck of around fifty cards that visually depicted emotions. After each active treatment session, participants received daily phone calls for a week and three in-person integration meetings.

As Danforth, Walker, Grob, and their colleagues reported in 2018 in *Psychopharmacology*, at the end of the trial, participants who had received therapy paired with MDMA had significantly greater reduction in their social anxiety symptoms compared to those who had received therapy and a placebo. In a six-month follow-up after the sessions, the social anxiety scores for people in the MDMA group had either remained at the same lowered level or improved slightly—results, Walker said, that "fit our most optimistic hypothesis."

Berra Yazar-Klosinski, MAPS PBC's chief scientific officer and a coauthor on the social anxiety study, said she was most heartened to hear personal stories from participants about how their lives had improved in the months and years after the trial. One individual who initially presented with obesity lost eighty pounds after treatment; another moved out from their parents' house, got married, and had kids; and another joined a soccer club and finished their college degree. One participant even attended a scientific conference with Danforth and gave a presentation about their experience in the trial. "The fact that this person went from having severe social anxiety to talking onstage is amazing," said Yazar-Klosinski, who has a brother on the autism spectrum. "It's really those kinds of events that are the true measure of improvement."

\*

AARON ALREADY CREDITS MDMA and other psychedelics with dramatically changing and improving his life. After his book came out, and as he continued to post about his experiences online, he began receiving more and more emails from other autistic people looking to compare notes and share their own stories about psychedelics. In response, in 2020 Aaron cofounded the Autistic Psychedelic Community, an online group for people interested in the intersection of psychedelics and neurodivergence. The group sponsors weekly Sunday Zoom discussions that have attracted some eighteen hundred attendees, including people from as far away as Australia, Kenya, and Israel. Around four thousand people have participated on the group's messaging forums, and Aaron also maintains an "Autistic Psychedelic Wiki" of peer-reviewed literature pertaining to psychedelics and autism. While education is important, Aaron's main goal, he said, "is really bringing autistics together to accept one another and to demonstrate radical acceptance outwardly, because most of us are acclimated to radical rejection."

Aaron is now collaborating as a coinvestigator with researchers at University College London to conduct a qualitative survey with autistic people about their use of psychedelics, and he is also working on an audio documentary on the same topic. Relatedly, in 2021 he published *Autistic Psychedelic*, a compilation of community essays and survey responses. Some of the stories people shared provided anecdotal support for the research findings about social anxiety and MDMA, and mirrored Aaron's own experiences. Shae, for example, described herself as a twenty-seven-year-old who thinks in colors, shapes, and sounds rather than words. When she tried MDMA, she said, she experienced "effortless and fluid verbal communication" for the first time in her life. Suzanne, a thirty-two-year-old who also has ADHD, wrote that MDMA made her feel "seen and understood by my neurotypical friends in a way that I hadn't experienced previously and vice versa. I learned more about actively listening to other people and that at the end of the day, neurodivergent and neurotypical people both want to connect, to be understood, and to love and be loved."

The valuable lessons MDMA can impart about communication, connection, and acceptance can apply just as well to people who are not on the spectrum, too. My neurotypical friend John Allison, for example, is the type of guy who isn't afraid to go to a bar by himself on a Friday night, because he knows he can just start a conversation with whoever is sitting next to him. He wasn't always like this, though. John described himself as being "not that well socially calibrated" growing up in Arkansas—a wallflower at parties and the quiet kid at school. "I wanted to be social and be able to make more friends, to have better connections and have a good time with other people," he said. "But I didn't really know how to get out of my shell."

As he got older John pushed himself to be more outgoing, but he still frequently felt anxious and awkward, especially in groups. When he was thirty-four, however, he tried Molly for the first time at a warehouse somewhere in Brooklyn and "just exploded," he said. "I could talk to anyone and express myself in ways I hadn't been able to before, and I could empathize more openly with strangers. I was surprised at how many different conversations I had, and how well they went. It was something I'd been trying to do, but I didn't know how to do it until Molly just brought it out of me." After the Molly-induced "jolt" to John's system, he started making a point of trying to access that version of himself in his sober life. When he did, he found that he got the same positive reactions from friends and strangers alike. As these experiences built, so too did John's confidence. Today, his practiced friendliness comes across as effortless and natural.

MDMA seems to be an especially effective tool for facilitating communication and overcoming social anxiety, Lieberman said, because it "resets your expectations about other people and the reaction you're going to get from them." The drug also changes how people express and respond to emotions, a feature that researchers think could help them identify the fundamental components of meaningful connection. "We can use MDMA as a tool to bottle that sense of deep, instant connection and study it in the lab, and also as a tool to directly improve people's lives," said Sonja Lyubomirsky, a social psychologist at UC Riverside who specializes in happiness. In 2022 Lyubomirsky published a paper proposing a new field of study, psychedelic social psychology, that would incorporate psychoactive substances like MDMA into research investigating topics varying from how to foster a connection to nature to how to reduce prejudice and intergroup conflict. This "exciting new frontier" is only in its infancy, Lyubomirsky wrote to her colleagues, and she fully expects "an avalanche of ideas for relevant research questions and paradigms to emerge."

Studies have already shown, for example, that individuals on MDMA are slower to pick up on angry facial expressions, but that they react with extra enthusiasm to happy expressions. The drug also lowers fear of being judged or rejected, freeing people up to experiment with different modes of interacting. There are hints that these lab-based findings might translate for some MDMA users into real-life gains. According to a 2023 analysis of data collected from 214,505 U.S. adults for the National Survey on Drug Use and Health, people who have taken MDMA at least once in their lives, compared to those who have never taken the drug, have lower odds of difficulty interacting with strangers; of difficulty engaging in social activities such as visiting with friends or going to parties; and of being prevented from being social due to a mental health issue. "A lot of social anxiety is about the idea of, if I put myself out there, I will be shamed, humiliated, and judged, and that's terrifying to think about," Lieberman said. "MDMA can move the needle on that by allowing you to have different experiences than you typically do." In best cases, he added, the drug can help "transform your understanding of yourself, the world, and your relationship to it, and give you new beliefs moving forward."

*

WHILE MDMA ON its own cannot fix societal-level drivers of loneliness and disconnection, on an individual basis it can make a difference. In certain cases, the drug may even be able to help people see through the fog of discrimination and fear that divides so many of us and is the cause of so much suffering today. MDMA does not seem to be able to magically rid people of prejudice, bigotry, or hate on its own. But some researchers have begun to wonder if it could be an effective tool for pushing people who are already somehow primed to reconsider their ideology toward a new way of seeing things.

Harriet de Wit, a professor of psychiatry and behavioral science at the University of Chicago, witnessed this potential application for MDMA firsthand—and completely by accident. It was February 2020, and de Wit was running an experiment on whether MDMA increased the pleasantness of social touch in healthy volunteers. The day was proceeding like any other Tuesday when Mike Bremmer, de Wit's research assistant, appeared at her office door with a concerned look on his face. The latest participant in the double-blind trial, a man named Brendan, had filled out a standard questionnaire at the end. Strangely, at the very bottom of the form, Brendan had written in bold letters: "This experience has helped me sort out a debilitating personal issue. Google my name. I now know what I need to do."

Seeing this cryptic message, both Bremmer and de Wit were worried. "We really have to look into this," de Wit said. They googled Brendan's name, and up popped a disturbing revelation: until just a couple of months before, Brendan had been the leader of the Midwest faction of Identity Evropa, a notorious white nationalist group rebranded in 2019 as the American Identity Movement. Two months earlier, members of Chicago Antifascist Action had exposed Brendan's identity, and he had lost his job.

De Wit was now very worried. She'd just given a drug to a disgraced white supremacist, she realized, and had apparently inspired him to do who knows what out in the world. "Go ask him what he means by 'I now know what I need to do,' " she instructed Bremmer. "If it's a matter of him picking up an automatic rifle or something, we have to intervene."

A murderous spree turned out to be the opposite of what Brendan had in mind. As he clarified to Bremmer, love is what he had just realized he had to do. "Love is the most important thing," he told the baffled research assistant. "Nothing matters without love."

When de Wit recounted this story to me nearly two years after the fact, she still could hardly believe it. "Isn't that amazing?" she said. "It's what everyone says about this damn drug, that it makes people feel love. To think that a drug could change somebody's beliefs and thoughts without any expectations—it's mind-boggling."

I wanted to hear more about what happened directly from the horse's mouth, so in December 2021 I paid Brendan a visit (he asked that his last name not be revealed, as he's trying to distance himself from his past). As I rode the elevator up to his apartment in a luxury high-rise overlooking Lake Michigan, I felt a flutter of nervousness. I was unsure of what kind of person I would be meeting, and had even half-jokingly texted a couple of friends to let them know where to come looking for me in case I disappeared. What I didn't expect was how ordinary the thirty-one-year-old who answered the door would appear to be: blue plaid button-up shirt, neatly cropped hair, and a friendly smile. After politely hanging up my coat, he explained that, back when he was a white nationalist leader, cultivating an air of ordinariness had been exactly the point. "I really wanted it to be for guys making a good amount of money, who are educated and who could feel comfortable joining these sorts of communities," he said. "I wanted to normalize it."

Brendan grew up in an affluent Chicago suburb in an Irish Catholic family. He leaned liberal in high school but got sucked into white nationalism at the University of Illinois Urbana-Champaign, where he joined a fraternity mostly composed of conservative Republican men, began reading antisemitic conspiracy books, and fell down a rabbit hole of racist, sexist content online. Brendan was further emboldened by the dehumanizing rhetoric Donald Trump used in his campaign and subsequent election to president. "His speech talking about Mexicans being rapists, the fixation on the border wall and deporting everyone, the Muslim ban—I didn't really get white nationalism until Trump started running for president," Brendan said.

Brendan joined Identity Evropa to connect with others who shared his views. He attended the notorious "Unite the Right" rally in Charlottesville and quickly rose up the ranks of his organization, first becoming the coordinator for Illinois and then the entire Midwest. He traveled to Europe and around the United States to meet other white nationalist groups, with the ultimate goal of taking the movement mainstream.

Brendan likely would have continued in this vein were it not for S., who asked me not to reveal his name to protect his identity as an antifascist activist. S. came to the States in the early 1990s as a three-year-old refugee whose family had fled the genocide in Bosnia. He grew up on stories of the massacres, ethnic cleansing, and wider crimes against humanity that devastated his country and claimed the lives of family, friends, and relatives. So when Trump rose to power on a platform of racist, nationalist rhetoric that turbocharged white supremacy groups, S. felt a sense of déjà vu. "I know what that did to my own country, what it looked like and the ramifications it entailed," he said.

S. felt he had to do something, so he began tracking and exposing members of white nationalist groups. He and his comrades revealed the names of more than a hundred people in Identity Evropa, but Brendan's identity was especially difficult to crack. S. wound up going undercover as someone who wanted to join the group. He posed as a Serbian nationalist, a member of the faction that had perpetrated the genocide in Bosnia; during the intense interview process, he had to improvise when Brendan brought along a real Serbian to grill him, in Serbian. Meeting the guy "threw me for quite a loop," S. said. "He started asking me questions about the war, and it became very emotional for me, but I tried to stick to the character as much as I could."

Once S. finally figured out who Brendan was, he and his colleagues released a dox containing, among other things, screenshots of Brendan's homophobic and misogynistic tweets; photos of his family's home; a list of his co-workers; and screenshots of him interviewing S. at his workplace. Brendan was immediately fired from his job and ostracized by his siblings and friends outside white nationalism.

When Brendan saw a Facebook ad in early 2020 for some sort of drug trial at the University of Chicago, he decided to apply just to have something to do and to earn a little money. At one of the visits, he was given a pill. He didn't know it, but he'd just taken 110 milligrams of MDMA from David Nichols's original batch. At the time, Brendan was "still in the denial stage" following his dox, he said. He was racked with regret—not over his bigoted views, which he still held, but over the missteps that had landed him in this predicament.

About thirty minutes after taking the pill, he started to feel peculiar. "Wait a second—why am I doing this? Why am I thinking this way?" he began to wonder. "Why did I ever think it was okay to jeopardize relationships with just about everyone in my life?"

Just then, Bremmer came to collect Brendan to start the experiment. Brendan slid into an MRI, and Bremmer started tickling his forearm with a brush and asked him to rate how pleasant it felt. "I noticed it was making me happier—the experience of the touch," Brendan recalled. "I started progressively rating it higher and higher." As he relished in the pleasurable feeling, a single, powerful word popped into his mind: *connection*.

It suddenly seemed so obvious: connections with other people were all that mattered. "This is stuff you can't really put into words, but it was so profound," Brendan said. "I conceived of my relationships with other people not as distinct boundaries with distinct entities, but more as we-are-all-one. I realized I'd been fixated on stuff that doesn't really matter, and is just so messed up, and that I'd been totally missing the point. I hadn't been soaking up the joy that life has to offer."

That night Brendan reached out to Chicago Antifascist Action and connected with S. "He messaged me via email months after the dox went live to say he was going through a trial at the University of Chicago for MDMA, and that he now understood why I did the things I did: because of radical love," S. said. "I was like, 'Well, yes, Brendan, this is kind of why I do the things I do!' "

At first, S. was skeptical when Brendan claimed that MDMA had made him want to prioritize connecting with other people above all else. But he was heartened when Brendan started taking steps that seemed to indicate his sincere commitment to change. Brendan hired a diversity, equity, and inclusion consultant, enrolled in therapy, began meditating, and started working his way through a list of educational books. S. still regularly communicates with Brendan and, for his part, thinks that Brendan is serious in his efforts to change. "It's been a couple years we've been working together, trying to disconnect him from things that were harmful and reconnect him with positive reinforcement and get him ideologically educated," S. said. "I think he is trying to better himself and work on himself, and I do think that experience with MDMA had an impact on him. It's been a touchstone for growth, and over time, I think, the reflection on that experience has had a greater impact on him than necessarily the experience itself."

Brendan is still struggling, though, to make the connections with others that he craves. When I visited him, he'd just spent Thanksgiving alone. He also has not completely abandoned his bigoted ideology, and is not sure that will ever be possible. He voted for Trump in 2020, and is still in touch with a few people from the movement. "There are moments when I have racist or antisemitic thoughts, definitely," he said. "But now I can recognize that those kinds of thought patterns are harming me more than anyone else."

\*

WHILE BRENDAN'S EXPERIENCE is outside the norm, it's not without precedent. In the 1980s, for example, an acquaintance of early MDMA-assisted therapy practitioner Requa Greer administered the drug to a pilot who had grown up in a racist home and had inherited those views. The pilot had always accepted his bigoted way of thinking as being a normal, accurate reflection of the way things were. MDMA, however, "gave him a clear vision that unexamined racism was both wrong and mean," Greer said.

Rare as they might be, stories such as these are worth examining for the implications they give about MDMA's potential ability to "influence a person's values and priorities," as de Wit and several coauthors wrote in a case study they published about Brendan in 2021 in *Biological Psychiatry*. If "extremist views [are] fueled by fear, anger and cognitive biases," the researchers posed, "might these be targets of pharmacological intervention?"

Encouraging stories of seemingly spontaneous change appear to be exceptions to the norm, however, and from a neurological point of view, this makes sense. Research shows that oxytocin—one of the key hormones that MDMA triggers neurons to release—drives a "tend and defend" response across the animal kingdom. The same oxytocin that causes a mother bear to nurture her newborn, for example, also fuels her rage when she perceives a threat to her cub, reported Hare and Woods. In people, oxytocin likewise strengthens caregiving tendencies toward liked members of a person's in-group and strangers perceived to belong to the same group, but it increases hostility toward individuals from disliked groups. In a 2010 study published in *Science*, for example, men who inhaled oxytocin were three times more likely to donate money to members of their team in an economic game, as well as more likely to harshly punish competing players for not donating enough.

Gül Dölen's findings about the critical period likewise indicate that without the proper set and setting, MDMA probably will not have a revelatory effect for ridding someone of bigoted beliefs. Anecdotal reports indicate that some members of the Taliban, for example, use MDMA to channel a connection to the divine during prayer chants. In the West, plenty of members of right-wing authoritarian political movements, including neo-Nazi groups, also have track records of taking MDMA and other psychedelics. This suggests, researchers write, that psychedelics are nonspecific, "politically pluripotent" amplifiers of whatever is going on in somebody's head, with no particular directional leaning "on the axes of conservatism-liberalism or authoritarianism-egalitarianism." So while people sometimes half-joke about spiking Donald Trump's Diet Coke with MDMA to make him more empathetic and compassionate toward humanity, there's no scientific or real-world basis to expect this kind of miraculous conversion to occur.

"Without the right context, all that would do is make Trump love people who love him more, and hate those who hate him more," Dölen said. "If you open that window of metaplasticity and you just think of things that reaffirm what you already believe to be true beforehand, then you haven't changed anything. You've just made those connections and pathways that much stronger."

Put another way by an interviewee in the 1994 ethnography of MDMA users, *Pursuit of Ecstasy*, "If you give this drug to shallow assholes, they will continue to be shallow assholes. They're not going to get any better."

That said, a growing body of scientific evidence indicates that the human capacity for compassion, kindness, empathy, gratitude, altruism, fairness, trust, and cooperation are core features of our natures and among the strongest of our behavioral tendencies—stronger than distrust, tribalism, and violence. If MDMA, with proper preparation, can nudge us toward embracing this natural state of being, then the idea of using the drug as an aid to help make the world a more loving, less hateful place may be more than just a pipe dream. As Emory University primatologist Frans de Waal wrote, "Empathy is the one weapon in the human repertoire that can rid us of the curse of xenophobia."

Natalie Ginsberg, MAPS's global impact officer, remembers standing next to the Washington Monument in D.C. at the Catharsis Festival right after the 2016 election, talking with Rick Doblin at one or two in the morning about the possibility of using MDMA to facilitate a dialogue between Republicans and Democrats. Ginsberg also envisions using the drug in workshops aimed at eliminating racism, or as a means of bringing people together from opposite sides of shared cultural histories to help heal intergenerational trauma. "I think all psychedelics have a role to play, but I think MDMA has a particularly key role because you're both expanded and present, heart-open and really able to listen in a new way," Ginsberg said. "That's something really powerful."

"If you give MDMA to hard-core haters on each side of an issue, I don't think it'll do a lot of good," Doblin added. "But if you start with open-minded people on both sides, then I think it can work. You can improve communications and build empathy between groups, and help people be more capable of analyzing the world from a more balanced perspective rather than from fear-based, anxiety-based distrust."

In 2021 Ginsberg and Doblin were coauthors on a study led by Leor Roseman at Imperial College London investigating the possibility of using ayahuasca in group contexts to bridge divides between Palestinians and Israelis, with positive findings. They hope to undertake a similar study using MDMA in the future. In the meantime, some informal underground groups of Israeli and Palestinian individuals have already started taking MDMA together, not with the overt purpose of conflict resolution and peace building but to harness serotonin's ancient role in mediating social behavior—specifically, that is, to encourage connection, spiritual growth, and healing.

MDMA is not going to end war, bigotry, and polarization any more than it will permanently transform antisocial octopuses into social butterflies. But there could be a role for it and other psychedelics to play to help people better see each other as fellow human beings. "I kind of have a fantasy that maybe as we get more reacquainted with psychedelics, there could be group-based experiences that build community resiliency and are intentionally oriented toward breaking down barriers between people, having people see things from other perspectives and detribalizing our society," said psychiatrist Franklin King at Massachusetts General Hospital and Harvard Medical School. "But that's not going to happen on its own. It would have to be intentional, and—if it happens—it would probably take multiple generations."

Based on his experience with extremism, Brendan agreed with expert takes that no drug, on its own, will spontaneously change the minds of white supremacists or end political conflict in the United States. "A lot of these guys who end up in these movements have a history of doing MDMA," he pointed out. But he does think that, with the right framing and mindset, MDMA could be useful for people who are already at least somewhat open to reconsidering their ideologies, just as it was for him. "It helped me see things in a different way that no amount of therapy or antiracist literature ever would have done," he said. "I really think it was a breakthrough experience."

# DESTIGMATIZATION

TUESDAY EVENINGS IN January are hardly big go-out nights, even in New York City. But on this particular Tuesday, a crowd of scientists, doctors, students, writers, tech bros, therapists, nerds, and others have packed the seats at Caveat, a cabaret-style theater in the Lower East Side that specializes in "smart entertainment." At seven o'clock sharp Sarah Rose Siskind, a tall blond with a penchant for bodybuilding, strides onto the stage to cheers and applause. "Thank you guys so much for coming out tonight, I do this show just so I can meet all of you people and pretend that I have friends," Siskind cracks. "I'm here to give you the deal about drugs—your drug dealer, if you will."

Siskind is a professional science comedian, and she's here tonight to present her latest installment of *Drug Test*, a show literally and figuratively on drugs, as she puts it. There's very little (if anything) Siskind won't do in service of drug education, or to win a few laughs. She's shown videos of herself running an ultramarathon on LSD, talking with her parents about her use of psychedelics, and undergoing a very intense ketamine infusion. To kick off tonight's show, she'll be inviting the crowd to participate in a game of Guess That Drug. She'll show a video clip of a VIP ("very inebriated person"), and the audience's job is to guess which drug the person is on.

The VIP tonight is a white-haired man named Paul who works in the artificial intelligence field. Sitting on a big gray couch with Siskind, the still-sober

Paul preps viewers for what they are about to see. "If there's anyone watching this or in the audience that is considering doing a drug," Paul says, "I'm glad that I'm helping demystify it."

A cut to three hours later shows Paul still calmly sitting on the couch, but now he is receiving a shoulder rub from Siskind. His eyes are closed and he is smiling. "I'm happy to go along—I'm just a leaf bobbing along the river of life," he says, his voice registering pure bliss. The video cuts again to clips of the two of them performing a series of experiments to test their coordination—assembling a puzzle, walking in a straight line, playing the piano—and Siskind taking measurements of Paul's temperature, heart rate, and pupil size.

The video ends, and Siskind pops back on stage. "I don't know if you guys could tell he was on drugs at all—but he was!" she says, grinning. But what drug *was* Paul on? Pulling up a PowerPoint, Siskind reviews a list of his symptoms:

- Faster HR
- Sweaty palms
- Dilated pupils
- No hallucinations
- No loss of coordination
- No lost reaction time
- Highly focused (on tasks other than what he was asked to do)

Honing in on the answer, one audience member asks if Paul drank a lot of water (he did); another asks if he was grinding his teeth (he was not). Yet another wonders if hugs felt very good (they did). The answer, of course, is MDMA. "You all get an A!" Siskind says, tossing Pop Rocks into the crowd over a blaring soundtrack of Tyga's "Molly."

Comedy comes naturally to Siskind. She grew up in a family where "the hierarchy was who's the funniest," she said, and she practiced comedy writing throughout college. After developing the specialized skill set needed to make science humorous yet accurate, she even served a stint as head comedy writer for Neil deGrasse Tyson. Drug-based comedy is something she stumbled into by accident, though, following a harrowing close call at Burning Man in 2018 that wasn't funny at all.

Siskind had been dealing with a dark bout of depression and had read somewhere that MDMA could help with PTSD, so she figured maybe it could help shake her out of her funk. She still wasn't feeling anything an hour after taking the drug, though, so a random Russian guy she'd just met on the playa gave her something he claimed would help it work. The booster he gave her turned out to be a mix of fentanyl and PCP, and Siskind wound up collapsing on a heap of bicycles and being taken to the hospital.

When Siskind came to, she was livid at the Russian man for almost killing her. But when she learned that he had taken the same nearly deadly concoction and had also had a close call, her anger dissipated. This experience hammered home for her that it's ignorance, not malice, that so often causes problems among drug users.

Siskind returned to New York City determined to do her part to help close the education gap on drugs—not just about minimizing their risks, but also about the politics, history, culture, pharmacology, and science surrounding them. As a comedian, Siskind knew that she could do this in a uniquely entertaining way. And she also knew she'd have more leeway in talking openly about drugs than others who might fear blowback from employers or society at large. "I can get more real, I can talk about my experience, and I don't have to censor myself," she told me. "Also, as a white lady, I haven't felt as intense a fear of incarceration or baggage from stereotypes like others have."

Even so, creating a wildly popular show that openly discusses illegal drug use—not to mention one that frequently shows videos of the host under the influence of said drugs—would have been inconceivable a few short years ago. Now, it's just another weekday night in the psychedelic renaissance. Taking a closer look at the cultural transformation that has brought us to this point can shine a light on just how far we've come, and how much further we still have to go.

*

WHEN I WAS interviewing experts in 2021 and the first half of 2022 about what they see as the key challenges for moving MDMA-assisted therapy forward and for coming up with more sensible approaches to drug policy and use in general, the word *destigmatization* frequently came up. People mentioned the stubborn resilience of the Ecstasy-causing-holes-in-the-brain myth, and even lingering 1960s-era bias against psychedelics.

The zeitgeist is shifting fast, though, and much of this comes down to communication. People like Siskind are helping to normalize conversations about banned substances, as well as educate the public about the science behind them. This includes not just disseminating new research findings, but also talking about drug taking itself in an honest, nonalarmist way. Scientists and mental health practitioners themselves are also helping this process along by increasingly coming out of the closet about trying or regularly using the drugs they study. Carl Hart at Columbia University is the most outspoken example of this, having written an entire book on the subject and urging fellow middle-class drug takers to stop concealing their use in order to effect societal-level positive change. Others agree with this strategy. "I believe, just like Harvey Milk, that if everyone who had ever benefited from a psychedelic stood up and said this, it would completely change drug policy and turn the tide," said psychiatrist and author Julie Holland. "If you want to be less oppressed, you have to stand up and out yourself."

More and more scientists are following Hart, Holland, and others' brave lead. While quite a few still demurred when I asked them about their use of MDMA, others were comfortable discussing it. "I used to have this line when the media would ask me that: 'Damned if I have, and damned if I haven't!' " said Charles Grob at Harbor-UCLA Medical Center. His thinking at the time, he said, was that if he hadn't tried MDMA, he could be accused of leading trial participants into a terrain he had never explored himself. Yet if he had tried the drug, his objectivity as a scientist could be questioned. That was twenty years ago, though, and "I think the world is a lot more receptive to hearing about people's firsthand accounts," Grob said. "At this point, I'd rather just be straightforward and open. It's like, why not?"

"Obviously, if you're going to devote your life to researching something, don't you think you would have tried it?" Holland added. "That 'I can neither confirm nor deny' adds to the stigma and shame."

It's understandable that some scientists may be hesitant about discussing their experiences openly, though, because some have faced very real repercussions for doing so, including relatively recently. In December 2017 psychiatrist Will Siu gave a presentation to doctors and scientists at NYU, where

274 I FEEL LOVE

he'd recently been hired as a junior faculty member. Siu was talking about MDMA-assisted therapy for PTSD, and rather than just present the standard data from the clinical trials, he spoke about his own experience undergoing the treatment as part of MAPS's training program for clinicians. He told the audience about viscerally revisiting the childhood memory of his father beating him with a belt, and of sitting in his room afterward, crying, feeling the welts on his body, and repeating over and over to himself, "Nobody loves me." He described how MDMA-assisted therapy had allowed him to identify these early experiences as the driver behind the loneliness he'd felt his entire life, and his need to overcompensate through academic excellence.

The talk seemed to be well received—quite a few people approached Siu afterward, and some had even been moved to tears. But when the department chair later called him into her office, Siu instinctively knew he was in trouble. The chair hadn't attended the talk, but she'd heard about it. "In twenty years, I have never had this many faculty tell me that a talk made them uncomfortable," she sternly reprimanded him.

"What's wrong with uncomfortable?" he ventured.

"It's inappropriate," the chair snapped back. Siu tried to defend himself, but she cut him off. "If you want to keep your job, you won't talk about your personal life in public," she said, and then slid a piece of paper across her desk. It was an official agreement stating that he'd keep such things to himself in the future.

"I signed, because I knew I was leaving," Siu said. As painful and disappointing as the experience at NYU was, it made him realize that he did not want to be part of a system built on a framework of suppression—suppression of patients' emotions by papering them over with pharmaceuticals, and suppression of uncomfortable truths from the doctors who treat them. "It's like the medical system has turned emotions into symptoms into diagnoses," Siu said. Instead of seeing emotions as normal human experiences, he continued, they're pathologized as something wrong to be gotten rid of, "thereby actually perpetuating the original state."

Recognizing this, Siu is now in private practice in Los Angeles and has dedicated his career to educating clients, fellow mental health practitioners, and society at large about the importance of emotional vulnerability and compassion in healing ourselves and our communities.

Siu's honesty about his experience with MDMA-assisted therapy perhaps would be met with less fear and hostility today. Universities are quickly coming around to psychedelic-based science and medicine, driven in large part because of student enthusiasm. "The interest is huge," said Charles Raison, a professor of psychiatry at the University of Wisconsin–Madison. At the 2021 Horizons conference, Raison estimated that 15 percent of current students planning to pursue a career in mental health express a specific interest in psychedelic medicine. "Every week, I get multiple emails from undergrads saying 'How can I get involved? How can I get involved?'" Raison said. "I see it from undergraduates all the way up through psychiatry residents."

Matthew Johnson at Johns Hopkins concurred: "Up until recently, people who ended up in psychedelics research kind of had to be a little bit of professional risk takers. That's gone now. Every year, there seems to be an order of magnitude more young people interested."

The sea change in demand has triggered the launch of new academic centers dedicated to basic and clinical psychedelic research, including at UC Berkeley and at Massachusetts General Hospital, the teaching hospital of Harvard Medical School. Major professional groups are also taking note. In late 2021 the American Psychiatric Association, for example, invited Holland and Rick Doblin to give a talk at their annual conference about "the psychedelic revolution in psychiatry," as the organizers put it. "I framed that letter and put it on my desk," Holland said. "It was a big validation of everything we've been talking about for thirty years now."

Yet another major landmark arrived in October 2021, when the NIH—breaking a fifty-year dry spell—issued its first grant in support of therapeutic psychedelic research, for a study Johnson is leading on psilocybin's use in treating tobacco addiction. Scientists think it's only a matter of time before the NIH issues a grant for MDMA. Psychedelic research- and therapy-related legislation has also passed in several states, even including Texas, which adopted a bill in June 2021 that supports the study of "alternative therapies" like MDMA to treat PTSD, depression, anxiety, bipolar disorder, chronic pain, and migraines. "What's happening now is just kind of amazing, especially to those of us who were around in the early 1980s," said Debby Harlow, Doblin's former codirector at Earth Metabolic Design Laboratories.

"Nobody really thought that psychedelic research would get off the ground the way it is now. I just hope the kids and younger researchers doing it now are having as much fun as we did."

In the clinical realm, a growing number of practitioners are also looking to psychedelic-assisted therapy as means to bring about a long-overdue shakeup of mental health care, both practically and culturally. "The embrace from the mental health community was at first puzzling and surprising," said journalist and author Michael Pollan. When Pollan published *How to Change Your Mind* in 2018, he expected to receive pushback from the psychiatric establishment. Instead, he was invited to give talks at psychiatric hospitals and at the headquarters of the American Psychological Association. "I came to understand it as a sign of their desperation for new tools," he said.

"Broken" is the word Thomas Insel, the former NIH director and author of *Healing: Our Path from Mental Illness to Mental Health*, uses to describe mental health care today. More people are on pharmaceutical drugs than ever before, yet serious mental health problems ranging from addiction to suicide are on the rise, and the treatment approach that psychiatry has developed over the past several decades has not worked. "The model we've had, which is the wrong model, has been infectious disease," Insel said. "It's built on an assumption that the cause is a simple bug, and the cure is a simple drug. That's a beautiful model for developing antibiotics or antiviral compounds, but it's irrelevant to what mental illness is, which is far more complicated."

The focus, too, has problematically become "all about reimbursement for hours spent, and not reimbursement for outcomes and progress," Insel continued. Care has also become fractured. A patient may see a psychiatrist for fifteen minutes to get prescribed medications, and if they have a therapist at all, their therapist may or may not be in contact with the psychiatrist—who likewise isn't in touch with their acupuncturist or family counselor. "All these people work independently, and the patients end up on kind of an assembly line, bouncing around," said psychiatrist and retired Brigadier General Stephen Xenakis.

Because of the way MDMA-assisted therapy breaks down the silos between psychiatry, psychology, and counseling—and because of how it helps a patient proactively address the root of what ails them rather than just dulling symptoms with pills—Insel, Xenakis, and others think its adoption could wind up transforming the entire field. "It fosters coordination and integration of medication and talk therapy," Xenakis said. MDMA-assisted therapy also opens up the possibility of bypassing focus on a particular "bug"—PTSD or social anxiety, for example—by working with the person's entire life experience. "This is the essence of healing—engaging the whole person beyond targeting treatments for a specific diagnosis," Xenakis said. "I think it is a game-changer, frankly."

This could happen quickly, because if and when MDMA-assisted therapy is approved by the FDA to treat PTSD, doctors will be able to start applying the treatment to other conditions through a commonly used legal loophole called off-label prescribing. According to the Agency for Healthcare Research and Quality, one in five prescriptions written in general in the United States today is for off-label use. "MAPS cannot advertise or promote off-label use because of regulatory requirements for the FDA, and whether there will be off-label use for people not diagnosed with PTSD is an open question," said Ismail Ali, director of policy and advocacy at MAPS. "But based on other trends in psychiatry, I think it's likely."

Ideally, MDMA- and other psychedelic-assisted therapy would eventually become just one available tool in a revamped, "integrative" approach—that is, mental health care that considers a suite of factors like diet, sleep, exercise, supplements, technology, and more to address the true drivers of a patient's problem. There are some signs that this shift is underway. "Inside of conventional settings, there are still people in psychiatry who don't even think of gut health or diet as a frame of reference," said Will Van Derveer, a psychiatrist in Niwot, Colorado, and cofounder of the Integrative Psychiatry Institute. "But I've also been approached by training directors at universities who want us to teach their psychiatry residents integrative medical approaches to resolving the root causes of symptoms. It's a quiet revolution that's happening in the background of global mental health care."

Another major cultural shift is occurring at the intersection of science and policy. More than a hundred U.S. cities and counties have decriminalized or are considering decriminalizing personal possession of certain drugs, and in 2020 Oregon voted for state-wide decriminalization for possession of small amounts of nearly all drugs. While the war-on-drugs approach prevails at the federal level, on the local level more and more voters are signaling their desire for change. And in instituting these changes, they're communicating to researchers that it's okay to acknowledge the political implications of their work and findings—something that the scientific establishment has previously been reluctant to do.

MAPS is one exception. At Doblin's insistence, the group has always been committed to broader drug policy reform and has not shied away from these discussions, even when doing so was unpopular and potentially counterproductive in the near term. For years, though, others in the psychedelic science sphere went to great lengths to distance themselves from any taint of talk about legalization of banned substances. Ethan Nadelmann, founder of the antiprohibition Drug Policy Alliance, recalled being invited to speak at the MAPS conference in San Jose in 2010—only to be disinvited when a couple of leading psilocybin researchers told Doblin they would not attend if Nadelmann was a speaker. The researchers were afraid that any association with advocacy would harm their chances of getting government funding. A few years later, the two psilocybin researchers again demanded that Nadelmann be excluded from the latest conference, and Doblin once again had to disinvite him. "I love Rick, so I accepted it," Nadelmann said. "But I felt embarrassed for him, torn between principle and accommodating the b.s. irrational fears of people he needed."

In 2017 the two researchers tried pulling the same stunt yet again, but this time Doblin put his foot down and told them that Nadelmann was coming. The conference ran smoothly, of course, and there were no negative repercussions from having scientists and policy advocates in the same room together. And to everyone's advantage, the situation has continued to improve since then.

"There's still fears, but people are relaxing and having more sophisticated conversations about the relationships between scientific research and the FDA approval route, on the one hand, and on the other the decriminalization of psychedelics via the political process through local and state ballot initiatives and legislation," Nadelmann said. There's also more talk about the ways in which psychedelics reform needs to be part and parcel of broader drug policy reform in the interest of social justice. "People increasingly get that there's something wrong about celebrating the psychedelic renaissance while a hundred thousand people a year are dying from fatal overdoses, mostly involving fentanyl, and hundreds of thousands of Americans are still being incarcerated for nonviolent drug offenses."

*

IN ALL THE MDMA-related talk about therapy and healing, science and policy, one thing that often gets glossed over or even looked down upon is drug taking for the sake of drug taking—that is, for partying and having a good time. "There's been a lot of sweeping under the rug of the culture of MDMA in favor of only discussing its value in medical contexts," said Kevin Balktick of Horizons. "It's come to overshadow the entire discussion in a way I think is unfair."

This isn't surprising or new. While mainstream Western society readily accepts taking a drug for medical reasons, doing so for pleasure has always been taboo—"except, of course, if the drug happens to be nicotine or alcohol," noted the British writer Nicholas Saunders. Harkening back to the friction between recreational and therapeutic MDMA users in the 1980s, some people within the community are calling for the drug to remain strictly in the realm of what they deem to be more lofty pursuits, such as personal growth. "There's this notion of, 'Oh, it must be justified! You need to be using it in a ceremony or for therapeutic use or for some medical application,'" said Keeper Trout, an independent scholar and author in Northern California. "I'd ask, why? How and when and where did recreation become a bad thing?"

Recreational use of MDMA today is vast and diverse, encompassing a global group of individuals who are far more varied than the stereotypical white college student attending an EDM festival. Vanja Palmers, for example, is a Zen priest in Switzerland who usually uses MDMA for meditation and for spending contemplative time in nature. But the last time he did the drug was at a party, and he considers this to be "a totally legitimate use," he said. "It can definitely be an ecstatic dancing experience."

MDMA is recreationally consumed in countries as disparate as South Africa, India, and Kazakhstan. In China, it's called "head-rocking pills," and in Afghanistan it's also a popular party drug, although not in the same sense as in the Western world. "Usually, Ecstasy is for friends gathering around the fire inside the house on a Friday night, drinking lots of tea and just chatting, laughing, crying, and sharing their feelings," said Murtaza Majeed, a drug rights activist in Kabul. "It's like a support group. It's interesting to see, because it's completely different than in the West."

MDMA has gained popularity among more varied demographic groups in the United States as well. In 2013, for example, Irina Aleksander reported for the *New York Times* about Molly being given out to party guests "at the elegant home" of a fiftysomething socialite in Brooklyn's Park Slope neighborhood. "MDMA has found a new following in a generation of conscientious professionals who have never been to a rave and who are known for making careful choices in regard to their food, coffee and clothing," Aleksander wrote.

While some people prefer to take their MDMA at Brooklyn brownstones, others opt for hip-hop clubs, where the drug has been taken up by Black users—a new cultural phenomenon. "I'm Black, a bunch of my friends are Black, but growing up in Miami, MDMA wasn't really a drug I heard much about, it just wasn't on our radar," said Khary Rigg, an associate professor of addiction research at the University of South Florida. "I associated it with white kids from suburbia, ravers, and gay men."

Around 2013 Rigg's interest was piqued, however, when he heard Miley Cyrus singing about "dancing with Molly" and put two and two together that this was the new name for Ecstasy. After making that connection, he suddenly felt like he was hearing the word "Molly" in every other song on the radio, including ones by Jay-Z, Kanye West, Lil Wayne, and French Montana. "It was like, 'Wait, he just said Molly! And this entire song is devoted to Molly!'" Rigg recalled.

MDMA had clearly penetrated hip-hop culture, which made Rigg suspect that it probably had also been taken up by Black users. When Rigg looked into the scientific literature, however, he found that it focused almost exclusively on white people, so he decided to fill that gap with research of his own. He secured a small grant and "basically, went out to bars and clubs in the Tampa Bay area and recruited for my study."

Confirming Rigg's hypothesis, 82 percent of one hundred Black heterosexual Molly users he surveyed cited hip-hop culture as influential in their decision to use the drug. In in-depth interviews with fifteen of the respondents about their motivations for taking Molly, ten mentioned using the drug to enhance their sex life, and eleven talked about taking it in conjunction with marijuana. Regardless of users' motivations, though, none said anything negative about Molly. "It was always, 'This drug is amazing!' " Rigg said.

Through this research, Rigg came to see MDMA as "one of the most fascinating drugs that's out there," he said, and he hoped to continue investigating how Black Americans are using it. But after his initial funding ran out, he struggled to find support for further studies. "The truth is, people aren't dying en masse because of MDMA, so no one's going to give me a million-dollar grant to look at MDMA use," he said. This is unfortunate, he added, because "it's important to do research on specific subgroups so we know what's going on—especially subgroups that have been ignored historically."

It's not just subgroups that are being ignored. Relatively little research or attention is directed toward recreational MDMA use at all, including among people who attend dance music festivals and raves. Balktick sees this as a major oversight. "The largest single population of Ecstasy users is probably still young people in music-focused environments, and for many of them, these are among their most treasured and beautiful life experiences," he said. "I think that deserves real attention."

There are people working to change this. Michelle Lhooq, a drugs and nightlife journalist in Los Angeles and author of *Weed: Everything You Want to Know but Are Always Too Stoned to Ask*, has devoted her career to shining a light on this important group of users through nuanced, compassionate, and enviably well-written coverage from the frontlines of the recreational drug world. Parties, festivals, and raves "are the places where people are actually viscerally experiencing these drugs and experimenting with them on their own terms," Lhooq pointed out. "Giving proper weight to the drug experiences of ravers matters because due to prohibition's curtailing of scientific research and clinical studies, personal testimonies from transformative dance floor experiences on MDMA have formed the bulwark of the collective wisdom around this drug for generations. Ravers have been, in effect, guinea pigs for both the promises and potential harms of MDMA-assisted healing."

Mainstream conversations that separate medical versus recreational use of psychedelics actually create false dichotomies, she added, because nonclinical use of MDMA and the attendant pleasure that accompanies it *does* have a strong healing potential. "That MDMA can only be administered in a clinical setting, under the supervision of two licensed therapists, in order to be 'legitimate,' I think leaves out a lot of people who want to use this substance with their friends or partners in environments that are comfortable to them—whether that's at home, in bed, or on a dance floor."

Lhooq grew up in Singapore, where drug laws are some of the harshest in the world and include mandatory death sentences for anyone convicted of trafficking even modest amounts of banned substances, including cannabis. "I don't think it's a coincidence that I come from Singapore and am obsessed with drugs," Lhooq said. "People who are the most repressed become the most obsessed."

Lhooq moved to New York City in 2007 for school and found herself transported "from my very traditional, strict Asian upbringing" into the heart of underground Kandi Kid culture. Nightlife, she learned, "is a place where pleasure is centered and not shameful"—and she loved it. On the dance floor, trading candy bracelets and hugs, she learned to find kinship with strangers and to trust and be open with friends in a way that she'd never experienced before. She developed a rave family, many of whom were lost or marginalized youths on the fringes of mainstream society. Ecstasy, of course, was an integral part of the formula for any night out.

"People interested in rave culture are also interested in drugs because the impulse is the same: a desire for extreme experiences and intensity," Lhooq said. "A lot of people are also predisposed to challenging mainstream frameworks of right and wrong, and of having visceral experiences that may be pleasurable or healing."

Lhooq has come to see raves as, at the most superficial level, a "release valve to capitalism"—a chance for weekend warriors to briefly escape the constraints of the nine-to-five crunch and express themselves on the dance floor. But raves can also serve more hallowed roles, including as spaces where oppression is lifted and where people who do not count themselves among the majority can find belonging. For some, the dance floor can also satisfy a craving for spirituality and ritual that's largely lacking in contemporary times. "Raves are this ancient tradition that have been modernized with software and things, but fundamentally, you're taking a substance and transcending into this communal realm with shamans or guides—DJs—who help you access that realm with music," Lhooq said. "That's the ultimate thing people are looking for, whether they know it or not."

Lhooq's assessment is in line with scholarship on this topic. In a 1979 paper, for example, social scientists described Grateful Dead and other rock concerts as being "one of the most popular and spectacular 'rituals of controlled drug use.' " Concert attendees turn to mind-altering drugs for "a closer communion with the performers," the researchers wrote, and to allow "the self to be more compellingly affected by the rhythms and imagery of the music and lyrics."

Researchers examined this observation from a biological point of view in 2008 by giving rats MDMA or a placebo and then exposing them to either music, white noise, or no added sound. Allison Feduccia, the lead author of the study and cofounder and CEO of Psychedelic Support, chose to expose the rodents to euphoric house—and by the end of the study, she said, "everyone hated that CD." But the rats on MDMA seemed to have enjoyed it. They had significantly higher levels of serotonin and dopamine in their nucleus accumbens than did rats that had been given a placebo or that had not been provided music to listen to while rolling.

Rats cannot tell researchers if the synergy of pleasure produced by pairing MDMA and music also inspires in them a sense of mysticism or oneness with other rats. But ravers can. In a 2021 study of 481 Brits who had attended a rave within the past five years, researchers found that those who took a classic psychedelic or MDMA and spent time dancing at the event were more likely to say that they experienced a sense of awe, and that awe, in turn, was associated with finding the experience to be personally transformative. Those who experienced awe were also more likely to report a strong sense of connection with others on the dance floor. According to lead author Martha Newson, a cognitive anthropologist at the University of Kent, the findings suggest that raves are just modern versions of what humans have been doing for at least tens of thousands of years: coming together for ritualized, nocturnal dancing and drug taking to promote social bonding. "Raves are an Indigenous practice, and that's not a misappropriation of the word," Newson said. "They're a grassroots response to the cultural need to fill this ritual gap."

Lhooq, like many hard-core ravers, wound up getting burned out on MDMA after a few years, and even became disillusioned with the drug for a while. Her original rave family drifted apart, and many of them wound up developing substance use problems with other drugs. Lhooq has most recently been experimenting with sobriety at parties, but in the past couple of years, she's also reevaluated her stance on MDMA. In 2021, for example, she attended the Electric Daisy Carnival in Las Vegas, and although she wasn't rolling, she was surrounded by people who were. "It was contagious," she said. "What I found to be so humbling was the complete innocence and childlike joy that people were able to experience. There's a lot of power in emotional healing and in not seeing the heart space as inferior, and that's what MDMA's about."

Lhooq will be keeping a close eye on, and chronicling through her work, how the recreational landscape changes after MDMA-assisted therapy presumably gains approval and as decriminalization and even legalization of the drug possibly follow. While greater accessibility might lessen some of MDMA's counterculture clout, Lhooq doesn't think the drug will ever be considered "uncool," no matter how normalized it becomes. "Being cool, to me, means genuinely caring about yourself and your community," Lhooq said. "So if anything, MDMA might become more cool in that sense of the word."

## 14
# FELLOW TRAVELERS

WILL MDMA SAVE the world?

Obviously, the answer is no. But I posed this somewhat tongue-in-cheek question as a closer in my interviews with dozens of sources, because it is worth considering how things could play out if MDMA becomes available not just as a therapeutic aid for specific maladies but also for well people's use. What might happen, in other words, if Rick Doblin's nearly forty-year-old plan—dreamed up one night on the beach at Big Sur—was finally realized?

Doblin, for one, has not wavered from this original goal. By 2035 he hopes to see licensed legalization of MDMA for adult use, and by 2050 he envisions the drug helping to usher in a "spiritualized humanity"—one that recognizes and celebrates commonalities and connection, and acts accordingly. "So many of the problems of the world today are mental. It's not that we lack technology to solve them, but just that we lack the will," Doblin said. "Psychedelics could help people deal with big issues like climate change, racism, and war by showing us how much we have in common, and by shaking us out of inaction."

In talking with various sources, I was surprised to find that quite a few see Doblin's vision for MDMA-assisted mass mental health not as a whimsical fantasy but as something nearing an imperative. Some, too, are not waiting for the rest of society to catch up. Through their underground efforts, they're creating a blueprint for what might come to pass, should we choose to make MDMA available to everyone.

*

THE SKY WAS hazy with smoke from nearby wildfires the day I met neurobiology professor David Presti at his home in Berkeley to talk about psychedelics' use for healing, learning, and growth. "As many of us now see, if we don't start doing something, we're not going to have a world we like living in," Presti told me over a cup of Darjeeling tea. This increasingly unavoidable observation is taking a toll. "Folks are way more in touch with existential anxiety now than they were twenty-five years ago," Presti said. "The nineteen-year-olds in my classes, they're scared."

Teaching is one tool Presti uses on a daily basis to try to broaden conversations and move humanity to a better place in terms of behavior, values, and ethics. He considers MDMA and other psychedelics to be potential means of working toward the same goal. Psychedelics can help people realize how interdependent we are on each other and on the planet for survival, he said. They can also bring back an element of spirituality, mysticism, and curiosity about the nature of the mind that's missing from Western culture's current worldview, which tends to disregard or dismiss what it can't understand scientifically, materially, and (ostensibly) objectively.

"That worldview has taken us very far in certain ways, but it's also bringing us to the brink of destruction of our planet because it has taken the sentience out of nature and supported an illusion of control and a process of exploitation," Presti said. "I think the conversation between science, religion, and psychedelics is one of the single most important engagements we can cultivate, in part because there are many reasons suggesting that only a radical expansion of our scientific paradigm will allow us to more deeply understand the role of mind in nature."

Poet and author Nicholas Powers, on the other hand, prefers to leave religion out of the equation. He views the magical or supernatural thinking that sometimes accompanies drug trips as a dead end or, at worst, a potential danger. "If you start thinking you're getting personal messages from Huitzilopochtli, Thor, Jesus, or Aphrodite, you may act out in very irresponsible ways," he said. "I think the emphasis should be that you're getting a message from your own unconscious."

To Powers, one of the greatest utilities of mind-altering drugs is their ability to serve as the metaphorical hot water to dissolve the psychological glue trapping us within the larger machine of capitalist society. Psychedelic drugs can help us break free of what Plato called the noble lie: that from birth until death, we are shackled to predefined roles based on external factors such as gender, race, socioeconomic status, or family history. "Psychedelics could literally pour acid on these attachments and help people transcend to get a larger view of themselves," Powers said. "The poor can realize they can let go of painting watercolors on their scar tissue, and the rich can dissolve some of their golden chains and realize they're the ones locking themselves into cages. Possibly, I think psychedelics could help us take a detour around the implicit 'us vs. them' narrative, regardless of what side you're on."

Psychedelics, Powers continued, can also reveal to people that the things assigned the greatest value in a modern capitalist society—wealth, status, and the "conveyor belt of materialism"—have in fact left us spiritually bereft, and that their pursuit has wrecked our planetary home in the process. "I think psyche-delics offer at least a possibility of trying to liberate people in a way that doesn't always depend on a militant class struggle that ends in civil war," Powers said. "That's a very utopian socialist path—and I want to acknowledge that that may not work—but sometimes social forces combine in ways that things that didn't seem possible before may have a brief window of possibility."

A crucial first step for enacting societal-level changes, though, is for people simply to feel better about themselves and others—for them not just to be free from infirmity but to enjoy *health*, what the World Health Organization's 1948 constitution defined as a state of "complete physical, mental and social well-being." If someone's well-being is compromised, it's unlikely that they'll have the energy or motivation to invest in improving things around them. "People tend to think they're not worth saving, and then extrapolate that to the world," said Berra Yazar-Klosinski at MAPS PBC. "They think, 'Why should I extend my narrow runway of life to saving the planet?'"

Especially in the wake of the Covid-19 pandemic, "a lot of people have come to realize how unnatural their lives feel," added Gül Dölen at Johns Hopkins. "More and more of them are asking, how do I restore my connection to others, how do I restore my connection to nature, how do I restore my connection to the world? If we want to return to a more natural way of existing, we may have to reset, return, and relearn."

Put another way by John Cacioppo and William Patrick in *Loneliness*, "the warmth of genuine connection frees our minds to focus on whatever challenges lie before us."

MDMA and other psychedelics are a potential tool for doing just that, and the personal transformations they usher in could, once again, result in much-needed global change if applied broadly enough. "It certainly feels like society needs a reorientation of just kind of paying attention to simple things, like what do I want out of life, what does all of this mean?" said Franklin King at Massachusetts General Hospital and Harvard Medical School. "Psychedelic drugs offer a window into accessing this stuff, and a lot of people, myself included, hope that they can be brought back into society in a way that goes beyond the mental health sphere."

Powers imagines a future in which psychedelic centers are established around the world, catering to people of varied backgrounds. After visiting such a center, clients would be put in touch with others who have gone through the same process. "You'd become part of something larger, so you don't feel these insights are things you have to squeeze back into the default world," Powers said. "People can integrate and join larger organizations and then cross-pollinate."

Presti sees such transformation, applied across populations, as a means "of deepening our connections and capacities to heal one another and the planet." In *The Immortality Key*, Brian Muraresku—pointing to evidence from ancient Greece—even goes so far as to wonder whether a society robbed of the mystical experience of psychedelics is one that is fundamentally flawed, its institutions lacking the shared vision that kept the world's first democracy afloat, its citizens unable to remember how to care for themselves, each other, and nature.

Transforming the world through psychedelics wouldn't necessarily require everyone getting high, though. "We know that when people have a profound psychedelic experience, it doesn't just change the way they feel—their loved ones also report that they interact with them differently," said Shelby Hartman, cofounder and editor in chief of *DoubleBlind*. "So conceivably, it would just need to happen on a large enough scale to change culture and how we regard one another." That said, she added, "all the MDMA in the world won't make a difference if many folks are still struggling to have their basic needs met, such as health care and housing."

In some places, and among some social circles, these changes are already quietly transpiring. I visited the leader of one such movement, a composer, musician, and former professor who asked me to call him Sebastian, at his New York City apartment, which he shares with some 350 musical instruments. Sebastian was first introduced to what he calls "supplements"— MDMA, LSD, magic mushrooms, and other psychedelics—around twenty-five years ago, and he found that they helped him work through the trauma of a childhood marred by years of violent civil war in his home country. "When I tried MDMA, it was incredible," he said. "The deep sense of compassion, of empathy, of the weight being lifted off me—MDMA is very deeply healing."

It's not just the drugs, though, that produce the healing effect. Through Sebastian's personal psychedelic explorations and field research conducted in more than forty countries, he came to see sound as being just as important as the supplements themselves, if not more so. "In the end, it's about harmony and acoustics," he said. "That's the reason why all shamanic and religious ceremonies always have sound or music. We're programmed to intuitively, subconsciously seek music to create an experience to unravel consciousness."

After fine-tuning his own use of sound and supplements for healing and growth—and after seeing others using psychedelics in what he considered to be flippant, ignorant, or even harmful ways—Sebastian decided to create a sound-based program he could share. "I became interested in bringing this to people because of compassion and empathy, and because of love," he said. Sebastian has spent the last two-plus decades perfecting the program, which he considers to be his life's work. He hosts both solo and group experiences, the latter of which can number up to one hundred attendees but usually average about twenty people.

Typically, the group experiences take place across several days, frequently in upstate New York but also sometimes in other states or countries. To get everyone on the same page, Sebastian begins with a keynote presentation that delves into Eastern philosophy, musical phenomenology, spirituality, consciousness, shamanism, psychedelic research, meditation, sound, and even quantum physics. He explains how he believes the various elements of sound, supplements, and the subconscious combine to allow people the opportunity to reevaluate their own narratives, let go of unhealthy emotions, and seek answers to existential questions. He also talks about responsible and safe use of the drugs, and preps attendees for what's coming. "A powerful tool needs a lot of knowledge, mastery, attention, and awareness to make it more effective," Sebastian explained. "Otherwise, it can cause more damage."

The morning after the lecture, the group members take their supplements—usually, MDMA and mushrooms—together in a safe, quiet setting. Everyone starts with a small dose and has the option of taking boosters, depending on how deep they wish to go. Sebastian does not speak much during the experience, noting that "a good facilitator is one who knows how to get out of the way." What he does do, though, is play an array of instruments with harmonic overtones, such as singing bowls, gongs, and bells, to assist the work people are doing internally.

"I don't call them medicine songs, and I don't have a power—I'm not a shaman," Sebastian clarified. "What I humbly believe is going on is that the experience is empowering the individual to tap into the self-healing capacity we all have inside us, the embodied knowledge of the heart that comes from within—what the Greeks called gnosis, or the Tibetan Buddhists call vidyā."

Michael Pollack, a former Wall Street executive and NYU professor turned social entrepreneur, credits Sebastian for helping him get over PTSD caused by surviving the 2008 terrorist attack on the Taj Mahal Hotel in Mumbai. Michael tried traditional talk therapy for close to a decade, but "there were just walls and barriers that I'd keep hitting," he said. "I'd become very attached to this weight that was pulling me down, to this impossible debt I felt obligated to pay for making it out when others didn't."

After a disastrous experience with underground psychedelic therapy—the licensed clinician he was working with gave him methamphetamine instead of MDMA—Michael found Sebastian. He's met with Sebastian eight times since 2018, first using MDMA and mushrooms together, and more recently just taking mushrooms on their own. Michael no longer has a diagnosis of PTSD and now uses the biannual sessions as a way to check in on how he's living and to remind himself of certain core truths, such as the inevitability of death and the connectedness of everyone and everything. Sebastian's music permits him to explore these fundamentals head on rather than retreat back into his ego, Michael said. "Music shapes the sound waves of the room, and when it's in perfect harmony, your body is vibrating with it and it enables you to go to a different place. It's not about the drugs—they're just an opening into oneself. It's about how deep you can go inside yourself with complete attentional focus on the sound."

Sebastian said he has guided some twenty-one thousand people over the years, including politicians, royalty, Hollywood stars, and leaders in tech, finance, art, and higher education. He has taught his method to hundreds of trainees, and he and his colleagues—who include leading researchers and psychiatrists—plan to take his work aboveground when they deem "the time to be right," as Sebastian put it. He ultimately hopes that experiences such as the ones he guides can help get us out of the reductionist, materialistic corner we've backed ourselves into as a species. "We're creating technology that's alienating us from ourselves, from our hearts, and from each other, and we have become the perfect parasitic force on the earth," he said. "We think that this is the best we can do, but we have blind spots galore. This is what happens when we're suffering."

*

AT NOON SHARP on the Saturday of Memorial Day weekend 2022, forty-four people gathered at a penthouse apartment in Williamsburg, Brooklyn, for a very special rooftop party. Some arrived with blankets, flowers, fruit, chips, and chewing gum; others pitched in with bubble wands, candy bracelets, and Tums. One person brought her little white dog; another, his healing crystals. Most were coming from various neighborhoods in New York City, but a few had traveled from as far as Rhode Island and Pittsburgh. Some of them had been friends for decades; others were strangers to all but the hosts. By the time the sun set that evening, though, all would share a special bond forged by a day spent doing MDMA together.

The event was organized by Charley and Shelley Wininger, a couple who may at first seem like unlikely hosts for large drug parties. Charley, seventy-three, is a licensed psychoanalyst and mental health counselor with a white goatee and curious eyes that beam out from behind black-framed glasses. Shelley, seventy-one, is a retired critical care nurse who is quick to smile and wears her gray hair bobbed, with a flare of pink in the front. They may look like innocuous grandparents, but for two decades Charley and Shelley have been figureheads in the New York City psychedelics community.

The Winingers' events—usually held in Prospect Park, but sometimes in private apartments when the weather doesn't cooperate—are attended by novices and veteran psychonauts alike. Several people at Heart in the Apartment, as they called their 2022 party, had never tried MDMA at all, or had not done it in years. One woman noted that she was looking forward to taking MDMA for the first time in four decades; another couple had only ever used the drug at home with each other as a relationship enhancer, and were excited to try it in a larger group setting. Some had come to get in touch with parts of themselves that were usually inaccessible, while others hoped to make new friends or take "a little vacation," as one woman put it. Attendees were as diverse generationally as they were in their intentions, ranging from twenty-two to seventy-five years of age. "I just want to celebrate the fact that we *can* be together again," one of the oldest participants declared. "I just want to celebrate today!"

Charley opened the event with a few ground rules. First and foremost, while attendees were welcome to share stories about the experience with whomever they wanted, he said, the names of those present were "only our business." He also reminded everyone to respect each other's boundaries, including asking for permission before hugging someone or attempting to comfort someone who might appear to be in distress. "They might need to cry, they might need to be alone, they might need to be upset," he pointed out. The final rule was a request to refrain from any other substances, including alcohol and marijuana, until the event was officially closed in an evening ceremony. "We find that the pure MDMA for the day is the best way to make this work," he said.

With the formalities out of the way, it was time to get the party started. Everyone took out their capsules and held them up in open palms. Another longtime attendee, Rich Orloff (who granted his permission to be named in this book), invited the group to take three deep breaths, and then said a short opening prayer that he had written:

I welcome you into my body and soul.

I welcome your teachings

your inspirations

your healings

And I welcome my self—all parts of myself that may rise
and visit me during this journey.

I welcome the place where I connect to more
than just the me I already know.

I welcome the place where I connect to others
and to a divine place I may not be able to define
but which I am open to knowing.

I invite all of me to participate in this journey.

And I welcome and bless my fellow travelers on this journey.

Then Orloff chanted, in Hebrew, the Shehecheyanu, a Jewish prayer that
marks meaningful occasions. He translated:

We give thanks to the Divine (however we define that)
for giving us life,
for sustaining us,
and for bringing us to this special moment.

And let us say, Amen.

"Amen," the group echoed, and everyone downed their pills.

The Winingers found both each other and MDMA somewhat late in life.
Charley was not a novice to drugs in general, though. As an active member
in the 1960s counterculture, he'd tried LSD many times back in the day. "We
loved calling it acid because it helped us burn through all the b.s.," he said.
"We would trip and look around us and realize not only just how sick and
warped society and culture was, but how ridiculous it was."

As time marched on, Charley watched in dismay, however, as many of his fellow former hippies turned more politically conservative and denigrated their years of activism and psychedelic drug taking as youthful folly. Charley bounced around between various jobs, from cabdriver to financial- and IT-sector recruiter, and for a while he developed a problematic relationship with cocaine. He felt like he was squandering his time and talents, and contributing nothing meaningful to the world. In 1989 he finally found his true calling as a psychotherapist. But his marriage to his first wife began to collapse around the same time, and he struggled to find a relationship of any substance in the aftermath.

Shelley, on the other hand, grew up in a "nice Jewish family," as she put it, and never did drugs. She recalled being offered a joint once at a party when she was nineteen and fleeing in terror. She enrolled in nursing school right out of high school and pursued a rewarding forty-year career. When she was forty-eight, however, she realized she was no longer happy in her eighteen-year marriage. She filed for a divorce, moved out, and got a cat. "That was it, you know, I was going to be the cat lady," she said. "Or the cat nurse."

Shelley and Charley met in 2000 at a lecture Charley was giving about relationships. Charley was smitten with "this cute and curvy lady," as he described his first impression of Shelley, and wound up calling her after she left her name and number on a sign-up sheet he'd passed around. After confirming that she wasn't going to be taking any more of his workshops or hiring him as a therapist, he asked her out. The relationship was going splendidly when, one night, a few months into dating, Shelley began detailing all the places she wanted to go and the things she wanted to try now that she was liberated from her former marriage. One of those things, she told Charley, was Ecstasy.

Charley had tried MDMA a few times before and wasn't that impressed, but he was happy to oblige Shelley. And he soon found out that, with her, it was totally different. The first time they did it, Shelley jubilantly ran naked through the warm summer rain at a friend's secluded upstate home, and the two spent the rest of the evening reveling in the world and each other.

Shelley and Charley have since taken MDMA together seventy-five times and counting, including at raves, botanic gardens, spas, music festivals, and in the bedroom ("We add a bit of cannabis and call it 'sextasy,' " Charley quipped). The best remedy for burnout, they've found, is to "stop, drop, and roll"—a strategy that grants them a rejuvenating chemical vacation from life's and aging's drudgeries. All told, MDMA adds an additional layer of indescribably scrumptious icing on an already happy relationship. "Every day we tell each other how grateful we are for each other," Shelley said. "Never in my wildest dreams did I expect my life to be like this after the age of fifty."

Charley and Shelley are judicious about their use of MDMA, taking it just a few times a year. "Otherwise, at our age, we'd be knocked on our asses," Charley noted. But they incorporate the lessons learned while rolling into their daily sober life, including about the importance of slowing down to savor the moment while there's still a moment to be had. As the years have passed, MDMA has helped to show the Winingers firsthand that vitality, wonder, and play are not things reserved only for the young. "MDMA is the antidote to feeling old: we become ageless for a day," Charley said. "It reminds me that society's view about aging as a decline does not serve me."

Their life as a couple has been further enriched by a community they've built of like-minded friends and acquaintances, all of whom share an interest in psychedelic substances. The group comes together at drug-free winter potlucks the couple have hosted at their home in Kensington, Brooklyn, since 2004, and at the annual "spring rolls" they've organized for the past twelve years.

For older people, these events provide a chance to connect with others their age who also enjoy getting high—a rare opportunity for some, given the taboo nature of drug taking. For younger attendees, they're an opportunity to benefit from the wisdom of those who have lived through different times. For everyone, they're a precious chance to mingle across generations and backgrounds, resulting "in new friendships and professional connections as we all continue to 'find the others,' " as Charley put it in the 2022 Heart in the Apartment invite.

Among those in the know, Charley and Shelley are well established "roll models," as they like to say, for recreational drug use in life's golden years. In 2020, though, they publicly came out of the chemical closet with the publication of *Listening to Ecstasy*, a book Charley authored about how MDMA helped him to become a better husband, therapist, and person. Writing the book was not an obvious decision. As a child of the 1960s, Charley had always been worried about getting busted and ostracized for drug use, and the couple had also been concerned about jeopardizing Shelley's job. Yet as he got older, Charley felt more compelled to share his experiences with MDMA. "I felt like this chemical was speaking to me, presenting a whole curriculum, and over time it was having a cumulative effect," he said. "I started realizing it was changing me in a very benign, gentle but profound way, and like a lot of psychonauts, I wanted to tell the world. Plus, I'm too old to not be everything I am, to hide who I am."

After Shelley retired, the couple agreed that the time was finally right. For Charley, writing the book became an opportunity to work through his internalized shame about drug use, and also to make a meaningful contribution to the cultural movement away from the war on drugs. Most important of all, though, he wanted his story to show people, especially fellow baby boomers, that there is hope in this time of hatred and chaos, and that MDMA can be a window through which to find meaning and optimism for the future. "I want them to know there is—however 'out there' it appears—a way home," he wrote. "One we can all have now, if we but find the gumption to claim it—in the name of each other, our children and of all living beings today and especially tomorrow."

Charley, like others, stresses that MDMA is not an absolute antidote to suffering, nor is it a replacement for the societal-level transformations needed to address things like global warming and inequity. But as he also notes, "extraordinary times call for extraordinary pleasures." If a critical mass of people begin thinking and acting in new ways, then that, in turn, could alter the world for the better. "MDMA helps me feel what it would be like to embody a better future, along with some of the boldness we'll all need to build one," Charley wrote. "Having a change of heart is the heart of change."

In 2021 Shelley was given a profound glimpse of what a more loving and compassionate future could look like when her thirty-nine-year-old son, Scott, unexpectedly died. The news arrived just nine days before the annual spring roll she and Charley were organizing, but she did not consider canceling. "I knew I had to go more than ever," she told me six weeks after it happened, her green eyes glistening.

It was a beautiful May day when Shelley and Charley arrived at their traditional spot at the park, and they were soon joined by forty friends. Shelley had shared with the group ahead of time about what had happened to Scott and had requested a healing circle. As it turned out, she wasn't alone in her grief. Another friend had lost his mom just days earlier, and two others had lost their sister and father in the year prior.

Someone had brought along a framed photo of Scott, and Shelley began to cry in a way she hadn't permitted herself to since his death. She felt hands gently touching her as the sobs shook her body, and when she finally looked up, she saw something remarkable: rows upon rows of her friends all around her, heads bowed and hands touching the shoulder of the person ahead of them. The group's loving energy was flowing directly into Shelley and everyone else there who needed it. "To know I wasn't alone, I wasn't alone," Shelley recounted, dabbing her eyes with Charley's handkerchief. "The MDMA allowed me to completely let out all that grief, and let in all that love and peace. That's when my healing began."

A year later, Shelley is still carrying that moment with her and still feels healed. At Heart in the Apartment, she paid that energy forward to other guests who joined a healing circle and shared the tragedies, challenges, and road bumps they'd experienced over the last year. Others chose to sit out that optional gathering, instead taking quiet time in different rooms, relaxing and chatting on colorful lawn chairs on the roof, or dancing barefoot to a mix of disco tunes. Numbers were exchanged, future plans were made, and new friendships were forged. As the sun set over Manhattan, casting the sky in shades of orange and gold, the group came together in a circle for one last silent ceremony, a Heart Wheel—a rotating chain through which each person wordlessly expressed gratitude to the person across from them with hugs, laughter, beaming smiles, and a few tears.

No one knew what the coming year would bring. But everyone in attendance could be sure, at least, that a community of both strangers and friends would be ready to commiserate and celebrate with them next spring. And that across their life's journey, should they choose, MDMA would be there to help them along the way.

# ACKNOWLEDGMENTS

Thanks, first and foremost, go to my agent, Jane Dystel, and to my editor, Ben Hyman, for believing in this project, and for believing in me.

This book would not have been possible without the many sources who generously shared their stories, insights, and time. In particular, thanks go to Rick Doblin, who, no matter how busy, always made himself available to assist with stray questions and difficult-to-find facts or email addresses; Gül Dölen, for being an early supporter of this book idea and for patiently getting me up to speed on all things neuroscience on numerous lengthy Zoom calls; David Carlson, for his generosity in sharing documents, notes, and contacts; Matthew Baggott, for being game to answer random questions I threw his way; Carina Leveriza-Franz, for a wonderful hike in Sedona; Sarah Rose Siskind, for the inside scoop on the who's who of drug culture; and Charley and Shelley Wininger, for welcoming me into their community. Special thanks also go to Wendy Tucker for making an interview with her mom possible; Emanuel Sferios for introducing me to Carl and Judith; and Paul Daley for a personal tour and chemistry lesson in Sasha's lab. Thank you, too, to Stephanie Schmitz at Purdue University for giving me a tutorial on how archives work, encouraging my visit, and helping me find resources I wouldn't have even known to ask for, and to Megan Mann at the U.S. District Court for the Middle District of Florida for assisting in tracking down case files nearly three decades old. Thanks are also due to all the experts who helped ensure my facts and language were straight, especially Bahar Gholipour, Graham Lee Brewer, and David Nichols. For help wrangling citations, my thanks go to Leah Foreman, Emily Carmichael, and Alejandra Arevalo.

Thank you, too, to the entire Bloomsbury team for a smooth and thorough production process.

I'm grateful, too, to all my friends in New York City, London, and Berlin for the group hugs and all-night dance sessions over the years that laid the foundations for this book. Special shout-outs go to Nathan Oglesby for an early brainstorming session and for keeping my classics in order; to Ryan Trekell for the inside scoop on Mormons and drugs; to Danielle Venton for her ever-encouraging Word Count Wednesdays; and to Amelia Nuwer and Camden Rouben for support when a veterinary crisis threatened to derail book writing. Thank you, Kit, for being my steadfast and loving writing companion through one final project; you will forever be my small orange baby. And as always, I'm eternally grateful to Paul Dix for subsidizing yet another book of mine, for honest and encouraging feedback on early chapter drafts, and for being my most devoted reader.

# NOTES

INTRODUCTION

5    Australia became the first country to officially recognize MDMA: Grace Browne, "MDMA and Psilocybin Are Approved as Medicines for the First Time," *Wired*, February 3, 2023, https://www.wired.com/story/australia-psilo cybin-mdma-approval/.

CHAPTER 1: THE FERRY TO SAUSALITO

11    Carl Resnikoff was in eighth grade: Carl Resnikoff, interview by the author, January 2022.

11    accounts of esoteric drug experiences: Emanuel Sferios, "Meet the First Person in the World to Take MDMA," with Carl Resnikoff and Ann Shulgin, August 21, 2018, *Drug Positive*, podcast, https://drugpositive.org/meet-the-first-person-in -the-world-to-take-mdma-that-we-know-of.

11    "mellow drug of America": Jerome Beck and Marsha Rosenbaum, *Pursuit of Ecstasy: The MDMA Experience* (New York: SUNY Press, 1994), 13.

12    intriguing 1969 article: Alexander Shulgin, Thornton Sargent, and Claudio Naranjo, "Structure-Activity Relationships of One-Ring Psychotomimetics," *Nature* 221 (1969): 537–41.

12    Hawaiian shirts and black sandals: Alexander Shulgin and Ann Shulgin, *PIHKAL: A Chemical Love Story* (San Francisco: Transform Press, 1990), 66.

12    towered over the class: Alexander Shulgin, *The Nature of Drugs: History, Pharmacology, and Social Impact*, vol. 1 (Berkeley, CA: Transform Press, 2021), 321.

13    "That's a fine idea": Sferios, "Meet the First Person."

14    "I knew he was in that world": Judith Gips, interview by the author, January 2022.

15    some forty-two years later: Emanuel Sferios, interview by the author, January 2022.

15    exists across the animal kingdom: Giorgio Samorini, *Animals and Psychedelics: The Natural World and the Instinct to Alter Consciousness* (Rochester, VT: Park Street Press, 2002).

15    "All the vegetable sedatives": Aldous Huxley, *The Door of Perception and Heaven and Hell* (New York: Harper Perennial Modern Classics, 1954), 62.

15    Mammoths still roamed: D. Duke et al., "Earliest Evidence for Human Use of Tobacco in the Pleistocene Americas," *Nature Human Behaviour* 6 (2022): 183–92, https://doi.org/10.1038/s41562-021-01202-9.

15    Cannabis might have been domesticated: David E. Presti, *Foundational Concepts in Neuroscience: A Brain-Mind Odyssey*, illustrated ed. (New York: W. W. Norton, 2015), 113.

15–16  Alcohol brewing was taking place: P. E. McGovern et al., "Fermented Beverages of Pre- and Proto-Historic China," *Proceedings of the National Academy of Sciences* 101 (2004): 17593–98, https://www.pnas.org/doi/10.1073/pnas.0407921102.

16    in the Caucasus Mountains in Georgia: P. E. McGovern et al., "Early Neolithic Wine of Georgia in the South Caucasus," *Proceedings of the National Academy of Sciences* 114 (2017): 10309–18, https://www.pnas.org/doi/10.1073/pnas.1714728114.

16    Armenia started making wine: Brian Muraresku, *The Immortality Key: The Secret History of the Religion with No Name* (New York: St. Martin's Press, 2020), 203.

16    Ritual use of peyote: Michael Pollan, *This Is Your Mind on Plants* (New York: Penguin Press, 2021), 170.

16    Sumerians: Presti, *Foundational Concepts in Neuroscience*, 104.

16    Ancient Taoist texts from China: Li Chen and Fan Pen, "Hallucinogen Use in China," *Sino-Platonic Papers*, no. 318 (2021).

16    took part in the Eleusinian Mysteries: F. J. Carod-Artal, "Psychoactive Plants in Ancient Greece," *Sociedad Española de Neurología Neurosciences and History* 1, no. 1 (2013): 23–38, https://nah.sen.es/vmfiles/abstract/NAHV1N1201328_38EN.pdf.

16    Women were the keepers: Muraresku, *Immortality Key*, 281, 248.

16    "At the moment of quitting": Elizabeth Pepper and John Wilcock, *Magical and Mystical Sites: Europe and the British Isles* (Grand Rapids, MI: Phanes Press, 2000), 62.

16    there must be benefits: Pollan, *Mind on Plants*, 8.

16    "I do think psychoactive drugs": Michael Pollan, interview by the author, October 2021.

16  "We have the accounts of artists": Sam Gandy et al., "Psychedelics as Potential Catalysts of Scientific Creativity and Insight," *Drug Science, Policy and Law* 8 (2022): 1–16, https://doi.org/10.1177/20503245221097649.

17  millennia-old, women-led ceremonies: Muraresku, *Immortality Key*, 21.

17  still an illegal cult: Muraresku, 220.

17  "the Eucharist simply *had* to involve": Muraresku, 247.

17  mystical core at the heart of countless religions: Muraresku, 9.

17  cultures around the world have traditionally valued psychedelic substances: Osiris Sinuhé González Romero, interview by the author, March 2022.

17  complex ceremonies to prevent abuse: F. J. Carod-Artal, "Hallucinogenic Drugs in Pre-Columbian Mesoamerican Cultures," *Neurología* (English ed.) 30, no. 1 (2015): 42–49, https://doi.org/10.1016/j.nrleng.2011.07.010.

17  "God's bouncers": Muraresku, *Immortality Key*, 94.

17  "If anyone with the right ingredients": Muraresku, 249.

17  knowledge of psychoactive substances was kept alive: Muraresku, 21.

18  religious authorities began aggressively persecuting: Ben Sessa, "The History of Psychedelics in Medicine," *Handbuch Psychoaktive Substanzen* (2016): 1–26, https://doi.org/10.1007/978-3-642-55214-4_96-1.

18  Over the span of three hundred years: Charles Grob, "Psychiatric Research with Hallucinogens: What Have We Learned?" *Heffter Review of Psychedelic Research* 1 (1998): 8.

18  "tools of Satan": Grob, "Psychiatric Research with Hallucinogens," 8.

18  sacred mushrooms, morning glory, and peyote: Kristina Lazdauskas, "Peyote and Diabolism in New Spain," 2018, https://emh30.ace.fordham.edu/2018/12/09/peyote-and-diabolism-in-new-spain/.

18  "herbs and roots": Grob, "Psychiatric Research with Hallucinogens," 9.

18  "the Church sought to eliminate": Grob, 8.

18  German pharmacologist Louis Lewin: Grob, 9.

18  Arthur Carl Wilhelm Heffter: Sessa, "History of Psychedelics."

18  The first ever psychedelic substance: Presti, *Foundational Concepts in Neuroscience*, 110.

19  MDMA's official story begins: David Adam, "Origins of Ecstasy an Urban Myth," *Nature* 5 (October 2006): 806.

19  a patent application for "methylsafrylamin": Roland W. Freudenmann, Florian Öxler, and Sabine Bernschneider-Reif, "The Origin of MDMA (Ecstasy) Revisited: The True Story Reconstructed from the Original Documents," *Addiction* 101 (2006): 1241–45, https://doi.org/10.1111/j.1360-0443.2006.01511.x.

20  a drug to promote blood clotting: Adam, "Origins of Ecstasy."

20  chemist named Max Oberlin: Freudenmann, Öxler, and Bernschneider-Reif, "Origin of MDMA."

20  "some insinuations of a cooperation": Freudenmann, Öxler, and Bernschneider-Reif.

20  "In the Merck archives is a file card": Torsten Passie, interview by the author, January 2022.

20  "was not tested in humans": Freudenmann, Öxler, and Bernschneider-Reif, "Origin of MDMA."

20  "their records are incomplete": David Carlson, interview by the author, September 2021.

21  "available at request": Freudenmann, Öxler, and Bernschneider-Reif, "Origin of MDMA."

21  Under the dark cloud of the Cold War: John Marks, interview by the author, February 2022.

21  "definitive book on the experiments": Tim Weiner, "Sidney Gottlieb, 80, Dies; Took LSD to C.I.A.," *New York Times*, March 10, 1999, https://www .nytimes.com/1999/03/10/us/sidney-gottlieb-80-dies-took-lsd-to-cia .html.

21  at least eighty-six universities and institutions: *Project MKULTRA: The CIA's Program of Research in Behavioral Modification*, Joint Hearing before the Select Committee on Intelligence and the Subcommittee on Health and Scientific Research of the Committee of Human Resources, 96th Cong. 7 (1977) (statement of Edward M. Kennedy, Chairman).

21  Hundreds of drugs were tested: Martin A. Lee and Bruce Shlain, *Acid Dreams: The Complete Social History of LSD; The CIA, the Sixties, and Beyond* (New York: Grove Press, 1994), 41.

21  some seven thousand soldiers: "Edgewood/Aberdeen Experiments," U.S. Department of Veterans Affairs, https://www.publichealth.va.gov/exposures /edgewood-aberdeen/index.asp.

21  experiments had been useless: Weiner, "Sidney Gottlieb Dies."

22  special interest of the Nazis: Lee and Shlain, *Acid Dreams*, 5–6.

21  "to eliminate the will": Torsten Passie and Udo Benzenhöfer, "MDA, MDMA, and Other 'Mescaline-Like' Substances in the US Military's Search for a Truth Drug (1940s to 1960s)," *Drug Testing and Analysis* 10 (2018): 72–80, https://doi .org/10.1002/dta.2292.

21  After learning of the Nazis' work: John D. Marks, *The Search for the "Manchurian Candidate": The CIA and Mind Control; The Secret History of the Behavioral Sciences* (New York: W. W. Norton, 1991), 5–6.

22  code-named EA-1475: Ulrich Braun, A. Shulgin, and G. Braun, "Centrally Active N-Substituted Analogs of 3,4-Methylenedioxyphenylisopropylamine (3,4-Methylenedioxyamphetamine)," *Journal of Pharmaceutical Sciences* 69, no. 2 (February 1980): 192–95.

22  five or six newly synthesized mescaline derivatives: James S. Ketchum and Harry Salem, "Incapacitating Agents," in *Medical Aspects of Chemical Warfare*, ed. Shirley D. Tourinsky (Washington, D.C.: Office of the Surgeon General, 2008), 411–39.

22  a well-respected mental health hospital: Passie and Benzenhöfer, "MDA, MDMA, and other 'Mescaline-Like' Substances."

22  "for offensive use as sabotage weapons": Barrett v. United States, 660 F. Supp. 1291 (S.D. New York 1987).

22  "very apprehensive": *Barret.*

22  "a guinea pig in an experiment": Arnold H. Lubasch, "$700,000 Award Is Made in '53 Secret Test Death," *New York Times*, May 6, 1987.

22  As a result of the injections: Passie and Benzenhöfer, "MDA, MDMA, and other 'Mescaline-Like' Substances."

22  an injection of 450 milligrams of MDA: *Barret.*

22  he began sweating profusely: Lubasch, "Secret Test Death."

23  "a fatal coronary attack": Passie and Benzenhöfer, "MDA, MDMA, and other 'Mescaline-Like' Substances."

23  documents stamped "secret": Passie and Benzenhöfer.

23  "If you look at the timing": Matthew Baggott, interview by the author, January 2022.

23  one of the eight chemicals: H. Hardman, C. Haavik, and M. Seevers, "Relationship of the Structure of Mescaline and Seven Analogs to Toxicity and Behavior in Five Species of Laboratory Animals," *Toxicology and Applied Pharmacology* 25 (1973): 299–309.

23  none of the compounds, including MDMA: Alexander Shulgin, "Die frühe geschichte von MDMA," in *Ecstasy: Design für die Seele?*, ed. J. Neumeyer and H. Schmidt-Semisch, trans. David Carlson (Freiburg im Breisgau, Germany: Lambertus, 1997), 97–105.

23  "bizarre body attitudes": Hardman, Haavik, and Seevers, "Relationship of the Structure of Mescaline."

23 "difficulty in vision": E. Ross Hart, *Psychochemical Program (C) Status Report as of 31 December 1955*, Chemical Warfare Laboratories, Maryland, May 3, 1956.

23 obsessed with finding a definitive answer: Nicholas Denomme, interview by the author, February 2022.

24 escaping from a Bay Area military facility: Nicolas Rasmussen, email interview by the author, February 2022.

24 "is protected, intentionally or unintentionally": James Romano, email interview by the author, January 2022.

24 toxicity data for thirty-six compounds: Hart, *Psychochemical Program (C) Status Report*.

24 "the few Army records available": James R. Taylor and William N. Johnson, *Use of Volunteers in Chemical Agent Research* (Washington, D.C.: Office of the Inspector General, 1975).

25 "designer drug": Torsten Passie and Udo Benzenhöfer, "The History of MDMA as an Underground Drug in the United States, 1960–1979," *Journal of Psychoactive Drugs* 48, no. 2 (2016): 67–75, https://doi.org/10.1080/02791072.2015.1128580.

25 a mystery substance picked up by the Chicago police: V. R. Sreenivasan, "Problems in Identification of Methylenediony and Methoxy Amphetamines," *Journal of Criminal Law, Criminology & Police Science* 63, no. 2 (1972): 304–12.

25 confiscated nearly nine hundred grams: Passie and Benzenhöfer, "MDA, MDMA, and other 'Mescaline-Like' Substances."

26 "a very competent chemist": Shulgin, "Die frühe geschichte."

26 "Sorry, David, pass": David Obst, interview by the author, February 2022.

27 "dear, dear sprite": Shulgin and Shulgin, *PIHKAL*, 69.

27 "We'd listen to his stories": "Merrie Kleinman," interview by the author, February 2022.

28 In September 1976 he decided to finally see: Shulgin, "Die frühe geschichte."

CHAPTER 2: PENICILLIN FOR THE SOUL

29 all manner of chemical paraphernalia: "Shulgin Lab," 3D virtual tour on Matterport, https://my.matterport.com/show/?m=Z93pXf9jiWK.

30 "stepfather of MDMA": Alexander Shulgin and Ann Shulgin, *PIHKAL: A Chemical Love Story* (San Francisco: Transform Press, 1990), 186.

30 His family always called him: Udo Benzenhöfer and Torsten Passie, "Rediscovering MDMA (Ecstasy): The Role of the American Chemist Alexander T. Shulgin," *Addiction* 105 (2010): 1355–61, https://doi.org/10.1111/j.1360-0443.2010.02948.x.

30 To avoid practicing instruments: Shulgin and Shulgin, *PIHKAL*, 5–6.

30 Before surgery for a thumb infection: Shulgin and Shulgin, 11–13.

30 PhD in biochemistry: Peyton Jacob, "Another Side of Sasha Shulgin," submission to Transform Press.

30 "academic prostitute": Alexander Shulgin, "Psychedelics outside the Box," interview with David Healy, late 1990s, Samizdat Health Writer's Co-operative, https://samizdathealth.org/wp-content/uploads/2020/12/Shulgin1.pdf.

30 "a day that will remain blazingly vivid": Shulgin and Shulgin, *PIHKAL*, 16.

30 dreamed in black and white: Emanuel Sferios, "Meet the First Person in the World to Take MDMA," with Carl Resnikoff and Ann Shulgin, August 21, 2018, *Drug Positive*, podcast, https://drugpositive.org/meet-the-first-person-in-the-world-to-take-mdma-that-we-know-of.

30 "fraction of a gram of a white solid": Shulgin and Shulgin, *PIHKAL*, 16.

31 Two years after that formative experience: Benzenhöfer and Passie, "Rediscovering MDMA."

31 "sounds like a motor additive": Alexander Shulgin, *The Nature of Drugs: History, Pharmacology, and Social Impact*, vol. 1 (Berkeley, CA: Transform Press, 2021), 283.

31 Using the mescaline molecule: Shulgin, "Psychedelics outside the Box."

31 over the next thirty years: Shulgin and Shulgin, *PIHKAL*, ix.

31 "It was not profound chemistry": Solomon Snyder, interview by the author, December 2021.

31 starting at extremely low doses: Shulgin and Shulgin, *PIHKAL*, xvii.

31 "It saves a lot of mice and dogs": Shulgin and Shulgin, 143.

31 research group composed of nine to eleven trusted friends: Shulgin and Shulgin, xxvi.

31 "taking these substances to flourish": Erika Dyck, interview by the author, February 2022.

31 "completely convinced that there is a wealth of information": Shulgin and Shulgin, *PIHKAL*, xvi.

32 give anyone a clear route of entry: Shulgin and Shulgin, xvi.

32 it's up to the individual to choose: Shulgin and Shulgin, xvii.

32 "Do you know how an orchestra and a bull": Paul Daley, interview by the author, September 2021.

32 aka FNDs: Shulgin, *Nature of Drugs*, 321.

32 Terence McKenna, Carl Sagan, Daniel Ellsberg: Peyton Jacob, interview by the author by email, February 2022.

32 "I brought my girlfriend out": David Carlson, interview by the author, September 2021.

32 "some humble, privileged family": Shulgin, *Nature of Drugs*, 326.

32 "It was another world": David Nichols, interview by the author, June 2021.

32 By the mid-1960s: Shulgin and Shulgin, *PIHKAL*, 41.

33 "I worked for ten years before they finally realized": Shulgin, *Nature of Drugs*, 283.

33 twenty acres of property: Shulgin and Shulgin, *PIHKAL*, 160.

33 postgraduate studies in psychiatry: Shulgin, *Nature of Drugs*, 11.

33 paid the bills by lecturing: Shulgin, "Psychedelics outside the Box."

33 "One of our best friends was a top official": Ann Shulgin, interview by the author, September 2021.

33 "gung ho [about] working with the government": Etienne Sauret, dir., *Dirty Pictures*, 2010.

34 "the most beautiful Native American marriage ceremony": George Greer, interview by the author, June 2021.

34 "I feel absolutely clean inside": Shulgin and Shulgin, *PIHKAL*, 736–37.

34 the word *window* kept coming to mind: Alexander Shulgin, "Die frühe geschichte von MDMA," in *Ecstasy: Design für die Seele?*, ed. J. Neumeyer and H. Schmidt-Semisch, trans. David Carlson (Freiburg im Breisgau, Germany: Lambertus, 1997), 97–105.

34 the Reno Fun Train: Shulgin, "Die frühe geschichte."

34 "pleasant lightness of spirit": Shulgin and Shulgin, *PIHKAL*, 187.

34 closely matched the alcohol-induced intoxication: Shulgin and Shulgin, 72.

35 "The slight disinhibition of alcohol": Shulgin, "Psychedelics outside the Box."

35 "a low calorie martini": Alexander Shulgin and David Nichols, "Characterization of Three New Psychotomimetics," in *The Psychopharmacology of Hallucinogens*, ed. Richard C. Stillman and Robert E. Willette (St. Louis: Elsevier, 1978): 74–83, https://chemistry.mdma.ch/hiveboard/rhodium/shulgin-nichols.three.new.html.

35 more to this material than light, tipsy fun: Shulgin, "Die frühe geschichte."

35 resolved the trauma around his LSD experience: Shulgin and Shulgin, *PIHKAL*, 72.

35 "MDMA was perfectly suitable for use in psychotherapy": Shulgin, "Die frühe geschichte."

35 decided to introduce MDMA to Leo Zeff: Benzenhöfer and Passie, "Rediscovering MDMA."

35 "everyone's idea of what a grandfather": Shulgin and Shulgin, *PIHKAL*, 73.

35 Zeff stood at just five foot six: Myron Stolaroff, *The Secret Chief Revealed* (San Francisco: Multidisciplinary Association for Psychedelic Studies, 2004), 28.

35 overseen such trips for thousands of people: Stolaroff, *Secret Chief*, 56.

35 "something that might interest you": Sferios, "Meet the First Person."

36 "a special magic": Shulgin and Shulgin, *PIHKAL*, 74.

36 "I'm getting too old for this": Shulgin, "Psychedelics outside the Box."

36 Shulgin's phone rang: Shulgin and Shulgin, *PIHKAL*, 74.

36 following Albert Hofmann's discovery of LSD: John R. Neill, " 'More Than Medical Significance': LSD and American Psychiatry, 1953 to 1966," *Journal of Psychoactive Drugs* 19, no. 1 (1987): 39–45, https://doi.org/10.1080/02791072.1987 .10472378.

36 "Psychedelics were awfully important": David Healy, interview by the author, January 2022.

36 mescaline and MDA, as potential tools: Martin A. Lee and Bruce Shlain, *Acid Dreams: The Complete Social History of LSD; The CIA, the Sixties, and Beyond* (New York: Grove Press, 1994), 55.

36 "a new drug": Aldous Huxley, *The Door of Perception and Heaven and Hell* (New York: Harper Perennial Modern Classics, 1954), 65.

37 researchers began investigating LSD: Lee and Shlain, *Acid Dreams*, 49–50.

37 first public LSD clinic opened in 1953: Lee and Shlain, 56.

37 some *forty thousand* patients received LSD treatment: Ben Sessa, "From Sacred Plants to Psychotherapy: The History and Re-Emergence of Psychedelics in Medicine," paper presented at the Royal College of Psychiatrists Special Symposium on Psychosis, Psychedelics and the Transpersonal Journey, 2006.

37 everything from obsessive-compulsive disorder and depression: Ben Sessa, "The History of Psychedelics in Medicine," *Handbuch Psychoaktive Substanzen* (2016): 1–26, https://doi.org/10.1007/978-3-642-55214-4_96-1.

37 More than a thousand scientific papers: Neill, " 'More Than Medical Significance.' "

37 "comparable to the value the microscope has": Stolaroff, *Secret Chief*, 14.

37 In 1962 Congress enacted new rules: Lee and Shlain, *Acid Dreams*, 90–91.

37 it was "nonspecific": Neill, " 'More Than Medical Significance.' "

37 Most doctors were also highly resistant: Lee and Shlain, *Acid Dreams*, 90–91.

37 LSD's increasingly central role in the counterculture: Lee and Shlain, 128–33.

38 Lyndon Johnson and others in power: Lee and Shlain, 154.

38 LSD damages chromosomes: Neill, " 'More Than Medical Significance.' "

38 "Dionysian elements": Stolaroff, *Secret Chief*, 13.

38   "the haunting fear": Carl Hart, *Drug Use for Grown-Ups: Chasing Liberty in the Land of Fear* (London: Penguin, 2021), 118.

38   "We should not forget to assess the cost of sustained euphoria": Neill, " 'More Than Medical Significance.' "

38   "Let us never forget": Lyndon B. Johnson, "Statement by the President Upon Signing Relating to Traffic in or Possession of Drugs Such as LSD," transcript of speech delivered at Washington, D.C., October 25, 1968, https://www .presidency.ucsb.edu/documents/statement-the-president-upon-signing-bill -relating-traffic-or-possession-drugs-such-lsd.

38   "public enemy number one": "President Nixon Declares 'War' on Drugs," speech, June 17, 1971, https://www.encyclopedia.com/science/medical-magazines /president-nixon-declares-war-drugs.

39   "relentless warfare": Johann Hari, *Chasing the Scream: The First and Last Days of the War on Drugs* (New York: Bloomsbury, 2016), 7.

39   "Draconian drug laws": Matthew Oram, email to the author, February 2022.

39   set his sights on outlawing marijuana: Hari, *Chasing the Scream*, 7.

39   marijuana caused people to go insane: Hari, 15–17.

39   fears and prejudices of the American public: Hari, 26.

39   "A lot of law enforcement people": Keeper Trout, interview by the author, December 2021.

39   "had two enemies": Dan Baum, "Legalize It All: How to Win the War on Drugs," *Harper's Magazine*, April 2016, https://harpers.org/archive/2016/04/legalize-it-all/.

40   "a far more powerful administrative regulatory apparatus": Joseph F. Spillane, "Debating the Controlled Substances Act," *Drug and Alcohol Dependence* 76 (2004): 17–29.

40   this new system would stifle research: Spillane, "Controlled Substances Act."

40   drowned out by mainstream media hysteria: Lee and Shlain, *Acid Dreams*, 150–53.

40   "a tragic loss for psychiatry": Stolaroff, *Secret Chief*, 15.

40   forbidden "medicines": Stolaroff, 40.

41   "the chief of a secret tribe": Mariavittoria Mangini, interview by the author, November 2021.

41   "secret chief": Torsten Passie and Udo Benzenhöfer, "The History of MDMA as an Underground Drug in the United States, 1960–1979," *Journal of Psychoactive Drugs* 48, no. 2 (2016): 67–75, https://doi.org/10.1080/02791072.2015.1128580.

41   150 or so underground therapists: Stolaroff, *Secret Chief*, 59.

41   "decided not to sacrifice the well-being": Stolaroff, 16.

41 "What are you exposing yourself": Stolaroff, 61.

41 "completely enraptured": Stolaroff, 18.

41 "a proselytizer of MDMA": Passie and Benzenhöfer, "History of MDMA."

41 "I kept him supplied with the drug": Shulgin, "Psychedelics outside the Box."

41 hundreds of fellow therapists: Passie and Benzenhöfer, "History of MDMA."

41 "I think it was inevitable": Matthew Baggott, interview by the author, January 2022.

41 *empathogen* sounded too close to *pathogen*: David Nichols Papers, box 1, folder 5, Purdue University, West Lafayette, IN, https://archives.lib.purdue.edu/repositories/2/resources/531.

41 a mishmash of Greek and Latin: Nathan Oglesby, email interview by the author, February 2022.

42 Zeff just called the drug Adam: Stolaroff, *Secret Chief*, 86.

42 a near-anagram he coined: Julie Holland, ed., *Ecstasy: The Complete Guide; A Comprehensive Look at the Risks and Benefits of MDMA* (Rochester, VT: Park Street Press, 2001), 186.

42 "The profound simplicity of the Adam state": Ralph Metzner and Sophia Adamson, "Chapter 12: Using MDMA in Healing, Psychotherapy, and Spiritual Practice," in Holland, *Ecstasy*, 200–201.

42 most popular medicine at Zeff's group retreats: Stolaroff, *Secret Chief*, 98.

42 "The MDMA people liked to get up": Stolaroff, 81.

43 "told us he'd come across a new material": Requa Greer, interview by the author, November 2021.

44 the Greers treated around eighty people: George Greer Papers, box 1, folder 2, Purdue University, West Lafayette, IN, https://archives.lib.purdue.edu/repositories/2/resources/32.

45 Bob Sager, the DEA agent: Sauret, *Dirty Pictures*.

45 credit MDMA-assisted therapy with saving her life: Naomi Fiske, interview by the author, December 2021.

48 "MDMA is penicillin for the soul": Shulgin and Shulgin, *PIHKAL*, 74; Ann Shulgin confirmed by email in February 2022 that this quote, in full, is attributed to her.

CHAPTER 3: "Y'ALL DO X?"

49 Monica Greene arrived at the Starck Club: Monica Greene, interview by the author, March 2022.

50   The Starck Club's creators had set out: Michael Cain and Miles Hargrove, dirs., *The Starck Club*, 2014.

50   "They didn't close": Michael Cain, interview by the author, February 2022.

50   DJ Kerry Jaggers, a native Texan: Peter Simek, "Playboy: Ecstasy Was Legal in 1984, and It Was Glorious," MAPS, December 2, 2015, https://maps.org/news /media/playboy-ecstasy-was-legal-in-1984-and-it-was-glorious/.

51   "Y'all do X?" became a common refrain: Cain and Hargrove, *Starck Club*.

51   she recently retired and now lives "blissfully": Monica Greene, email to the author, February 2023.

51   In 1981 Analysis Anonymous: Torsten Passie and Udo Benzenhöfer, "The History of MDMA as an Underground Drug in the United States, 1960–1979," *Journal of Psychoactive Drugs* 48, no. 2 (2016): 67–75, https://doi.org/10.1080 /02791072.2015.1128580.

51   spiritually minded New Age types: Jerome Beck and Marsha Rosenbaum, *Pursuit of Ecstasy: The MDMA Experience* (New York: SUNY Press, 1994), 37.

51   to assist with transcendence: Beck and Rosenbaum, *Pursuit of Ecstasy*, 40–41.

52   the first ethnographic survey of MDMA users: Jerome Beck et al., *Exploring Ecstasy: A Description of MDMA Users*, final report to the National Institute on Drug Abuse (San Francisco: Institute for Scientific Analysis, 1989).

52   "A surprisingly difficult part of this phase of research": Beck and Rosenbaum, *Pursuit of Ecstasy*, 164.

52   Their sample included interviews with postal workers: Beck and Rosenbaum, 171–73.

52   educated professionals in their thirties and forties: Beck and Rosenbaum, 34–36.

52   Gay clubgoers at places like the Saint: Simek, "Ecstasy Was Legal."

52   Deadheads constituted another early user group: Beck and Rosenbaum, *Pursuit of Ecstasy*, 48–49.

52–53 everyone from conservative Southern Methodist University students: Beck and Rosenbaum, 42–43.

53   Dancers at Dallas topless bars: Beck and Rosenbaum, 76–77.

53   the fact that MDMA was legal: Beck and Rosenbaum, 43–45.

53   "It was a fascinating scene in Texas": Jerome Beck, interview by the author, January 2022.

53   spas that offered MDMA massages: Beck and Rosenbaum, *Pursuit of Ecstasy*, 74.

53   overwhelmingly used Ecstasy for enjoyment: Beck and Rosenbaum, 80–86.

54  Darrell Lemaire, for example, was a lanky cowboy type: *Hamilton's Pharmacopeia*, dir. Hamilton Morris, season 1, episode 6, "The Lazy Lizard School of Hedonism," aired December 7, 2016.

54  the Boston Group, made more modestly sized batches: Beck and Rosenbaum, *Pursuit of Ecstasy*, 19.

54  "this is where I chose to do my chipping": Beck and Rosenbaum, *Pursuit of Ecstasy*, 17.

54  trips to places like Thailand and Bali: Debby Harlow, interview by the author, January 2022.

55  recalled "the Moon Man": Mariavittoria Mangini, interview by the author, November 2021.

55  Echoing disagreements among LSD distributors: Beck and Rosenbaum, *Pursuit of Ecstasy*, 17.

56  "I am about interviewed out": Michael Clegg, email to the author, February 2021.

56  "Seeker" was the word Clegg once used: Satyam Nadeen, "From Onions to Pearls: Peeling the Gem," interview by Elaine Smitha, *Evolving Ideas with Elaine Smitha*, aired September 18, 1997, https://archive.org/details/From OnionsToPearls.PeelingTheGem.

56  Raised in an Irish Catholic family: Simek, "Ecstasy Was Legal."

56  "wanted to somehow find God": United States v. Clegg, 92-70 (S4) -CR-J-20 (M.D. Fla. 1994).

56  he also earned two convictions: United States v. Clegg, CR 5-92-042 PVT (N.D. Cal. 1992).

56  "My eyes opened up in a way": *Clegg*, M.D. Fla. 1994.

56  "It was like Moses on the mountain": *Peter Jennings Reporting: Ecstasy Rising*, ABC News documentary, 43:27, aired April 1, 2014.

56  "I finally had a way to help the whole world": *Clegg*, M.D. Fla. 1994.

56  In 1983 a knock came to the door: Bob McMillen, interview by the author, March 2022.

57  McMillen sold five thousand pills in four days: Bob McMillen, "Forbidden Fruit in Changing Times" (unpublished manuscript, 2001), Microsoft Word file, 220.

58  "It came to me: It was pure ecstasy": Simek, "Ecstasy Was Legal."

58  Clegg linked up with the Boston Group: Beck and Rosenbaum, *Pursuit of Ecstasy*, 19.

58  he claimed to various people to have been given it: Nadeen, "From Onions to Pearls."

58  or to have bought it: "Karl Janssen," interview by the author, September 2021.

58  "This was the happiest period of my life": *Clegg*, M.D. Fla. 1994.

58 a beeper with the number 1-800-ECSTASY: McMillen, "Forbidden Fruit," 231.

59 Ecstasy "was discreetly slipped into rich Sanyassins' drinks": Hugh Milne, *Bhagwan: The God That Failed* (New York: St. Martin's Press, 1986), 290.

59 "you've got to tip toe through the tulips": McMillen, "Forbidden Fruit," 216.

59 "Their lives were totally touched": Jennings, *Ecstasy Rising*.

59 putting MDMA out on consignment: Testimony of Special Agent Robert C. Chester Jr., U.S. Department of Justice, Drug Enforcement Administration, docket 84–48, April 25, 1985, https://maps.org/wp-content/uploads/1988/11/0020.pdf.

59 "He brought it to the discotheque": Torsten Passie, interview by the author, January 2022.

59 "this hippy-type atmosphere": Phil Jordan, interview by Michael Cain, 2013.

60 "that kiddie drug": Simek, "Ecstasy Was Legal."

61 "Everybody knew that it was inevitable": George Greer, interview by the author, June 2021.

### CHAPTER 4: RICK KEPT GOING

62 thirteen-year-old Rick Doblin woke up disappointed: Rick Doblin, interview by the author, October 2021.

66 Debby Harlow had two thoughts: Debby Harlow, interview by the author, January 2022.

66 "There was something about Esalen": Howard Kornfeld, interview by the author, January 2022.

68 five hundred doses of MDMA to distribute among Soviet scientists: Robert K. Elder, "Psychedelics: The Newest Tool in Nuclear Negotiations?" *Bulletin of the Atomic Scientists*, December 17, 2021, https://thebulletin.org/2021/12/psychedelics-the-newest-tool-in-nuclear-negotiations/.

68 send world leaders LSD: Martin A. Lee and Bruce Shlain, *Acid Dreams: The Complete Social History of LSD; The CIA, the Sixties, and Beyond* (New York: Grove Press, 1994), 181.

68 Brother David Steindl-Rast told *Newsweek*: Tom Shroder, *Acid Test: LSD, Ecstasy, and the Power to Heal* (New York: Penguin, 2014), 175.

69 commissioned animal toxicity studies: Charles H. Frith, "28-Day Oral Toxicity Report of MDMA in Dogs," Division of Laboratory Animal Medicine, University of Arkansas for Medical Sciences, 1985, https://maps.org/research-archive/dea-mdma/pdf/0069.pdf.

70  "has unquestioned medical utility": Alexander Shulgin, letter to administrator of Drug Enforcement Administration, U.S. Department of Justice, Drug Enforcement Administration, docket 84–48, August 29, 1984.

70  "will suffer both professionally and economically": George Greer, letter to administrator of Drug Enforcement Administration, docket 84–48, August 22, 1984.

70  "very naive indeed": David E. Nichols, letter to administrator of Drug Enforcement Administration, docket 84–48, August 17, 1984.

70  a scheduling hearing was now required by law: Richard Cotton, letter to administrator of Drug Enforcement Administration, docket 84–48, September 12, 1984.

70  "We were surprised, really": Frank Sapienza, interview by the author, December 2021.

70  Torsten Passie recalled Ralph Metzner: Torsten Passie, interview by the author, January 2022.

71  he'd responded by upping operations: Jerome Beck and Marsha Rosenbaum, *Pursuit of Ecstasy: The MDMA Experience* (New York: SUNY Press, 1994), 21.

72  "hated the term 'Ecstasy' ": Paul Daley, interview by the author, September 2021.

73  "Well, guess what, we've got another drug": Phil Donahue, *Donahue on Ecstasy*, Multimedia Entertainment, 1985.

73  announced to hundreds of thousands of viewers: Carolyn McGuire, " 'Donahue' Ratings High in New York," *Chicago Tribune*, January 19, 1985.

74  "a 99 percent chance": Shroder, *Acid Test*, 196.

75  the DEA invoked emergency measures: Jerome Beck et al., *Exploring Ecstasy: A Description of MDMA Users*, final report to the National Institute on Drug Abuse (San Francisco: Institute for Scientific Analysis, 1989).

75  the DEA pointed to Schuster's rat study: G. Ricaurte et al., "Hallucinogenic Amphetamine Selectively Destroys Brain Serotonin Nerve Terminals," *Science* 35, no. 4717 (1985): 986–88, doi:10.1126/science.4023719.

75  "selectively destroys": Beck and Rosenbaum, *Pursuit of Ecstasy*, 21.

75  The United Nations also fell in line: "Documents from the DEA Scheduling Hearing of MDMA, United Nations," docket 84–48, 1985.

75  just eight emergency room admissions: Beck and Rosenbaum, *Pursuit of Ecstasy*, 114.

75  one death in 1979: David Nichols Papers, box 11, folder 2, Purdue University, West Lafayette, IN, https://archives.lib.purdue.edu/repositories/2/resources/531.

75 nearly twice as much MDMA as MDA: Torsten Passie and Udo Benzenhöfer, "MDA, MDMA, and Other 'Mescaline-Like' Substances in the US Military's Search for a Truth Drug (1940s to 1960s)," *Drug Testing and Analysis* 10 (2018): 72–80, https://doi.org/10.1002/dta.2292.

75 roughly three to five times higher: Ricaurte et al., "Hallucinogenic Amphetamine."

76 "MDMA abuse has become a nationwide problem": "U.S. Will Ban 'Ecstasy,' A Hallucinogenic Drug," *New York Times*, June 1, 1985.

76 "We've had people locked in fetal positions": Joe Klein, "The New Drug They Call 'Ecstasy,' " *New York*, May 20, 1985.

76 "There were articles written in *Time*": David Nichols, interview by the author, June 2021.

76 "epidemic of MDMA abuse": Richard Seymour, *MDMA* (San Francisco: Haight-Ashbury, 1986), 60.

76 "The illegality and all the press": "Karl Janssen," interview by the author, September 2021.

76 Sixteen witnesses—twelve of whom were psychiatrists: Richard Cotton, "Memorandum for Interested Parties RE: Brief on MDMA Scheduling," docket 84–48, January 17, 1986.

77 "is guilty by association": Testimony of June E. Riedlinger, docket 84–48, April 1985.

77 countered the DEA's assertion: Testimony of Richard Seymour, docket 84–48, April 22, 1985.

77 "was kind of a nonissue": Richard Seymour, interview by the author, December 2021.

77 "in cases of severe emotional distress": Testimony of Philip E. Wolfson, docket 84–48, April 24, 1985.

77 "In rejecting the absurd notion promoted by some": Testimony of Lester Grinspoon, docket 84–48, April 18, 1985.

77 street use of MDMA had escalated: Declaration of Ronald K. Siegel, docket 84–48, April 1985.

77 "those trafficking 'Ecstasy' in the Dallas area": Testimony of Special Agent Robert C. Chester Jr., docket 84–48, April 25, 1985, https://maps.org/wp-content/uploads/1988/11/0020.pdf.

78 "MDMA has no currently accepted medical use": Testimony of Frank L. Sapienza, docket 84–48, April 25, 1985.

78 listened attentively to all of the arguments: Nichols Papers, box 11, folder 2.

78   "You know, I just want to see to it": Nichols Papers, box 11, folder 2.

78   After a couple of rounds of rebuttal testimony: Richard Cotton, "Memorandum for Interested Parties RE: Brief on MDMA Scheduling," docket 84–48, January 17, 1986.

78   three months to issue his seventy-one-page ruling: "Opinion and Recommended Ruling, Findings of Fact, Conclusions of Law and Decision of Administrative Law Judge," docket 84–48, May 22, 1986.

79   "This opinion represents an extraordinary vindication": Nichols Papers, box 2, folder 4.

79   "We won!": Nichols Papers, box 2, folder 4.

79   "The Administrative Law Judge has systematically disregarded": "Government's Exceptions to the Opinion and Recommended Ruling, Findings of Fact, Conclusions of Law and Decisions of the Administrative Law Judge," docket 84–48, June 13, 1986.

79   "the Grinspoon window": Julie Holland, ed., *Ecstasy: The Complete Guide; A Comprehensive Look at the Risks and Benefits of MDMA* (Rochester, VT: Park Street Press, 2001), 15.

79   "a few people were released from prison": Lester Grinspoon, interview by David Healy, "Marijuana and Psychopharmacological Boundaries," Samizdat Health Writer's Co-operative, April 2002.

80   "It was dreadful": Ann Shulgin, interview with the author, September 2021.

80   "Oh god, it was horrible": Requa Greer, interview by the author, December 2021.

80   "facilitat[e] MDMA research right now": Nichols Papers, box 2, folder 5.

## CHAPTER 5: GOOD CHEMISTRY

83   "We touched millions of people": Carina Leveriza-Franz, interview by the author, February 2022.

83   In November 1981: Carina Leveriza, statement for the defense, United States v. Carlson, 87 F.3d 440 (11th Cir. 1996).

83   Several months later, in April 1982: Leveriza, statement.

84   intended for industrial use: Leveriza.

84   In March 1985 Clegg called Carina: Leveriza.

84   ushered up the steps of a Cessna jet: Peter Simek, "Playboy: Ecstasy Was Legal in 1984, and It Was Glorious," MAPS, December 2, 2015, https://maps.org/news/media/playboy-ecstasy-was-legal-in-1984-and-it-was-glorious/.

84   Clegg had brought along clippings: Leveriza, statement.

84–85  They settled on a hundred thousand dollars: Leveriza.

86  "the Mecca of the drug Ecstasy": Michael Cain and Miles Hargrove, dirs., *The Starck Club*, 2014.

86  "The floor of the place looked like a pharmacy": Cain and Hargrove, *Starck Club*.

87  "Early British dance culture detonated a huge explosion": Matthew Collin, email interview by the author, April 2022.

87  Bob McMillen was regularly shipping pills: Bob McMillen, interview by the author, March 2022.

87  After Soft Cell's Marc Almond and Dave Ball: Matthew Collin, *Altered State: The Story of Ecstasy and Acid House* (London: Serpent's Tail, 2010), 36–37.

87  The pivotal moment for Ecstasy culture: Collin, *Altered State*, 52–53.

87  Bes, the Phoenician god of music and dance: Matthew Collin, *Rave On: Global Adventures in Electronic Dance Music* (Chicago: University of Chicago Press, 2018), 100.

87  an annual summer pilgrimage destination: Collin, *Altered State*, 51.

87  "XTC island": Jerome Beck and Marsha Rosenbaum, *Pursuit of Ecstasy: The MDMA Experience* (New York: SUNY Press, 1994), 50.

87  expat devotees of Bhagwan Shree Rajneesh: Collin, *Rave On*, 104.

87  House had first emerged: Collin, *Altered State*, 17.

87  inspired other DJs in the gay Black scene: Collin, 18–21.

88  The average heart rate: Russell Newcombe, interview by the author, November 2021.

88  "almost like a religious experience": Collin, *Altered State*, 53.

88  "All four of us changed that night": Emma Warren, "The Birth of Rave," *Guardian*, August 12, 2007, https://www.theguardian.com/music/2007/aug/12/electronicmusic.

88  Clubs closed early: Collin, *Altered State*, 55–56.

88  "homo shit": Collin, 59.

88  "There's this kind of mythical boys' holiday": Peder Clark, interview by the author, February 2022.

88  "Ecstasy makes you think": Collin, *Rave On*, 106.

89  MDMA had been an illegal Class A drug: Peder Clark, "Ecstasy: A Synthetic History of MDMA," in *Routledge Handbook of Intoxicants and Intoxication*, ed. G. Hunt, T. M. J. Antin, and V. A. Frank (Oxfordshire: Routledge, 2023), 127–40.

89  most people there had never heard of Ecstasy: Collin, *Altered State*, 65.

89 Rampling and his wife, Jenni, started hosting Shoom: Tim Pilcher, *E: The Incredibly Strange History of Ecstasy* (Philadelphia: Running Press, 2008), 104.

89 a free, invite-only, all-night weekly dance party: Warren, "Birth of Rave."

89 named for the feeling of coming up on Ecstasy: Pilcher, *E*, 104.

89 They developed their own terminology: Collin, *Altered State*, 62–64.

89 In April 1988 Oakenfold launched his own party: Pilcher, *E*, 106–7.

89 Ecstasy and the all-house soundtrack: Collin, *Altered State*, 59.

90 Known as the "Second Summer of Love": Collin, 78.

90 "the most vibrant, diverse and long-lasting": Collin, vii.

90 "The Ecstasy phenomenon literally exploded": Steve Rolles, interview by the author, October 2021.

90 "I'd literally be one of the only people drinking alcohol": Mandi James, interview by the author, January 2022.

91 seeing men hugging in public: Nicholas Saunders, *E for Ecstasy* (self-pub., Amazon Digital Services, 1993), 33.

91 a role in reducing violence at British football matches: Geoff Pearson, interview by the author, December 2021.

91 in response to restrictive laws: Collin, *Altered State*, 162.

91 empty lots off London's M25: Clark, "Ecstasy."

91 "If they were lieutenants in a military outfit": Collin, *Altered State*, 106–7.

91 The colossal cost of sending police out: Collin, 126.

92 leaflets featuring humorous cartoons: Linnell Communications, "Safer Dancing," https://michaellinnell.org.uk/michael_linnell_archive/safer_dancing/safer _dancing.html.

92 "Rave Research Bureau": Saunders, *E for Ecstasy*, 108.

92 ten-point harm reduction strategy: Russell Newcombe, "The Use of Ecstasy and Dance Drugs at Rave Parties and Clubs: Some Problems and Solutions," paper presented at symposium on Ecstasy, Leeds, UK, November 1992.

92 research at several major Liverpool clubs: Russell Newcombe, "Monitoring and Surveillance of Quadrant Park Nightclub, Bootle, Merseyside," November 2017, https://www.researchgate.net/publication/320910812_Monitoring_and _surveillance_of_Quadrant_Park_Nightclub_Bootle_Merseyside.

92 Bhagwan Shree Rajneesh follower who brought a thousand Ecstasy tablets: Saunders, *E for Ecstasy*, 125.

92–93 "He was traveling around with a bunch of pills": Philippus Zandstra, interview by the author, February 2022.

93    on the dance floor at a nightclub they ran in Amsterdam: David Hillier, "Did the Cult from 'Wild Wild Country' Introduce MDMA to Ibiza?" *Vice*, December 10, 2021, https://www.vice.com/en/article/g5qvyb/wild-wild-country-cult-mdma-ibiza.

93    a genre invented by Black DJs in post-industrial Detroit: Collin, *Altered State*, 21.

93    "We listened intensely": Collin, *Rave On*, 59.

93    Berlin-based DJ duo called System 01: Henry Ivry, "An Outstanding Compilation from Two Forgotten Pioneers of Berlin Techno," review of *1990–1994*, album by System 01, January 2022, *Resident Advisor*, February 3, 2022, https://ra.co/reviews/34628.

93    "Drugs Work" and "Any Reality Is an Opinion": System 01, *1990–1994*, Mannequin MNQ 150, limited edition vinyl record, January 26, 2022.

93    up to a million participants marched down Strasse des 17. Juni: Clark, "Ecstasy."

93    the Nazis once used for their demonstrations: Collin, *Rave On*, 66.

94    awarded a patent for a new technology: Carina T. Leveriza and Russell A. Morgan, "Silicone containing resists," U.S. Patent 4,764,247, filed August 16, 1988.

94    gotten into a costly lawsuit: Syn Labs, Inc. v. Superior Court of California, 670 471 Supreme Court S015983 (1990).

95    Carina and Walt sold MDMA directly to Pauline Clegg: Carina Leveriza, statement for the defense, United States v. Carlson, 87 F.3d 440 (11th Cir. 1996).

95    In seventeenth-century England, people drank sassafras tonic and tea: Bellarmine University, "Sassafras," https://www.bellarmine.edu/faculty/drobinson/sassafras.asp.

96    "All drink of the sassafras root": Jack London, *The Son of the Wolf* (Leipzig, Austria: Bernhard Tauchnitz, 1914), 107.

96    safrole, a root-beer-smelling essential oil: Bruce Eisner, *Ecstasy: The MDMA Story* (Berkeley, CA: Ronin, 1993), 139.

96    "I asked if she wanted to do some MDMA": Karl Janssen, interview by the author, September 2021.

96    The DEA had been aware of Clegg's involvement: United States v. Clegg, CR 5-92-042 PVT (N.D. Cal. 1992).

96    "this group you're calling the Texas Group": James Klindt, interview by the author, May 2022.

97    Weber made recorded phone calls: *Clegg*, N.D. Cal. 1992.

97    more than 2,200 pounds of MDMA: *Clegg*.

97    Agents nabbed Clegg on March 11, 1992: *Clegg*.

97  a fake ID identifying him as an ordained minister: *Clegg*.

97  Clegg "almost immediately" began cooperating: *Clegg*.

98  "He turned in everybody he knew": Bob McMillen, interview by the author, March 2022.

98  finally caught up to him on March 20, 1992: *Clegg*, N.D. Cal. 1992.

98  ten days after Carina's arrest, he was pulled over: *Clegg*.

99  "open[s] up the channel": *Clegg*.

99  "Mr. Clegg took this case in great part himself": *Clegg*.

100  a sentence of eighty-seven months in prison: *Clegg*.

100  putting together a joint appeal: *Clegg*.

100  make the same case to a Texas judge: *Clegg*.

100  In Manchester especially, gangs got involved: Collin, *Altered State*, 173.

100  Novice users sometimes accidentally took: Collin, 307.

101  Britain saw its first Ecstasy-related death in June 1988: Collin, 80.

101  More deaths sporadically followed: Russell Newcombe, "Ecstasy Deaths and Other Fatalities Linked to Dance Drugs and Dance Parties in UK, 1980–96," *3D Research Bureau*, January 1997.

101  "taking Ecstasy is like playing Russian roulette": Collin, *Altered State*, 311.

101  STOP THIS HELL FOR OUR KIDS: David Nichols Papers, box 1, folder 5, Purdue University, West Lafayette, IN, https://archives.lib.purdue.edu/repositories/2 /resources/531.

101  a 1992 poll conducted for the BBC: Charles S. Grob, "Deconstructing Ecstasy: The Politics of MDMA Research," *Addiction Research* 8, no. 6 (2000): 549–88, http://dx.doi.org/10.3109/16066350008998989.

101  sociologist Andrew Thompson calculated: Saunders, *E for Ecstasy*, 28.

102  in 1990 British lawmakers raised penalties: Saunders, *E for Ecstasy*, 125.

102  the Criminal Justice and Public Order Act: Criminal Justice and Public Order Act 1994, c. 33 (UK), https://www.legislation.gov.uk/ukpga/1994/33/introduction /enacted.

102  The bill also made it a criminal rather than civil offense: Pilcher, *E*, 118.

102  an estimated twenty thousand ravers and civil rights advocates: Collin, *Altered State*, 247–250.

102  By mid-1996, police had made more than a thousand arrests: Collin, 258.

102  large-scale outdoor raves had effectively been eradicated: Clark, "Ecstasy."

103  the longest sentences were given not for "hard drugs": Ruth Runciman, *Drugs and the Law: Report of the Independent Inquiry into the Misuse of Drugs Act 1971* (London: Police Foundation, 2000).

103 "If you're selling heroin": David Nutt, interview by the author, October 2021.

103 hundreds of "outlaw sound systems": Collin, *Altered State*, 259.

104 "I had a tremendous breakthrough": Satyam Nadeen, "From Onions to Pearls: Peeling the Gem," interview by Elaine Smitha, *Evolving Ideas with Elaine Smitha*, aired September 18, 1997, https://archive.org/details/FromOnionsToPearls .PeelingTheGem.

104 "deliverance" from "the preconditioned ego personality": Nadeen, "From Onions to Pearls."

CHAPTER 6: THE NEUROTOXICITY PUZZLE

106 "modifies the expected state of a living thing": Alexander Shulgin, *The Nature of Drugs: History, Pharmacology, and Social Impact*, vol. 1 (Berkeley, CA: Transform Press, 2021), 25.

106 things that affect the entire organism: Shulgin, *Nature of Drugs*, 196.

106 imperfectly imitating the structure of natural signaling chemicals: Carl Hart, *Drug Use for Grown-Ups: Chasing Liberty in the Land of Fear* (London: Penguin, 2021), 45.

106 "all affective states, from emotion to stimulation": Shulgin, *Nature of Drugs*, 195.

107 serotonin—a jack-of-all-trades neurotransmitter: David E. Presti, *Foundational Concepts in Neuroscience: A Brain-Mind Odyssey*, illustrated ed. (New York: W. W. Norton, 2015), 79.

107 moved into neurons by specialized proteins: Presti, *Foundational Concepts in Neuroscience*, 64.

107 dumping up to 80 percent of their stored serotonin: Brian Hare and Vanessa Woods, *Survival of the Friendliest: Understanding Our Origins and Rediscovering Our Common Humanity* (New York: Random House, 2020), 71.

107 the two fundamental questions of the neurotoxicity puzzle: Rick Doblin, "MAPS Newsletter, August 29, 1988," *Newsletter of the Multidisciplinary Association for Psychedelic Studies*, 1988, https://maps.org/news-letters /v01n1/.

108 In experiments with forty rats: Charles H. Frith, "28-Day Oral Toxicity Report of MDMA in Dogs" (Division of Laboratory Animal Medicine, University of Arkansas for Medical Sciences, 1985), https://maps.org/research-archive/dea -mdma/pdf/0069.pdf.

108 Dogs given daily MDMA doses: Tom Shroder, *Acid Test: LSD, Ecstasy, and the Power to Heal* (New York: Penguin, 2014), 224.

108 studies that looked more closely at the brains of rats: Donna M. Stone et al., "The Effects of 3,4-methylenedioxymethamphetamine (MDMA) and 3,4-methylenedioxyamphetamine (MDA) on Monoaminergic Systems in the Rat Brain," *European Journal of Pharmacology* 128, nos. 1–2 (August 1986): 41–48, https://www.doi.org/10.1016/0014-2999(86)90555-8.

108 David Nichols at Purdue: David Nichols Papers, box 1, folder 13, Purdue University, West Lafayette, IN, https://archives.lib.purdue.edu/repositories/2/resources /531.

108 "The fears of neurotoxicity": Rick Doblin, interview by the author, October 2021.

108 Doblin even went to Ricaurte's wedding: Shroder, *Acid Test*, 263.

109 "famous for using government grants": Alexander Shulgin, "Psychedelics Again," interview by Claus Langmaack, July 11, 2001, Samizdat Health Writer's Co-operative, Inc., https://samizdathealth.org/wp-content/uploads/2020/12 /Shulgin-2.pdf.

109 "even one dose of MDMA": Charles S. Grob, "Deconstructing Ecstasy: The Politics of MDMA Research," *Addiction Research* 8, no. 6 (2000): 549–88, http://dx .doi.org/10.3109/16066350008998989.

109 Ricaurte gave the monkeys: G. A. Ricaurte et al., "Toxic Effects of MDMA on Central Serotonergic Neurons in the Primate: Importance of Route and Frequency of Drug Administration," *Brain Research* 446 (1988): 165–68.

109 usually around 1.7 mg/kg: Shroder, *Acid Test*, 263.

109 NEW DATA INTENSIFY THE AGONY OVER ECSTASY: Deborah M. Barnes, "New Data Intensify the Agony over Ecstasy," *American Association for the Advancement of Science* 239, no. 4842 (February 1988): 864–66, https://www .doi.org/10.1126/science.2893452.

110 a single new data point didn't justify an entire paper: Grob, "Deconstructing Ecstasy," 563.

110 cerebrospinal fluid: Una D. McCann et al., "Serotonin Neurotoxicity after (+/-) 3,4-Methylenedioxymethamphetamine (MDMA; 'Ecstasy'): A Controlled Study in Humans," *Neuropsychopharmacology* 10, no. 2 (April 1994): 129–38, https://www.doi.org/10.1038/npp.1994.15.

110 the thirty control participants had been chronic pain patients: Grob, "Deconstructing Ecstasy," 571.

110 low serotonin levels could have led to MDMA use: Shroder, *Acid Test*, 266.

110 a $161,416 grant: National Institute of Mental Health, "MDMA Neurotoxicity in Humans–Occurrence and Consequence," project 1R01DA005938-01 (1989),

https://reporter.nih.gov/search/advaRWVqZEiAilAly6NlGg/project-details
/3212534.

110 The government agency went on to provide Ricaurte: National Institutes of
Health, "Search Results: George Ricaurte," https://reporter.nih.gov/search
/advaRWVqZEiAilAly6NlGg/projects.

110 $14.6 million in grants: "Ricaurte MDMA Research Controversy," Multidisci-
plinary Association for Psychedelic Studies, https://maps.org/research-archive
/mdma/studyresponse.html.

110 making his lab one of the most influential and well funded in the world: Grob,
"Deconstructing Ecstasy," 563.

111 "sexually vigorous" male rats: Wayne A. Dornan, Jonathan L. Katz, and George A.
Ricaurte, "The Effects of Repeated Administration of MDMA on the Expression
of Sexual Behavior in the Male Rat," *Pharmacology Biochemistry and Behavior* 39,
no. 3 (July 1991): 813–16, https://doi.org/10.1016/0091-3057(91)90171-W.

111 "That MDMA neurotoxicity generalizes to humans": National Institute of
Mental Health, "MDMA Neurotoxicity."

111 Ronald Reagan had scaled up: German Lopez, "The War on Drugs, Explained,"
*Vox*, updated May 8, 2016, https://www.vox.com/2016/5/8/18089368/war-on
-drugs-marijuana-cocaine-heroin-meth.

111 "number one problem": "Just Say No," History.com, updated August 21, 2018,
https://www.history.com/topics/1980s/just-say-no.

111 Shulgin even became a target of the war on drugs: Erowid, "DEA Raid of Shulgin's Laboratory on October 27, 1994," Vaults of Erowid, updated February 4, 2015,
https://erowid.org/culture/characters/shulgin_alexander/shulgin_alexander
_raid.shtml.

111 "Dr. Shulgin apparently was a pretty good chemist": Frank Sapienza, interview
by the author, December 2021.

112 "The problem was, we didn't find that many problems": Marsha Rosenbaum,
interview by the author, January 2022.

112 NIDA funds nearly 90 percent: Hart, *Drug Use for Grown-Ups*, 86.

112 "Those questions just aren't asked": Ethan Nadelmann, interview by the author,
December 2021.

112 "As an academic, if you can't get grants": David Nichols, interview by the author,
June 2021.

112 Shulgin mailed Doblin a letter: Charles Grob, Gary Bravo, and Roger
Walsh, "Second Thoughts on 3,4-Methylenedioxymethamphetamine (MDMA)
Neurotoxicity," *Archives of General Psychiatry* 47, no. 3 (March 1990): 288–89.

112 "I'm sitting in my office": Charles Grob, interview by the author, September 2021.

113 The four doctors collaborated: Mitchell B. Liester et al., "Phenomenology and Sequelae of 3,4 Methylenedioxymethamphetamine Use," *The Journal of Nervous and Mental Disease* 180, no. 6 (June 1992): 345–52.

113 graduating from New College sixteen years after enrolling: Shroder, *Acid Test*, 233.

114 "The masterstroke": Jerome Beck, interview by the author, January 2022.

114 reviewing psychedelic protocols: Richard E. Doblin, "Regulation of the Medical Use of Psychedelics and Marijuana" (PhD diss., Harvard University, 2000), https://maps.org/wp-content/uploads/2014/11/chapter2.pdf.

115 "certain death": Nichols Papers, box 12, folder 7.

115 clinical hold: "IND Application Procedures: Clinical Hold," U.S. Food and Drug Administration, updated October 9, 2015, https://www.fda.gov/drugs/investigational-new-drug-ind-application/ind-application-procedures-clinical-hold.

115 "the kiss of death": Jennifer M. Mitchell, "A Psychedelic May Soon Go to the FDA for Approval to Treat Trauma," *Scientific American*, February 1, 2022, https://www.scientificamerican.com/article/a-psychedelic-may-soon-go-to-the-fda-for-approval-to-treat-trauma/.

115 "it is invidious": Doblin, "Regulation of the Medical Use of Psychedelics," 71.

115 Pilot Drug Evaluation Staff approved: Doblin, 72–73.

115 "like persistent turtles": Nichols Papers, box 12, folder 7.

115 the FDA decided to convene a meeting: Doblin, "Regulation of the Medical Use of Psychedelics," 78.

116 Shulgin made the room laugh: Doblin, 80.

116 In front of TV crews and reporters: Doblin, 82.

116 If a pharmaceutical company created a drug: Bruce Eisner, *Ecstasy: The MDMA Story* (Berkeley, CA: Ronin, 1993), 172.

117 the FDA officially gave Grob the green light: Doblin, "Regulation of the Medical Use of Psychedelics," 91.

117 PROOF THAT ECSTASY DAMAGES THE BRAIN: Jeremy Laurance, "Proof that Ecstasy Damages the Brain," *Independent*, October 30, 1998, https://www.independent.co.uk/news/proof-that-ecstasy-damages-the-brain-1181512.html.

117 "holes in the brain": Donald G. McNeil Jr., "Research on Ecstasy Is Clouded by Errors," *New York Times*, December 2, 2003, https://www.nytimes.com/2003/12/02/science/research-on-ecstasy-is-clouded-by-errors.html.

117 glossed over by Oprah: Shroder, *Acid Test*, 282.

117 "pattern of flawed research methodologies": Charles Grob, "The Politics of Ecstasy," *Journal of Psychoactive Drugs* 34, no. 2 (April–June 2002): 143–44, https://www.tandfonline.com/doi/abs/10.1080/02791072.2002.10399948.

117 "subtle, but significant, cognitive deficits": Una D. McCann et al., "Cognitive Performance in (+/-) 3,4-Methylenedioxymethamphetamine (MDMA, "Ecstasy") Users: A Controlled Study," *Psychopharmacology* 143, no. 4 (April 1999): 417–25, https://www.doi.org/10.1007/s002130050967.

117 polydrug users: Julie Holland, ed., *Ecstasy: The Complete Guide: A Comprehensive Look at the Risks and Benefits of MDMA* (Rochester, VT: Park Street Press, 2001), 108.

118 "highly suspect": Grob, "Deconstructing Ecstasy," 574–75.

118 imported by British expats: Jerome Beck and Marsha Rosenbaum, *Pursuit of Ecstasy: The MDMA Experience* (New York: SUNY Press, 1994), 53.

118 "They wanted to check you out": Paul Dix, interview by the author, April 2022.

119 "it was like being in preschool again": Matthew Lieberman, interview by the author, April 2022.

119 in 2001 alone, nearly two million Americans: Shroder, *Acid Test*, 173.

119 an estimated ten million: McNeil, "Research on Ecstasy."

120 From at least 1997 until his arrest in 2000: "DEA Investigation Leads to Successful Extradition of Ecstasy Kingpin Fugitive from Spain to the United States," U.S. Drug Enforcement Administration, April 16, 2003, https://www.dea.gov/sites/default/files/pubs/states/newsrel/nyc041603.html.

120 a two-hundred-pound Israeli fugitive: Lisa Sweetingham, *Chemical Cowboys: The DEA's Secret Mission to Hunt Down a Notorious Ecstasy Kingpin*, reprint (New York: Ballantine, 2010), 91.

120 "Fat Man": Sweetingham, *Chemical Cowboys*, 220.

120 formerly dealt in heroin, cocaine, and marijuana: Sweetingham, 92–93.

120 strippers, Hasidic students, and intellectually disabled people: Andy Newman, "Man Extradited on Ecstasy Smuggling Charge," *New York Times*, April 17, 2003, https://www.nytimes.com/2003/04/17/nyregion/metro-briefing-new-york-brooklyn-man-extradited-on-ecstasy-smuggling-charge.html.

120 Tuito's signature "Tweety" pills: Sweetingham, *Chemical Cowboys*, 246.

120 only an estimated 40 percent: Grob, "Deconstructing Ecstasy," 558.

120 a DEA PowerPoint presentation from 1999: Nichols Papers, box 12, folder 9.

120 cut with a wide variety of adulterants: Grob, "Politics of Ecstasy."

120 "macho ingestion syndrome": Grob, "Deconstructing Ecstasy," 557.

120 "all tragic": Grob, "Politics of Ecstasy."

120  the "time bomb" theory: Grob, "Deconstructing Ecstasy," 579.

120  Echoing claims from the late 1960s: Doblin, "Regulation of the Medical Use of Psychedelics," 89.

121  "What we don't know": Beck and Rosenbaum, *Pursuit of Ecstasy*, 149–50.

121  at risk for Parkinson's disease: Jeanie L. Davis, "One Night of Ecstasy Can Damage Brain," WebMD, September 26, 2002.

121  "There are people who say": Howard Kornfeld, interview by the author, January 2022.

121  "MDMA neurotoxicity just hasn't happened": Ben Sessa, interview by the author, October 2021.

121  overuse usually occurs: Andrew Smirnov et al., "Young Adults' Trajectories of Ecstasy Use: A Population Based Study," *Addictive Behaviors* 38, no. 11 (November 2013): 2667–74, https://doi.org/10.1016/j.addbeh.2013.06.018.

121  "I've been in private practice": Julie Holland, interview by the author, December 2021.

122  when people did overuse the drug: Beck and Rosenbaum, *Pursuit of Ecstasy*, 127.

122  average ravers in Toronto had a "shelf-life": Timothy R Weber, "Raving in Toronto: Peace, Love, Unity and Respect in Transition," *Journal of Youth Studies* 2, no. 3 (1999): 317–36, https://doi.org/10.1080/13676261.1999.10593045.

122  80 percent of Ecstasy users: Kirsten Von Sydow et al., "Use, Abuse and Dependence of Ecstasy and Related Drugs in Adolescents and Young Adults—a Transient Phenomenon? Results from a Longitudinal Community Study," *Drug and Alcohol Dependence* 66, no. 2 (April 2002): 147–59, https://doi.org/10.1016/S0376-8716(01)00195-8.

122  her "ally," MDMA: Ann Shulgin, interview by the author, September 2021.

123  Phase 1 trial results: Charles Grob, "MDMA Research: Preliminary Investigations with Human Subjects," *International Journal of Drug Policy* 9 (1998): 119–24.

124  The Pilot Drug Evaluation Staff had been dissolved: Doblin, "Regulation of the Medical Use of Psychedelics," 110–11.

124  Grob finally received an answer: Doblin, 116.

125  "stripping bare" serotonin nerve terminals: Nichols Papers, box 12, folder 9.

125  more heavily punished, dose by dose: Shroder, *Acid Test*, 283.

125  Joe Biden, a preeminent crusader in the war on drugs: Tim Pilcher, *E: The Incredibly Strange History of Ecstasy* (Philadelphia: Running Press, 2008), 138–41.

125  a startling paper published in the prestigious journal *Science*: George Ricaurte et al., "Severe Dopaminergic Neurotoxicity in Primates after a Common

Recreational Dose Regimen of MDMA ("Ecstasy")," *Science* 297, no. 5590 (September 2002): 2260–63, https://www.science.org/doi/abs/10.1126/science .1074501.

126 "When that paper was submitted": David Nutt, interview by the author, October 2021.

126 "It looks like their tech stole the MDMA": Matthew Baggott, interview by the author, January 2022.

126 *Science* issued a startling retraction: George Ricaurte et al., "Retraction," *Science* 301, no. 5639 (September 2003): 1479, https://doi.org/10.1126/science.301.5639.1479b.

127 the dead animals should have sent up a red flag: McNeil, "Research on Ecstasy."

127 RTI, the chemical manufacturing company: Shroder, *Acid Test*, 292.

128 an acute but temporary depletion of serotonin: Grob, "Deconstructing Ecstasy," 561.

128 Long-term heavy MDMA users: Shroder, *Acid Test*, 293.

128 "If I'm interested in the therapeutic effects": John Halpern, interview by the author, January 2022.

128 "avoid substances that are harmful": Church of Jesus Christ of Latter-day Saints, "Church Policies & Guidelines," in *General Handbook: Serving in The Church of Jesus Christ of Latter-day Saints* (Salt Lake City, UT: Intellectual Reserve, 2022).

129 found no significant difference: John H. Halpern et al., "Residual Neurocognitive Features of Long-Term Ecstasy Users with Minimal Exposure to Other Drugs," *Addiction* 106 (2011): 777–86, https://doi.org/10.1111/j.1360-0443.2010.03252.x.

## CHAPTER 7: A SPLINTER IN THE MIND

130 Lori Tipton woke up on Monday: Lori Tipton, interview by the author, December 2021.

131 "the only mama they ever had": "Patricia Tipton Obituary," *Times-Picayune*, July 17, 2005, https://obits.nola.com/us/obituaries/nola/name/patricia-tipton -obituary?id=15666144.

133 *trauma* derives from the Greek term for "wound": Gabor Maté, *The Myth of Normal: Trauma, Illness, and Healing in a Toxic Culture* (New York: Avery, 2022), 16.

133 one in five American children is sexually molested: Bessel van der Kolk, *The Body Keeps the Score: Brain, Mind, and Body in the Healing of Trauma*, reprint ed. (New York: Penguin, 2015), 1.

133 one in five women and one in thirty-eight men: Centers for Disease Control and Prevention, "Fast Facts: Preventing Sexual Violence," updated June 22, 2022, https://www.cdc.gov/violenceprevention/sexualviolence/fastfact.html.

133 "Turn on the news": Rachel Yehuda, interview by the author, July 2021.

133 an estimated 7 percent: Rachel Nuwer, "A Balm for Psyches Scarred by War," *New York Times*, May 29, 2022, https://www.nytimes.com/2022/05/29/health/mdma-therapy-ptsd.html.

133 fifteen million people suffering from the condition: Jennifer M. Mitchell, "A Psychedelic May Soon Go to the FDA for Approval to Treat Trauma," *Scientific American*, February 1, 2022, https://www.scientificamerican.com/article/a-psychedelic-may-soon-go-to-the-fda-for-approval-to-treat-trauma/.

134 the symptoms of PTSD have long been recognized: Judith L. Hehrman, *Trauma and Recovery: The Aftermath of Violence—from Domestic Abuse to Political Terror* (New York: Basic Books, 1997), 10–26.

134 "post-Vietnam syndrome": Matthew J. Friedman, "Post-Vietnam Syndrome: Recognition and Management," *Psychosomatics* 22, no. 11 (November 1981): 931–34, 941–42, https://doi.org/10.1016/S0033-3182(81)73455-8.

134 a new diagnosis, PTSD: Van der Kolk, *Body Keeps the Score*, 19.

134 "bible of psychiatry": Van der Kolk, 29.

134 finally legitimized a serious condition: Hehrman, *Trauma and Recovery*, 28.

134 It took the women's liberation movement: Hehrman, 28.

134 a landmark paper on racial trauma: Robert T. Carter, "Racism and Psychological and Emotional Injury: Recognizing and Assessing Race-Based Traumatic Stress," *Counseling Psychologist* 35, no. 1 (January 2007): 13–105, https://doi.org/10.1177/0011000006292033.

134 "The experience of African Americans": Joseph McCowan, interview by the author, December 2021.

135 "When people come to me with racial trauma": Monnica Williams, interview by the author, December 2021.

135 despite a growing body of scientific evidence: Hehrman, *Trauma and Recovery*, 8.

135 PLEASE KEEP YOUR TROUBLES TO YOURSELF: David Nichols Papers, box 1, folder 5, Purdue University, West Lafayette, IN, https://archives.lib.purdue.edu/repositories/2/resources/531.

135 "People who have been traumatized": Stephen Xenakis, interview by the author, July 2021.

136 nervous system becomes "stuck": Van der Kolk, *Body Keeps the Score*, 307.

136 "PTSD is about reorganization of your brain and mind": Bessel van der Kolk, interview by the author, November 2021.

136 their nervous systems have been fundamentally altered: Van der Kolk, *Body Keeps the Score*, 17, 53.

136 higher levels of stress hormones like adrenaline: Van der Kolk, 30.

136 activity decreases in Broca's area: Van der Kolk, 43.

136 activity lights up in parts of the visual cortex: Van der Kolk, 44.

136 significantly lower activity in self-sensing areas: Van der Kolk, 93–94.

136 a sense of feeling embodied: Van der Kolk, 249.

136 The earlier and more severe the trauma: Maté, *Myth of Normal*, 29.

136 can snowball into other physiological problems: Van der Kolk, *Body Keeps the Score*, 53, 100, 149.

137 women with severe PTSD had twice the risk: Maté, *Myth of Normal*, 42.

137 "There's a huge link between trauma and medical problems": Gabor Maté, interview by the author, December 2021.

137 "far from being the arbiters": Maté, *Myth of Normal*, 61.

137 The ability to flexibly: Rachel Yehuda and Amy Lehrner, "Intergenerational Transmission of Trauma Effects: Putative Role of Epigenetic Mechanisms," *World Psychiatry* 17, no. 3 (October 2018): 243–57, https://doi.org/10.1002/wps.20568.

138 the adult children of Holocaust survivors: Rachel Yehuda et al., "Low Cortisol and Risk for PTSD in Adult Offspring of Holocaust Survivors," *American Journal of Psychiatry* 157, no. 8 (August 2000): 1252–59, https://ajp.psychiatryonline.org/doi/full/10.1176/appi.ajp.157.8.1252.

138 pregnant and in New York City during 9/11: Rachel Yehuda et al., "Transgenerational Effects of Posttraumatic Stress Disorder in Babies of Mothers Exposed to the World Trade Center Attacks during Pregnancy," *Journal of Clinical Endocrinology and Metabolism* 90, no. 7 (July 2005): 4115–18, https://pubmed.ncbi.nlm.nih.gov/15870120/.

138 impact entire peoples or nations: Maté, *Myth of Normal*, 36.

138 630,000 permutations: Isaac R. Galatzer-Levy and Richard A. Bryant, "636,120 Ways to Have Posttraumatic Stress Disorder," *Perspectives on Psychological Science* 8, no. 6 (November 2013): 651–62, https://doi.org/10.1177/1745691613504115.

138 trauma affects many more people: Maté, *Myth of Normal*, 43.

138 Childhood trauma in particular: Van der Kolk, *Body Keeps the Score*, 157–61.

138 "if doctors can't agree": Van der Kolk, 167.

140 to treat phobias: Van der Kolk, 222.

140 until they realize they are in fact safe: Van der Kolk, 77.

141 one third of all PTSD patients: Van der Kolk, 223.

141 "CBT alone is OK": Jennifer Mitchell, interview by the author, September 2021.

142 the need for effective treatments: Rick Doblin, interview by the author, October 2021.

142 "I never doubted the vision": David Presti, interview by the author, September 2021.

143 "I was catching the tail end": Michael Mithoefer, interview by the author, October 2021.

143 As van der Kolk summarized: Van der Kolk, *Body Keeps the Score*, 27, 36.

144 accompany psychotic clients to the grocery store: Annie Mithoefer, interview by the author, October 2021.

145 "protect the rights and welfare of humans": U.S. Food and Drug Administration, "Institutional Review Boards (IRBs) and Protection of Human Subjects in Clinical Trials," updated September 11, 2019, https://www.fda.gov/about-fda /center-drug-evaluation-and-research-cder/institutional-review-boards-irbs -and-protection-human-subjects-clinical-trials.

145 "Ecstasy" being used to treat PTSD: Rachel Zimmerman, "FDA Permits First Test of Ecstasy as Treatment for Stress Disorder," *Wall Street Journal*, November 6, 2001.

146 psychedelic research center: Barbara E. Bauer, "The Medical University of South Carolina Is Launching a Psychedelic Research Center," *Psychedelic Science Review*, January 24, 2020, https://psychedelicreview.com/the-medical-university -of-south-carolina-is-launching-a-psychedelic-research-center/.

146 Mithoefer received a letter: William C. Jacobs to Michael C. Mithoefer, September 6, 2002, Multidisciplinary Association for Psychedelic Studies, https://maps.org/wp-content/uploads/2002/09/wirbrescind.pdf.

146 turned out to be Una McCann: Michael Mithoefer, *MDMA-Assisted Therapy in the Treatment of Posttraumatic Stress Disorder (PTSD): A Third Update on the Approval Process* (San Jose, CA: Multidisciplinary Association for Psychedelic Studies, 2003), https://maps.org/news/bulletin/mdma-assisted -psychotherapy-in-the-treatment-of-posttraumatic-stress-disorder-ptsd-a -third-update-on-the-approval-process/.

147 banned his book: Steph Solis, "Copernicus and the Church: What the History Books Don't Say," *Christian Science Monitor*, February 19, 2013, https://www .csmonitor.com/Technology/2013/0219/Copernicus-and-the-Church-What -the-history-books-don-t-say.

152   56 percent of the group: Michael C. Mithoefer et al., "MDMA-Assisted Psycho-therapy for Treatment of PTSD: Study Design and Rationale for Phase 3 Trials Based on Pooled Analysis of Six Phase 2 Randomized Controlled Trials," *Psychopharmacology* 236, no. 9 (May 2019): 2735–45, https://doi.org/10.1007/s00213-019-05249-5.

153   Twelve months or more after completing the trial: Lisa Jerome et al., "Long-Term Follow-Up Outcomes of MDMA-Assisted Psychotherapy for Treatment of PTSD: A Longitudinal Pooled Analysis of Six Phase 2 Trials," *Psychophar-macology* 237, no. 8 (June 2020): 2485–97, https://doi.org/10.1007/s00213-020-05548-2.

155   clinical psychologist in New York City: "Xena," interview by the author, November 2021.

156   two million U.S. service members: Watson Institute for International and Public Affairs, "U.S. Veterans & Military Families," updated August 2021, https://watson.brown.edu/costsofwar/costs/human/veterans.

156   Studies reveal that 15 to 19 percent of soldiers: Charles W. Hoge, "Measuring the Long-Term Impact of War-Zone Military Service across Generations and Changing Posttraumatic Stress Disorder Definitions," *JAMA Psychiatry* 72, no. 9 (September 2015): 861–62, https://www.doi.org/10.1001/jamapsychiatry.2015.1066; Charles W. Hoge et al., "The Prevalence of Post-traumatic Stress Disorder (PTSD) in US Combat Soldiers: A Head-to-Head Comparison of DSM-5 versus DSM-IV-TR Symptom Criteria with the PTSD Checklist," *Lancet Psychiatry* 1, no. 4 (August 2014): 269–77, https://doi.org/10.1016/S2215-0366(14)70235-4.

156   more than thirty thousand U.S. active-duty personnel: Thomas H. Suitt, *High Suicide Rates among United States Service Members and Veterans of the Post 9/11 Wars* (Providence, RI: Watson Institute for International and Public Affairs, 2021), https://watson.brown.edu/costsofwar/files/cow/imce/papers/2021/Suitt_Suicides_Costs%20of%20War_June%2021%202021.pdf.

156   low relative use of those services: Hoge, "Measuring the Long-Term Impact."

156   "soldiers don't like to reveal": Elspeth Cameron Ritchie, interview by the author, April 2021.

157   fewer than one in ten: Karen H. Seal et al., "VA Mental health Services Utiliza-tion in Iraq and Afghanistan Veterans in the First Year of Receiving New Mental Health Diagnoses," *Journal of Traumatic Stress* 23, no. 1 (February 2010): 5–16, https://onlinelibrary.wiley.com/doi/10.1002/jts.20493.

157   at best half of veterans: Maria M. Steenkamp et al., "Psychotherapy for Military-Related PTSD: A Review of Randomized Clinical Trials," *Journal of the*

*American Medical Association* 314, no. 5 (August 2015): 489–500, https://www
.doi.org/10.1001/jama.2015.8370.

157 "I have been working for twenty years": Eric Vermetten, email interview by the
author, March 2021.

157 nearly 414,000 American service members: U.S. Department of Veteran
Affairs, "VA Research on Traumatic Brain Injury (TBI)," Office of Research and
Development, updated February 16, 2022, https://www.research.va.gov/topics
/tbi.cfm#major.

157 30 percent of veterans: Carla Zelaya, James M. Dahlhamer, and Yu Sun,
"Quick Stats: Percentage of Adults Aged ≥ 20 Years Who Had Chronic Pain, by
Veteran Status and Age Group—National Health Interview Survey, United States,
2019," *Morbidity and Mortality Weekly Report* 69, no. 47 (November 2020): 1797,
http://dx.doi.org/10.15585/mmwr.mm6947a6external icon.

158 "Killing civilians": Robert Koffman, interview by the author, May 2021.

158 "The guilt, the shame, and the anger": Rakesh Jetly, interview by the author,
October 2021.

158 John Reissenweber: John Reissenweber, interview by the author, June 2021.

160 "How do you not love a man": Stacy Turner, interview by the author,
June 2021.

162 the results of the first Phase 3 trial: Jennifer M. Mitchell et al., "MDMA-Assisted
Therapy for Severe PTSD: A Randomized, Double-Blind, Placebo-Controlled
Phase 3 Study," *Nature Medicine* 27 (May 2021): 1025–33.

162 "the first-ever, late-stage clinical trial": Jennifer M. Mitchell, "A Psychedelic May
Soon Go to the FDA for Approval to Treat Trauma," *Scientific American*,
February 1, 2022, https://www.scientificamerican.com/article/a-psychedelic
-may-soon-go-to-the-fda-for-approval-to-treat-trauma/.

163 participants who had eating disorder scores: Timothy D. Brewerton et al.,
"MDMA-Assisted Therapy Significantly Reduces Eating Disorder Symptoms
in a Randomized Placebo-Controlled Trial of Adults with Severe PTSD,"
*Journal of Psychiatric Research* 149 (May 2022): 128–35, https://www.doi.org/10
.1016/j.jpsychires.2022.03.008.

164 "But they pulled it off": Thomas Insel, interview by the author, January 2022.

164 "To finally have all the data": Albert Garcia Romeu, email interview by the
author, March 2021.

164 "The study is well done": Allen Francis, email interview by the author, March 2021.

165 "I give Rick Doblin a lot of credit": Frank Sapienza, interview by the author,
December 2021.

165 Starting in July 2023: Grace Browne, "MDMA and Psilocybin Are Approved as Medicines for the First Time," *Wired*, February 3, 2023, https://www.wired.com/story/australia-psilocybin-mdma-approval/.

165 In Brazil, pilot studies: Alvaro V. Jardim et al., "3,4-methylenedioxymethampheta mine (MDMA)-Assisted Psychotherapy for Victims of Sexual Abuse with Severe Post-Traumatic Stress Disorder: An Open Label Pilot Study in Brazil," *Brazilian Journal of Psychiatry* 43, no. 2 (2021), https://doi.org/10.1590/1516-4446-2020-0980.

165 "In Brazil, we don't have the same big issue": Eduardo Schenberg, interview by the author, December 2021.

165 being finalized in Armenia: Sergey Vardanyan, interview by the author, November 2021.

165 "We're really at a tipping point": Chris Stauffer, Horizons Veterans and Families Forum, November 2021.

166 "Pictures of the Buddha": Ben Sessa, interview by the author, October 2021.

## CHAPTER 8: A CRITICAL PERIOD

167 Alexander Fleming had just returned: F. W. Diggins, "The Discovery of Penicillin: So Many Get It Wrong," *Biologist* (London) 47, no. 3 (June 2000): 115–19, https://pubmed.ncbi.nlm.nih.gov/11190242/.

167 intriguingly clear of bacterial growth: Siang Y. Tan and Yvonne Tatsumura, "Alexander Fleming (1881–1955): Discoverer of Penicillin," *Singapore Medical Journal* 56, no. 7 (2015): 366–67, https://www.doi.org/10.11622/smedj.2015105.

167 clinical trials with 170 patients: Mariya Lobanovska and Giulia Pilla, "Penicillin's Discovery and Antibiotic Resistance: Lessons for the Future?" *Yale Journal of Biology and Medicine* 90 (2017): 135–45, https://pubmed.ncbi.nlm.nih.gov/28356901/.

167 this "miracle drug" saved thousands: Annie Tête, "Posts Tagged 'Penicillin,'" National WWII Museum New Orleans, updated September 24, 2013, http://www.nww2m.com/tag/penicillin/.

168 nearly four decades after Fleming's initial revelation: Bessel van der Kolk, *The Body Keeps the Score: Brain, Mind, and Body in the Healing of Trauma*, reprint ed. (New York: Penguin, 2015), 264.

168 finally teased apart the exact mechanism: Donald J. Tipper and Jack L. Strominger, "Mechanism of Action of Penicillins: A Proposal Based on Their Structural Similarity to Acyl-D-Alanyl-D-Alanine," *Proceedings of the National Academy of Sciences of the United States of America* 54 (October 1965): 1133–41, https://www.doi.org/10.1073/pnas.54.4.1133.

168 "a softening and opening up": Eric Vermetten, email interview by the author, March 2021.

168 "why this short experience": Rachel Yehuda, interview by the author, July 2021.

168 the human brain: David E. Presti, *Foundational Concepts in Neuroscience: A Brain-Mind Odyssey*, illustrated ed. (New York: W. W. Norton, 2015), xiv.

169 "That's how I've been lured into science": Gül Dölen, interview by the author, June 2021.

170 several hundred billion cells: Presti, *Foundational Concepts in Neuroscience*, 7.

171 "the rules and regulations were much more lax": Solomon Snyder, interview by the author, December 2021.

171 greylag gosling he named Martina: Tania Munz, "My Goose Child Martina: The Multiple Uses of Geese in the Writings of Konrad Lorenz," *Historical Studies in the Natural Sciences* 41, no. 4 (2011): 405–46, https://pubmed.ncbi.nlm.nih .gov/22363967/.

171 later earned him a Nobel Prize: "The Nobel Prize in Physiology or Medicine 1973," NobelPrize.org., 2022, https://www.nobelprize.org/prizes/medicine/1973 /summary/.

171 psychologist William James: William James, "Habit," ch. 4 of *The Principles of Psychology* (1890), Classics in the History of Psychology, Christopher D. Green, York University, Toronto, 1997, https://psychclassics.yorku.ca/James/Principles /prin4.htm.

172 "This goes way back to Aristotle": Takao Hensch, interview by the author, January 2022.

172 We lose behavioral flexibility: Brian Hare and Vanessa Woods, *Survival of the Friendliest: Understanding Our Origins and Rediscovering Our Common Humanity* (New York: Random House, 2020), 91.

173 Cochlear implants likewise work best: Vincenzo Vincenti et al., "Pediatric Cochlear Implantation: An Update," *Italian Journal of Pediatrics* 40, no. 72 (September 2014), https://www.doi.org/10.1186/s13052-014-0072-8.

174 hormone is a necessary component: Gül Dölen et al., "Social Reward Requires Coordinated Activity of Nucleus Accumbens Oxytocin and Serotonin," *Nature* 501 (September 2013): 179–84, https://www.doi.org/10.1038/nature12518.

177 findings about MDMA and the social reward learning critical period: Romain Nardou et al., "Oxytocin-Dependent Reopening of a Social Reward Learning Critical Period with MDMA," *Nature* 569, no. 7754 (May 2019): 116–20, https://www.doi.org/10.1038/s41586-019-1075-9.

178 "very, very exciting": David Nutt, interview by the author, October 2021.

179  "one of the cleanest stories": Frederick Barrett, interview by the author, December 2021.

179  Plasticity: Presti, *Foundational Concepts in Neuroscience*, xiii.

180  "The work is cutting edge enough": Jennifer Mitchell, interview by the author, September 2021.

180  giving mice ketamine: Alessandro Venturino et al., "Microglia Enable Mature Perineuronal Nets Disassembly upon Anesthetic Ketamine Exposure or 60-Hz Light Entrainment in the Healthy Brain," *Cell Reports* 36, no. 1 (July 2021): 109313, https://www.doi.org/10.1016/j.celrep.2021.109313.

180  "We came from a completely different angle": Sandra Siegert, interview by the author, January 2022.

182  "As I was coming down off the medicine": David Nickles and Lily Kay Ross, "Open Heart Surgery," *Cover Story*, podcast, March 1, 2022, https://podcasts .apple.com/us/podcast/cover-story/id1594675355?i=1000552567394.

183  "there was a certain type of character": Martin A. Lee and Bruce Shlain, *Acid Dreams: The Complete Social History of LSD; The CIA, the Sixties, and Beyond* (New York: Grove Press, 1994), 186, 195.

184  "an unbelievably powerful idea": Steven Zeiler, interview by the author, December 2021.

184  "It's fascinating to think": Michael Silver, interview by the author, December 2021.

CHAPTER 9: THE ADDICT'S NEED

185  "we got on like a house on fire": Dave Pounds, interview by the author, October 2021.

187  for decades Native Americans have held peyote ceremonies: Michael Pollan, *This Is Your Mind on Plants* (New York: Penguin Press, 2021), 163.

187  Western medicine in the 1950s likewise discovered: Martin A. Lee and Bruce Shlain, *Acid Dreams: The Complete Social History of LSD; The CIA, the Sixties, and Beyond* (New York: Grove Press, 1994), 49–55.

188  Bill Wilson: Charles Grob, "Psychiatric Research with Hallucinogens: What Have We Learned?" *Heffter Review of Psychedelic Research* 1 (1998): 8–20.

188  after Osmond gave him tabs to try: Ben Sessa, "The History of Psychedelics in Medicine," *Handbuch Psychoaktive Substanzen* (2016): 1–26, https://doi.org/10 .1007/978-3-642-55214-4_96-1.

188  a study using psilocybin to help longtime smokers: Matthew W. Johnson et al., "Pilot Study of the 5-HT2AR Agonist Psilocybin in the Treatment of Tobacco Addiction," *Journal of Psychopharmacology* 28, no. 11 (September 2014): 983–92, https://www.doi.org/10.1177/0269881114548296.

188  followed up on their psilocybin subjects: Matthew W. Johnson, Albert Garcia-Romeu, and Roland R. Griffiths, "Long-Term Follow-up of Psilocybin-Facilitated Smoking Cessation," *American Journal of Drug and Alcohol Abuse* 43, no. 1 (July 2016): 55–60, https://www.doi.org/10.3109/00952990.2016.1170135.

188  Sessa's interest in MDMA and other psychedelic drugs: Ben Sessa, interview by the author, October 2021.

188  In 2004 Sessa wrote what is likely the first paper: Ben Sessa, "Can Psychedelics Have a Role in Psychiatry Once Again?" *British Journal of Psychiatry* 186, no. 6 (June 2005): 457–58, https://doi.org/10.1192/bjp.186.6.457.

189  An estimated 237 million men and 46 million women: Vladimir Poznyak and Dag Rekve, eds., *Global Status Report on Alcohol and Health 2018* (Geneva: World Health Organization, 2018), https://www.who.int/publications/i/item/9789241565639.

189  top five causes of years of life lost: Tesfa Mekonen et al., "Treatment Rates for Alcohol Use Disorders: A Systematic Review and Meta-Analysis," *Addiction* 116, no. 10 (October 2021): 2617–34, https://doi.org/10.1111/add.15357.

189  addiction entails any behavior a person engages in: Gabor Maté, *In the Realm of Hungry Ghosts: Close Encounters with Addiction*, illustrated ed. (Berkeley, CA: North Atlantic, 2010), 224.

189  can be a highly effective strategy for banishing pain: Maté, *In the Realm of Hungry Ghosts*, 207.

189  gross misconceptions about the condition prevail: Gabor Maté, *The Myth of Normal: Trauma, Illness, and Healing in a Toxic Culture* (New York: Avery, 2022), 225.

189  While the disease label can capture various aspects of addiction: Gabor Maté, interview by the author, December 2021.

189  there has never been a single addiction gene found: Maté, *Myth of Normal*, 231.

190  taking any drug by itself will produce an addiction: Maté, *In the Realm of Hungry Ghosts*, 140.

190  70 percent or more of regular drug users: Carl Hart, *Drug Use for Grown-Ups: Chasing Liberty in the Land of Fear* (London: Penguin, 2021), 11.

190 a whopping 20 percent of those serving in Vietnam: Maté, *In the Realm of Hungry Ghosts*, 142.

190 "Under certain conditions of stress": Maté, 146.

190 all addictions do have a biological dimension: Maté, 137.

190 Addiction causes neurological changes tied to either dopamine: Maté, 152.

190 or to the brain's natural opiate systems: Maté, *Myth of Normal*, 298.

190 "people become addicted to their own brain chemicals": Maté, *In the Realm of Hungry Ghosts*, 226.

190 chemical, physical, and epigenetic alterations: Maté, 153–54.

191 addictions arise to generate feelings that a healthy brain: Maté, *Myth of Normal*, 232.

191 Common reasons Maté encounters: Maté, 216–17.

191 Emotional pain, stress, and social disconnection are the central drivers: Maté, 304.

191 Up to 63 percent of veterans with PTSD: Srabani Banerjee and Carolyn Spry, *Concurrent Treatment for Substance Use Disorder and Trauma-Related Comorbidities: A Review of Clinical Effectiveness and Guidelines* (Ottowa, ON: Canadian Agency for Drugs and Technologies in Health, 2017), https://www.ncbi.nlm.nih.gov/books/NBK525683.

191 adolescents with histories of abuse: Maté, *Myth of Normal*, 223.

191 An estimated one third of people with major depression: Addiction Center, "Depression," updated August 8, 2022, https://www.addictioncenter.com/addiction/depression-and-addiction/.

192 9.2 million Americans have a co-occurring substance dependency: Substance Abuse and Mental Health Services Administration, "Co-Occurring Disorders and Other Health Conditions," updated April 21, 2022, https://www.samhsa.gov/medication-assisted-treatment/medications-counseling-related-conditions/co-occurring-disorders.

192 Just as no gene exists for addiction: Maté, *Myth of Normal*, 251.

192 "There is tremendous drive to find some biochemical marker": Alexander Shulgin, *The Nature of Drugs: History, Pharmacology, and Social Impact*, vol. 1 (Berkeley, CA: Transform Press, 2021), 260.

192 "I have a strong inclination to agree with Gabor Maté": Howard Kornfeld, interview by the author, July 2022.

192 "there are legitimate, fundamental questions": Jay Joseph and Carl Ratner, "The Fruitless Search for Genes in Psychiatry and Psychology: Time to Reexamine a Paradigm," in *Genetic Explanations: Sense and Nonsense*, ed. S. Krimsky and J. Gruber (Cambridge, MA: Howard University Press, 2013).

192  "being raised about their assumptions and validity": Jay Joseph, *The Trouble with Twin Studies: A Reassessment of Twin Research in the Social and Behavioral Sciences* (New York: Routledge, 2015).

193  "Genes affect how sensitive one is": Richard C. Lewontin, *Biology as Ideology: The Doctrine of DNA* (New York: Harper Perennial, 1991), 30.

193  researchers examined blood samples from 489 children: Charlie L. J. D. van den Oord et al., "DNA Methylation Signatures of Childhood Trauma Predict Psychiatric Disorders and Other Adverse Outcomes 17 Years after Exposure," *Molecular Psychiatry* (2022), https://doi.org/10.1038/s41380-022-01597-5.

193  sensitive people are often more aware: Maté, *Myth of Normal*, 250.

193  has likened the deeply feeling children: W. Thomas Boyce, *The Orchid and the Dandelion: Why Some Children Struggle and How All Can Thrive* (New York, Knopf, 2019), 2.

193  scientific evidence for conditions as diverse as: Maté, *Myth of Normal*, 248–70.

194  "The evidence of a link": Richard Bentall, "Mental Illness Is a Result of Misery, Yet Still We Stigmatise It," *Guardian*, February 26, 2016, https://www.theguardian.com/commentisfree/2016/feb/26/mental-illness-misery-childhood-traumas.

194  "Our major finding is your history of relational health": Oprah Winfrey and Bruce D. Perry, *What Happened to You? Conversations on Trauma, Resilience, and Healing* (New York: Flatiron, 2021).

194  "this very pervasive, core sense of being damaged goods": Bessel van der Kolk, interview by the author, November 2021.

194  They will be more reactive to stress throughout their lives: G. Maté, "Beyond the Medical Model," ch. 37 of *Evaluating the Brain Disease Model of Addiction*, ed. N. Heather et al. (New York: Routledge, 2022).

198  about 1.5 million people are arrested on drug charges: David Farber, *The War on Drugs* (New York: New York University Press, November 2021).

198  about half of the federal prison population is there: Sentencing Project, "Criminal Justice Facts," https://www.sentencingproject.org/criminal-justice-facts/.

198  Black men compose 40 percent of the prison population: Hart, *Drug Use for Grown-Ups*, 204.

198  Black men are ten times more likely to be imprisoned: Johann Hari, *Chasing the Scream: The First and Last Days of the War on Drugs* (New York: Bloomsbury, 2016), 207.

198  An estimated 65 percent of the U.S. prison population: Sentencing Project, "Criminal Justice Facts."

198  do not like to take responsibility for our own failings: Maté, *In the Realm of Hungry Ghosts*, 218.

200  Phase 2a safety and tolerability pilot study: Ben Sessa et al., "First Study of Safety and Tolerability of 3,4-Methylenedioxymethamphetamine-assisted Psychotherapy in Patients With Alcohol Use Disorder," *Journal of Psychopharmacology* 35, no. 4 (February 2021): 375–83, https://doi.org/10.1177/0269 881121991792.

200  carried out an observational study: Ben Sessa et al., "How Well Are Patients Doing Post-Alcohol Detox in Bristol? Results from the Outcomes Study," *Journal of Alcoholism, Drug Abuse and Substance Dependence* 6, no. 21 (December 2020): doi.org/10.24966/ADSD-9594/100021.

201  He has since developed a "reverence": Maté, *Myth of Normal*, 454.

201  Some of Maté's patients, but not all: Maté, 457.

## CHAPTER 10: GROWING PAINS

204  Merck's patent on the molecule: Nicholas Saunders, *E for Ecstasy* (self-pub., Amazon Digital Services, 1993), 14.

204  "the destructive nature of the use of patents": Rick Doblin, interview by the author, October 2021.

204  a 1957 article in *Life* magazine: K. Gerber et al., "Ethical Concerns about Psilocybin Intellectual Property," *ACS Pharmacology and Translational Science* 4, no. 2 (January 2021): 573–77, doi.org/10.1021/acsptsci.0c00171.

204  "Rick can come across as a wide-eyed hippie": Gül Dölen, interview by the author, June 2021.

204  pharmaceutical companies currently practice: Johann Hari, *Lost Connections: Why You're Depressed and How to Find Hope* (New York: Bloomsbury, 2018), 22.

205  "The nonprofit public benefit model of drug development": Michael Mithoefer, interview by the author, November 2021.

206  an ad campaign sponsored by the Heartland Institute: Rachel Nuwer, "Global Warming Ad Quickly Dropped," *New York Times*, May 5, 2012, https://www.nytimes.com/2012/05/06/us/heartland-institute-pulls-its-global-warming-ad.html.

206  a libertarian organization supported by Charles Koch's charitable foundation: Stephanie Pappas, "Documents Reveal Koch-Funded Group's Plot to Undermine Climate Science," *Christian Science Monitor*, February 15, 2012, https://www

.csmonitor.com/Science/2012/0215/Documents-reveal-Koch-funded-group-s -plot-to-undermine-climate-science.

206 hugely influential role in pushing conservative agendas: A. Hertel-Fernandez, C. Tervo, and T. Skocpol, "How the Koch Brothers Built the Most Powerful Rightwing Group You've Never Heard Of," *Guardian*, September 26, 2018, https://www.theguardian.com/us-news/2018/sep/26/koch-brothers-americans -for-prosperity-rightwing-political-group.

206 waging a disinformation campaign against climate change: Jane Mayer, " 'Koch-land' Examines the Koch Brothers' Early, Crucial Role in Climate-Change Denial," *New Yorker*, August 13, 2019, https://www.newyorker.com/news/daily -comment/kochland-examines-how-the-koch-brothers-made-their-fortune -and-the-influence-it-bought.

206 fighting to repeal the Affordable Care Act: Jeremy W. Peters, "Patience Gone, Koch-Backed Groups Will Pressure G.O.P. on Health Repeal," *New York Times*, March 5, 2017, https://www.nytimes.com/2017/03/05/us/politics/koch-brothers -affordable-care-act.html.

206 and block a major election reform bill: Jane Mayer, "Inside the Koch-Backed Effort to Block the Largest Election-Reform Bill in Half a Century," *New Yorker*, March 29, 2021, https://www.newyorker.com/news/news-desk/inside-the-koch -backed-effort-to-block-the-largest-election-reform-bill-in-half-a-century.

206 working to quash labor unions: Josh Eidelson, "Koch Brothers-Linked Group Declares New War on Unions," *Bloomberg*, June 27, 2018, https://www.bloomberg .com/news/articles/2018-06-27/koch-brothers-linked-group-declares-new-war -on-unions.

207 is a skill she has been cultivating nearly her entire life: Elizabeth Koch, inter-view by the author, December 2021.

207 "A child who does not experience himself": Gabor Maté, *The Myth of Normal: Trauma, Illness, and Healing in a Toxic Culture* (New York: Avery, 2022).

210 "new drug product exclusivity": FDA, "Small Business Assistance: Frequently Asked Questions for New Drug Product Exclusivity," https://www.fda.gov /drugs/cder-small-business-industry-assistance-sbia/small-business-assistance -frequently-asked-questions-new-drug-product-exclusivity.

210 "a very traditional, very aggressive grab": Nicole Howell, interview by the author, January 2022.

212 "This revenue financing allows for sharing": Andrew "Mo" Septimus, interview by the author, April 2022.

212 "a bouquet of options": Federico Menapace, interview by the author, April 2022.

213 "really strong positive responses": Joy Sun Cooper, interview by the author, April 2022.

213 greater risk of developing a suite of physical and mental health conditions: Maté, *Myth of Normal*, 317.

213 "an opportunity for a new wave of engagement": Joseph McCowan, interview by the author, December 2021.

213 "raises deeper seated questions": Albert Garcia-Romeu, interview by the author, December 2021.

214 "The drug war has left people very reticent": Nicholas Powers, interview by the author, December 2021.

214 "'I want to make sure the Black people get it, too'": Monnica Williams, interview by the author, December 2021.

215 remembers going into her MDMA-assisted therapy session: Sara Reed, interview by the author, January 2022.

215 "Some of the moments of feedback": Monnica T. Williams, Sara Reed, and Jamilah George, "Culture and Psychedelic Psychotherapy: Ethnic and Racial Themes From Three Black Women Therapists," *Journal of Psychedelic Studies* 4, no. 3 (September 2020): 125–38, https://doi.org/10.1556/2054.2020 .00137.

217 surveyed more than three hundred BIPOC respondents: Monnica T. Williams et al., "People of Color in North America Report Improvements in Racial Trauma and Mental Health Symptoms Following Psychedelic Experiences," *Drugs: Education, Prevention and Policy* 28, no. 3 (December 2021): 215–26, https://doi.org/10.1080/09687637.2020.1854688.

218 "The bad news is": Julie Holland, Horizons conference presentation, New York, December 2021.

218 "it was mostly private salons and secret meetings": Kevin Balktick, interview by the author, November 2021.

218 "Now you're also dealing with venture capital bros": Matthew Johnson, interview by the author, December 2021.

219 "There's a sense we need to make up for lost time": Charles Grob, interview by the author, September 2021.

219 7 to 12 percent admitted to having had erotic contact: J. L. Alpert et al., "Sexual Boundary Violations: A Century of Violations and a Time to Analyze," *Psychoanalytic Psychology* 34, no. 2 (2017): 144–50, doi.org/10.1037/pap0000094.

219 people who have experienced sexual trauma as children: Alpert et al., "Sexual Boundary Violations."

219 "It's unfortunately very common": Julie Holland, interview by the author, November 2021.

220 Given the lopsided power dynamic between therapists and patients: Laura Mae Northrup, interview by the author, December 2021.

220 Ingrasci told a patient with cancer that having sex with him: Alison Bass, "Therapist Accused of Sex Abuse of Clients," *Boston Globe*, March 5, 1989, https://willhall .net/files/BostonGlobeCoverPsychedelicIngrasciAbuseMDMAMarch1989.pdf.

220 a "way of partial fulfillment of [her] oedipal wishes": DiLeo v. Nugent, 592 A.2d 1126 (88 Md. App. 59 1991).

220 "prominent leader in psychedelics research for many decades": Will Hall, "Ending The Silence around Psychedelic Therapy Abuse," *Mad in America*, September 25, 2021, https://www.madinamerica.com/2021/09/ending-silence -psychedelic-therapy-abuse/.

220 Yensen addressed the issue of sexual abuse by therapists: David Nickels, "Cautionary Tales: MDMA & MDA in Psychotherapy—A Talk with Richard Yensen and Donna Dryer (Part 1 of 2)," lecture video, YouTube, May 28, 2019, 45:01, https://www.youtube.com/watch?v=9GNRoVIOI0M&t=1749s.

221 childhood abuse and a violent rape: Olivia Goldhill, "Psychedelic Therapy Has a Sexual Abuse Problem," *Quartz*, March 3, 2020, https://qz.com/1809184 /psychedelic-therapy-has-a-sexual-abuse-problem-3/.

221 what she saw then as a complicated but overall positive experience: Meaghan Buisson, "Psychedelic Series #1: Over the Mountain," *Mad in America*, October 7, 2019, removed at request of the author.

221 "I learnt how much I craved as much as I feared touch": David Nickles and Lily Kay Ross, "Open Heart Surgery," *Cover Story*, podcast, March 1, 2022 https:// podcasts.apple.com/us/podcast/cover-story/id1594675355.

221 Buisson filed a civil court claim: Goldhill, "Psychedelic Therapy."

221 Buisson additionally filed ethics complaints: Russell Hausfeld, "As Legal Psychedelic Therapy Emerges, Ethicists Urge for More Comprehensive Frameworks to Address Sexual Abuse," *Psymposia*, November 21, 2019, https://www.psymposia .com/magazine/psychedelic-therapy-ethics-sexual-abuse/.

222 MAPS released a public statement: MAPS, "Public Announcement of Ethical Violation by Former MAPS-Sponsored Investigators," https://maps.org/2019/05 /24/statement-public-announcement-of-ethical-violation-by-former-maps -sponsored-investigators/.

222 On Twitter, Buisson characterized these types of statements: Meaghan Buisson, "Twitter / @MeaghanBuisson: What I survived at @MAPS MDMA drug

trial is horrific," March 1, 2022, https://twitter.com/MeaghanBuisson/status/1498537116120190980.

223 "The problem is much larger in scale": Lily Kay Ross, email interview by the author, April 2022.

224 "Not that regulation fixes everything": Franklin King, interview by the author, October 2021.


CHAPTER 11: THE PROBLEM WITH PROHIBITION

226 "Your daughter is gravely ill": Anne-Marie Cockburn, *5,742 Days: A Mother's Journey Through Loss* (Oxford, UK: Infinite Ideas, 2013), 17.

226 "I was calling to her in the same tone": Cockburn, *5,742 Days*, 7.

227 Anne-Marie pieced together the circumstances: Anne-Marie Cockburn, interview by the author, October 2021.

227 all drugs have a two-faceted nature: Michael Pollan, *This Is Your Mind on Plants* (New York: Penguin, 2021), 6.

227 "So many of the drug harms we deal with": Steve Rolles, interview by the author, October 2021.

228 the risk of death associated with Ecstasy use: Russell Newcombe and Sally Woods, "How Risky Is Ecstasy? A Model for Comparing the Mortality Risks of Ecstasy Use, Dance Parties and Related Activities," paper presented at Club Health 2000, Amsterdam, 2000.

228 life, in general, "is a riskful thing": Wim van den Brink, interview by the author, December 2021.

228 analyzed a suite of twenty legal and illegal drugs: D. J. Nutt, L. King, and L. D. Phillips, "Drug Harms in the UK: A Multi-Criterion Decision Analysis," *Lancet* 376 (2010), https://www.researchgate.net/publication/285843262_Drug_harms_in_the_UK_A_multi-criterion_decision_analysis.

229 "Equasy—An Overlooked Addiction": D. J. Nutt, "Equasy—An Overlooked Addiction with Implications for the Current Debate on Drug Harms," *Journal of Psychopharmacology* 23, no. 1 (2009): 3–5, https://journals.sagepub.com/doi/10.1177/0269881108099672.

229 Nutt's paper was not well received: David Nutt, *Nutt Uncut* (Sherfield Gables, UK: Waterside Press, 2021), 109.

229 "The right-wing press went absolutely ape": David Nutt, interview by the author, October 2021.

229 "Professor Nutt's comments earlier this year": Daniel Cressey, "Nutt Dismissal in Britain Highlights Diverging Drug Views," *Nature* (December 2009), https://www.nature.com/articles/nm1209-1337.pdf/.

229 between nine and thirty-five million people worldwide: UNODC, *World Drug Report 2021*, United Nations, June 2021, https://www.unodc.org/res/wdr2021/field/WDR21_Booklet_4.pdf.

229 7.3 percent of Americans over twelve years old have tried Ecstasy: "2019 NSDUH Detailed Tables," Substance Abuse and Mental Health Services Administration, September 11, 2020, https://www.samhsa.gov/data/report/2019-nsduh-detailed-tables.

230 Ecstasy use in North America and Europe is stable: UNODC, *World Drug Report 2021*.

230 "not just an increase, but a *large* increase in use": Mitchell Gomez, interview by the author, January 2022.

230 quadrupling since 2011: UNODC, *World Drug Report 2021*.

230 67 percent of MDMA users around the world: Steve Rolles, Harvey Slade, and James Nicholls, *How to Regulate Stimulants: A Practical Guide* (Bristol, UK: Transform Drug Policy Foundation, 2020).

230 American party promoters felt they needed to distance themselves: Matthew Collin, *Rave On: Global Adventures in Electronic Dance Music* (Chicago: University of Chicago Press, 2018), 156.

230 commodified by the mainstream and rebranded as EDM: Matthew Collin, *Altered State: The Story of Ecstasy and Acid House* (London: Serpent's Tail, 2010), 295.

230 EDM as a violation of all they stood for: Collin, *Rave On*, 161.

230–31 "'Rave' had become a bad word": Joseph Palamar, interview by the author, November 2021.

231 mistakenly thought Molly was a new drug: Michaelangelo Matos, *The Underground Is Massive: How Electronic Dance Music Conquered America* (New York: Dey Street, 2016), 347.

231 generated at least €18.9 billion in revenue: P. Tops et al., *The Netherlands and Synthetic Drugs: An Inconvenient Truth* (The Hague: Eleven International, 2018), https://www.politieacademie.nl/kennisenonderzoek/Onderzoek/Documents/Synthetic_herdruk_def.pdf.

231 as far as Australia, Brazil, and Japan: J. Mounteney et al., *Recent Changes in Europe's MDMA/Ecstasy Market: Results from an EMCDDA Trendspotter Study* (Lisbon:

European Monitoring Centre for Drugs and Drug Addiction, 2016), https://www
.emcdda.europa.eu/publications/rapid-communications/2016/mdma_en.

232 "a logical evolution": Philippus Zandstra, interview by the author, February
2022.

232 "When the police enter a lab": Tim Surmont, interview by the author, January
2022.

232 "Within a single club, you can have pills": Russell Newcombe, interview by the
author, November 2021.

233 The composition of that mystery powder has shifted over time: J. J. Palamar
and A. Salomone, "Shifts in Unintentional Exposure to Drugs among People
Who Use Ecstasy in the Electronic Dance Music Scene, 2016–2019," *American
Journal on Addictions* 13086 (2021): 49–54, doi.org/10.1111/ajad.13086.

234 confiscated more than thirty-three U.S. tons of safrole oil: Steve Rolles, Harvey
Slade, and James Nicholls, *How to Regulate Stimulants: A Practical Guide*
(Bristol, UK: Transform Drug Policy Foundation, 2020).

234 the roots of illegally felled *mreah prew phnom* trees: Rebecca Foges, "Huge
Seizure of 'Ecstasy Oil' in Cardamom Mountains," news release, Flora & Fauna
International, June 24, 2009, https://www.fauna-flora.org/news/huge-seizure-of
-ecstasy-oil-in-cardamom-mountains/.

234 a potentially lethal condition called serotonin syndrome: Rolles, Slade, and
Nicholls, *How to Regulate Stimulants*.

235 labs in China responded just as quickly: Mounteney et al., *Recent Changes*.

235 engineering baker's yeast to biosynthesize propane alkaloids: Prashanth Srini-
vasan and Christina D. Smolke, "Biosynthesis of Medical Tropane Alkaloids
in Yeast," *Nature* 585 (2020): 614–19, doi.org/10.1038/s41586-020-2650-9.

235 cheap, top-notch Ecstasy to come surging back: Collin, *Rave On*, 113.

236 MDMA tablets ranged around 50 to 80 milligrams: Mounteney et al., *Recent
Changes*.

236 the average tablet in Europe was 180 milligrams: European Monitoring Centre
for Drugs and Drug Addiction, "European Drug Report 2020: Trends and
Developments," Publications Office of the European Union, 2020.

236 "Blue Punisher" tablet seized at a club in Manchester: Max Daly, "World's
'Strongest-Ever' Ecstasy Pill Found in English Nightclub," *Vice*, November 16,
2021.

236 reaching a height of 131 in 2020: "Deaths related to Drug Poisoning in England
and Wales: 2020 Registrations," Office for National Statistics, August 3, 2021,
https://www.ons.gov.uk/peoplepopulationandcommunity/birthsdeathsandmar

riages/deaths/bulletins/deathsrelatedtodrugpoisoninginenglandandwales
/2020.

236 Coroners in the States: Carl Hart, *Drug Use for Grown-Ups: Chasing Liberty in the Land of Fear* (London: Penguin, 2021), 64.

236 didn't even list the drug in question on the death certificate: H. Jalal et al., "Changing Dynamics of the Drug Overdose Epidemic in the United States from 1979 through 2016," *Science* 361, no. 6408 (2021), doi.org/10.1126/science .aau1184.

236 a number of countries already provide such services: Hart, *Drug Use for Grown-Ups*, 68.

237 witnessed a spate of serious medical problems: Wendy Allison, interview by the author, December 2021.

237 places where festivals take a zero tolerance approach to drugs: Rolles, Slade, and Nicholls, *How to Regulate Stimulants*.

238 significantly less likely to say they still intended to use their drugs: Sarah Saleemi et al., "Who is 'Molly'? MDMA Adulterants by Product Name and the Impact of Harm-reduction Services at Raves," *Journal of Psychopharmacology* 31, no. 8 (July 2017): 1–5, https://doi.org/10.1177/0269881117715596.

238 publicly voiced his support: B. Flahive, "Independent Drug-Testing Tents at Festivals 'a Fantastic Idea,' Says Police Minister Stuart Nash," *Stuff*, January 2, 2019, https://www.stuff.co.nz/national/health/109699570/independent-drugtesting -tents-at-festivals-a-fantastic-idea-says-police-minister-stuart-nash.

238 in stark contrast to the United States, United Kingdom, and most other countries: Hart, *Drug Use for Grown-Ups*, 68.

239 The Loop provides on-site testing services: Hart, 81–82.

240 "Give me what Martha took": Cockburn, *5,742 Days*, 90.

241 she and a friend took around 80 milligrams of Ecstasy: Nutt, *Nutt Uncut*, 104.

241 Leah's dad was a former police officer: Collin, *Altered State*, 319.

241 Leah wasn't dancing or sweating: Nutt, *Nutt Uncut*, 104.

241 hyponatremia, a condition that occurs when excess water dilutes the blood: Julie Holland, ed., *Ecstasy: The Complete Guide: A Comprehensive Look at the Risks and Benefits of MDMA* (Rochester, VT: Park Street Press, 2001), 75–76.

241 Especially in young women: Nutt, *Nutt Uncut*, 105.

241 Her family met with Prime Minister Tony Blair: Nutt, 105.

241 on antidrug billboards published at fifteen hundred locations: Collin, *Altered State*, 320.

241 the multimillion-pound advertising campaign had been paid for: Nutt, *Nutt Uncut*, 105.

241 MDMA was linked to 44 deaths in the United Kingdom: Rolles, Slade, and Nicholls, *How to Regulate Stimulants*.

242 "The core principle, to my mind, of drug policy reform": Ethan Nadelmann, interview by the author, December 2021.

243 the U.S. government is actually violating the fundamental rights of its citizens: Hart, *Drug Use for Grown-Ups*, 31.

243 "Our right to make decisions": Hart, 54.

243 American taxpayers spent approximately thirty-five billion dollars: Hart, 19.

243 more than 560,000 pounds of waste from MDMA: Eline Schaart, "Breaking Brabant: Drug Labs Blight a Dutch landscape," *Politico EU*, July 22, 2019, https://www.politico.eu/article/brabant-dutch-drug-labs-blight-the-landscape/.

245 quantify the best approach for reducing harms and risks: Jan van Amsterdam et al., "Developing a New National MDMA Policy: Results of a Multi-decision Multi-criterion Decision Analysis," *Journal of Psychopharmacology* 35, no. 5 (February 2021): 537–46, https://doi.org/10.1177/0269881120981380.

245 the British government passed the Psychoactive Substances Act: Psychoactive Substances Act 2016, May 26, 2016, https://www.legislation.gov.uk/ukpga/2016 /2/contents/enacted.

246 research and medicalization "changes peoples' understanding of the risk-benefit": Rick Doblin, interview by the author, October 2021.

246 "[MDMA's] risks in pure form": Allen Frances, email interview by the author, May 2021.

246 likened the current state of the battle to end the war on drugs: Johann Hari, *Chasing the Scream: The First and Last Days of the War on Drugs* (New York: Bloomsbury, 2016), 295–96.

CHAPTER 12: THE SOCIAL SPECIES

248 A five-hundred-million-year evolutionary gulf: Rachel Nuwer, "Rolling Under the Sea: Scientists Gave Octopuses Ecstasy to Study Social Behavior," *Scientific American*, December 1, 2018, https://www.scientificamerican.com /article/rolling-under-the-sea-scientists-gave-octopuses-ecstasy-to-study -social-behavior/.

248 Most neuroscience research is done on mice: Gül Dölen quoted in Rachel Nuwer, "An Octopus Could Be the Next Model Organism," *Scientific American*,

March 1, 2021, https://www.scientificamerican.com/article/an-octopus-could-be-the-next-model-organism/.

249  "he was really just having a good time": Gül Dölen, interview by the author, February 2021.

250  other researchers who had sequenced the octopus genome: C. B. Albertin et al., "Genome and Transcriptome Mechanism Driving Cephalopod Evolution," *Nature Communications* 13, no. 2427 (2022), doi.org/10.1038/s41467-022-29748-w.

250  the octopus study, published in 2018 in *Current Biology*: E. Edsinger and G. Dölen, "A Conserved Role for Serotonergic Neurotransmission in Meditating Social Behavior in Octopus," *Current Biology Report* 28 (2018): 3136–42, https://pubmed.ncbi.nlm.nih.gov/30245101/.

251  significantly contributed to our eventual dominant role on Earth: Matthew D. Lieberman, *Social: Why Our Brains Are Wired to Connect* (New York: Crown, 2013), 7–9.

251  "When *Homo sapiens* diverged from our closest ancestors": Brian Hare and Vanessa Woods, *Survival of the Friendliest: Understanding Our Origins and Rediscovering Our Common Humanity* (New York: Random House, 2020), xix.

251  a tipping point about fifty thousand years ago: Hare and Woods, *Survival of the Friendliest*, 63.

251  evolved to become friendlier: Hare and Woods, 28.

251  As our communities became denser, innovation accelerated: Hare and Woods, 98.

251–52  scientists now know often precedes depression and anxiety: Johann Hari, *Lost Connections: Why You're Depressed and How to Find Hope* (New York: Bloomsbury USA, 2018), 77.

252  "feelings of loneliness told them when those protective bonds were endangered": John T. Cacioppo and William Patrick, *Loneliness: Human Nature and the Need for Social Connection* (New York: W. W. Norton, 2009), 7.

252  our biological need to feel a sense of love and belonging: Lieberman, *Social*, 43.

252  "The price for our species' success at connecting": Lieberman, 48.

252  the same regions of the brain's dorsal anterior cingulate: Cacioppo, *Loneliness*, 8.

252  social pain also carries the risk of very real repercussions: Cacioppo, 5–12.

252  risk of death equivalent to smoking fifteen cigarettes per day: J. Holt-Lunstad, Timothy B. Smith, and J. Bradley Layton, "Social Relationships and Mortality Risk: A Meta-analytic Review," *PLOS Medicine* 10, no. 1371 (2010), doi.org/10.1371/journal.pmed.1000316.

252  health risks equivalent to being obese: Hari, *Lost Connections*, 75.

252  or having dangerously high blood pressure: Cacioppo, *Loneliness*, 5.

252   social isolation inhibits the immune system: Maté, *Myth of Normal*, 294.

252   "Think of all those lonely people": Julie Holland, *Good Chemistry: The Science of Connection, from Soul to Psychedelics* (New York: Harper Wave, 2020), 11.

253   delivers tangible benefits: Cacioppo, *Loneliness*, 12–19.

253   the well-being equivalent of making an extra hundred thousand dollars a year: Lieberman, *Social*, 247.

253   associated with a 50 percent reduced risk of early death: Holt-Lunstad, Smith, and Layton, "Social Relationships and Mortality Risk."

253   "Regardless of one's sex, country or culture of origin": Julianne Holt-Lunstad, Theodore Robles, and David A. Sbarra, "Advancing Social Connection as a Public Health Priority in the United States," *American Psychology* 72, no. 6 (September 2017): 517–30, https://doi.org/10.1037/amp0000103.

253   kicked off during the dawn of the industrial revolution: Cacioppo, *Loneliness*, 53–54.

253   compared to just a few decades ago: R. D. Putnam, *Bowling Alone: The Collapse and Revival of American Community* (New York: Simon & Schuster, 2000).

253   the percentage of Americans who said they are lonely: Maté, *Myth of Normal*, 295.

254   taking at least one drug for a psychiatric problem: Hari, *Lost Connections*, 10.

254   people living alone to changes in work structures and growing inequality: Hari, 121.

254   Materialism encouraged by a consumer society: Maté, *Myth of Normal*, 292–96.

254   the association between materialism and negative mental health: Hari, *Lost Connections*, 96.

254   people who overvalue money: Hari, 93.

254   "diminished the quality of interpersonal exchanges": Holt-Lunstad, Robles, and Sbarra, "Advancing Social Connection as a Public Health Priority."

254   people check their phones an average of: Hari, *Lost Connections*, 87.

254   "Social media ends up serving as a very temporary distraction": Matthew Lieberman, interview by the author, April 2022.

255   "being online and being physically among people": Hari, *Lost Connections*, 89.

255   more likely to experience high levels of loneliness: Dawn Ee et al., "Loneliness in Adults on the Autism Spectrum," *Autism in Adulthood* 1, no. 3 (2019): 182–93, doi.org/10.1089/aut.2018.0038.

255   7 percent of the general adult U.S. population: American Psychiatric Association, "What Are Anxiety Disorders?" https://psychiatry.org/patients-families/anxiety-disorders/what-are-anxiety-disorders.

255 one in four autistic adults do: S. Bejerot, J. M. Eriksson, and E. Mörtberg, "Social Anxiety in Adult Autism Spectrum Disorder," *Psychiatry Research* 220, nos. 1–2 (2014): 705–7, doi.org/10.1016/j.psychres.2014.08.030.

255 four times more likely to suffer from depression: Cheryl Platzman Weinstock, "The Deep Emotional Ties Between Depression and Autism," *Spectrum News*, July 31, 2019, https://www.spectrumnews.org/features/deep-dive/the -deep-emotional-ties-between-depression-and-autism/.

255 "When our negative social expectations elicit behaviors from others": Cacioppo, *Loneliness*, 179.

255 autistic adults are less likely to be lonely: K. Umagami et al., "Loneliness in Autistic Adults: A Systematic Review," *National Autism Society* 6, no. 684 (2022), doi.org/10.1177/13623613221077721.

255 "overly performative and needing to take over a situation": Aaron Paul Orsini, interview by the author, December 2021.

256 Aaron felt his mind go still: Aaron Paul Orsini, *Autism on Acid: How LSD Helped Me Understand, Navigate, Alter and Appreciate My Autistic Perceptions* (self-pub., 2019), 8.

257 "We're a diverse bunch": Nick Walker, interview by the author, January 2022.

258 data she collected from autistic individuals: Alicia Lynn Danforth, "Courage, Connection, and Clarity: A Mixed-Methods Collective-Case Study of MDMA (Ecstasy) Experiences of Autistic Adults" (PhD diss., Sofia University, 2013).

258 guided participants through various methods: MAPS, "Charles Grob & Alicia Danforth: MDMA-Assisted Therapy for Social Anxiety in Autistic Adults," YouTube, April 26, 2017, 46:48, https://www.youtube.com/watch?v=eINBXdq TfOQ.

258 significantly greater reduction in their social anxiety symptoms: Alicia L. Danforth et al., "Reduction in Social Anxiety after MDMA-Assisted Psychotherapy with Autistic Adults: A Randomized, Double-Blind, Placebo-Controlled Pilot Study," *Psychopharmacology* 235 (2018): 3137–48, https://doi.org/10.1007 /s00213-018-5010-9.

259 "The fact that this person went from having severe social anxiety": Berra Yazar-Klosinski, interview by the author, September 2021.

259 "Autistic Psychedelic Wiki": Aaron Paul Orsini, Autistic Psychedelic Wiki, https://www.autismonacid.com/research.

260 "effortless and fluid verbal communication": Aaron Paul Orsini, *Autistic Psychedelic: The Self-Reported Benefits and Challenges of Experiencing LSD,*

*MDMA, Psilocybin and Other Psychedelics As Told by Neurodivergent Adults Navigating . . . Depression and Other Conditions* (self-pub., 2021), 61–62.

260 "seen and understood by my neurotypical friends": Orsini, *Autistic Psychedelic*, 171.

260 "not that well socially calibrated": John Allison, interview by the author, April 2022.

261 "We can use MDMA as a tool": Sonja Lyubomirsky, interview by the author, December 2021.

261 a paper proposing a new field of study: Sonja Lyubomirsky, "Toward a New Science of Psychedelic Social Psychology: The Effects of MDMA (Ecstasy) on Social Connection," *Perspectives on Psychological Science* 10, no. 1177 (2022), doi .org/10.1177/17456916211055369.

261 are slower to pick up on angry facial expressions: Margaret C. Wardle and Harriet de Wit, "MDMA Alters Emotional Processing and Facilitates Positive Social Interaction," *Psychopharmacology* 231, no. 21 (October 2014): 4219–29, doi:10.1007/s00213-014-3570-x.

261 lowers fear of being judged or rejected: Matthew J. Baggott et al., "Effects of 3,4-Methylenedioxymethamphetamine on Socioemotional Feelings, Authenticity, and Autobiographical Disclosure in Healthy Volunteers in a Controlled Setting," *Journal of Psychopharmacology* 20, no. 4 (2016): 378–87, https://doi.org /10.1177/0269881115626348.

261 people who have taken MDMA at least once: Grant Jones, Joshua Lipson, and Erica Wang, "Examining associations between MDMA/ecstasy and classic psychedelic use and impairments in social functioning in a U.S. adult sample," *Scientific Reports* 13 (February 2023), https://www.nature.com/articles/s41598 -023-29763-x.

262 whether MDMA increased the pleasantness of social touch: Harriet de Wit and Anya K. Bershad, "MDMA Enhances Pleasantness of Affective Touch," *Neuropsychopharmacology* 45 (2020): 217–39, https://doi.org/10.1038/s41386-019-0473-x.

262 "We really have to look into this": Harriet de Wit, interview by the author, November 2021.

263 "I really wanted it to be for guys": Brendan (last name withheld), interview by the author, December 2021.

263 the dehumanizing rhetoric Donald Trump used: Hare and Woods, *Survival of the Friendliest*, 181.

264 "I know what that did to my own country": "S.," interview by the author, December 2021.

266 "gave him a clear vision that unexamined racism": Requa Greer, interview by the author, November 2021.

266 "influence a person's values and priorities": Harriet de Wit et al., "Can MDMA Change Sociopolitical Values? Insights From a Research Participant," *Biological Psychiatry* 89, no. 11 (April 2021): e61–e62, https://doi.org/10.1016/j.biopsych .2021.01.016.

266 drives a "tend and defend" response across the animal kingdom: Hare and Woods, *Survival of the Friendliest*, 109.

267 men who inhaled oxytocin were three times more likely: C. K. W. De Dreu et al., "The Neuropeptide Oxytocin Regulates Parochial Altruism in Intergroup Conflict among Humans," *Science* 328, no. 5984 (2010): 1408–11, doi .org.10.1038/npp.2014.12.

267 members of the Taliban, for example, use MDMA: Murtaza Majeed, interview by the author, April 2022.

267 members of right-wing authoritarian political movements: Brian A. Pace and Neşe Devenot, "Right-Wing Psychedelia: Case Studies in Cultural Plasticity and Political Pluripotency," *Frontiers in Psychology* 12 (December 2021), https://www .frontiersin.org/articles/10.3389/fpsyg.2021.733185/full.

267 "If you give this drug to shallow assholes": Jerome Beck and Marsha Rosenbaum, *Pursuit of Ecstasy: The MDMA Experience* (New York: SUNY Press, 1994), 8.

267 a growing body of scientific evidence indicates: David E. Presti, *Foundational Concepts in Neuroscience: A Brain-Mind Odyssey*, illustrated ed. (New York: W. W. Norton, 2015), 4.

267 the human capacity for compassion, kindness, empathy: D. Keltner, J. Marsh, and J. A. Smith, *The Compassionate Instinct: The Science of Human Goodness* (New York: W. W. Norton, 2010), 6.

267 "Empathy is the one weapon in the human repertoire": Frans de Waal, "The Evolution of Empathy," *Greater Good Magazine*, September 1, 2005, https:// greatergood.berkeley.edu/article/item/the_evolution_of_empathy.

268 "I think all psychedelics have a role to play": Natalie Ginsberg, interview by the author, September 2021.

268 of using ayahuasca in group contexts: L. Roseman et al., "Relational Processes in Ayahuasca Groups of Palestinians and Israelis," *Frontiers in Pharmacology*, May 19, 2021, doi.org/10.3389/fphar.2021.607529.

268 "I kind of have a fantasy": Franklin King, interview by the author, October 2021.

CHAPTER 13: DESTIGMATIZATION

270 "smart entertainment": Alex Barasch, "Remote Comedy's Technical Difficulties," *New Yorker*, March 30, 2020.

271 "the hierarchy was who's the funniest": Sarah Rose Siskind, interview by the author, August 2022.

273 having written an entire book on the subject: Carl Hart, *Drug Use for Grown-Ups: Chasing Liberty in the Land of Fear* (London: Penguin, 2021).

273 "I believe, just like Harvey Milk": Julie Holland, interview by the author, December 2021.

273 "I used to have this line when the media would ask me that": Charles Grob, interview by the author, December 2021.

273 Will Siu gave a presentation to doctors and scientists at NYU: Will Siu, interview by the author, December 2021.

275 "The interest is huge": Charles Raison, Horizons conference presentation, New York, December 2021.

275 "Up until recently, people who ended up in psychedelics research": Matthew Johnson, interview by the author, December 2021.

275 its first grant in support of therapeutic psychedelic research: Marisol Martinez, "Johns Hopkins Receives First Federal Grand for Psychedelic Treatment Research in 50 Years," October 18, 2018, https://www.hopkinsmedicine.org/news/newsroom/news-releases/johns-hopkins-medicine-receives-first-federal-grant-for-psychedelic-treatment-research-in-50-years.

275 a bill in June 2021 that supports the study of "alternative therapies": A Bill to Be Entitled an Act, 87(R), Texas HB 1802 (2021).

275 "What's happening now is just kind of amazing": Debby Harlow, interview by the author, January 2022.

276 "The embrace from the mental health community": Michael Pollan, interview by the author, October 2021.

276 "The model we've had, which is the wrong model": Thomas Insel, interview by the author, January 2022.

276 "All these people work independently": Stephen Xenakis, interview by the author, July 2021.

277 "MAPS cannot advertise or promote off-label use": Ismail Ali, interview by the author, December 2021.

277 just one available tool in a revamped, "integrative" approach: Will Van Derveer, interview by the author, May 2022.

278 "I love Rick so I accepted it": Ethan Nadelmann, interview by the author, December 2021.

279 "There's been a lot of sweeping under the rug": Kevin Balktick, interview by the author, November 2021.

279 Western society readily accepts taking a drug for medical reasons: Nicholas Saunders, *E for Ecstasy* (self-pub., Amazon Digital Services, 1993), 17.

279 "There's this notion of, 'Oh, it must be justified!'": Keeper Trout, interview by the author, December 2021.

279 "It can definitely be an ecstatic dancing experience": Vanja Palmers, interview by the author, December 2021.

279 countries as disparate as South Africa, India: Matthew Collin, *Rave On: Global Adventures in Electronic Dance Music* (Chicago: University of Chicago Press, 2018), 193, 204.

279 Kazakhstan: UNODC, *World Drug Report 2021*, United Nations, June 2021, https://www.unodc.org/res/wdr2021/field/WDR21_Booklet_4.pdf.

279 In China, it's called "head-rocking pills": Julie Holland, ed., *Ecstasy: The Complete Guide: A Comprehensive Look at the Risks and Benefits of MDMA* (Rochester, VT: Park Street Press, 2001), 155.

279 "Ecstasy is for friends gathering around the fire": Murtaza Majeed, interview by the author, April 2022.

280 Molly being given out to party guests "at the elegant home": Irina Aleksander, "Molly: Pure, but Not So Simple," *New York Times*, June 21, 2013, https://nyti.ms/14bZZsU.

280 "I'm Black, a bunch of my friends are Black": Khary Rigg, interview by the author, February 2022.

280 Molly users he surveyed cited hip-hop culture: K. Khary Rigg and Amanda Sharp, "Nonmedical Prescription Drug Use among African Americans Who Use MDMA (Ecstasy/Molly): Implications for Risk Reduction," *Addictive Behaviors* 79 (2018): 159–65, https://doi.org/10.1016/j.addbeh.2017.12.024/.

280 In in-depth interviews with fifteen of the respondents: K. Khary Rigg, "Motivations for Using MDMA (Ecstasy/Molly) among African Americans: Implications for Prevention and Harm-Reduction Programs," *Journal of Psychoactive Drugs* 49, no. 3 (2017): 192–200, https://doi.org/10.1080/02791072.2017.1305518.

281 "the places where people are actually viscerally experiencing these drugs": Michelle Lhooq, interview by the author, January 2022.

283 social scientists described Grateful Dead and other rock concerts: John Neumeyer and Gregory Johnson, "Drug Emergencies in Crowds: An Analysis of 'Rock Medicine,' 1973–1977," *Journal of Drug Issues* 9, no. 2 (Spring 1979): 235–45.

283 giving rats MDMA or a placebo: Allison A. Feduccia and Christine L. Duvauchelle, "Auditory Stimuli Enhance MDMA-Conditioned Reward and MDMA-Induced Nucleus Accumbens Dopamine, Serotonin and Locomotor Responses," *Brain Research Bulletin* 77, no. 4 (October 22, 2008): 189–96, https://doi.org/10.1016/j.brainresbull.2008.07.007.

283 "everyone hated that CD": Allison Feduccia, interview by the author, October 2021.

283 more likely to say that they experienced a sense of awe: Martha Newson et al., "'I Get High With a Little Help From My Friends': How Raves Can Invoke Identity Fusion and Lasting Co-operation via Transformative Experiences," *Frontiers in Psychology* 12 (September 2021): 719596, https://doi.org/10.3389/fpsyg.2021.719596.

283 "Raves are an indigenous practice": Martha Newson, interview by the author, January 2022.

CHAPTER 14: FELLOW TRAVELERS

285 he envisions the drug helping to usher in a "spiritualized humanity": Rick Doblin, interview by the author, October 2021.

286 "As many of us now see, if we don't start doing something": David Presti, interview by the author, September 2021.

286 "If you start thinking you're getting personal messages": Nicholas Powers, interview by the author, December 2021.

287 "complete physical, mental and social well-being": John T. Cacioppo, *Loneliness: Human Nature and the Need for Social Connection* (New York: W. W. Norton, 2009), 92.

287 "People tend to think they're not worth saving": Berra Yazar-Klosinski, interview by the author, September 2021.

287 "a lot of people have come to realize how unnatural their lives feel": Gül Dölen, interview by the author, May 2021.

288 "the warmth of genuine connection frees our minds": Cacioppo, *Loneliness*, 269.

288 "It certainly feels like society needs a reorientation": Franklin King, interview by the author, October 2021.

288 whether a society robbed of the mystical experience: Brian Muraresku, *The Immortality Key: The Secret History of the Religion with No Name* (New York: St. Martin's Press, 2020), 75.

288 "We know that when people have a profound psychedelic experience": Shelby Hartman, interview by the author, December 2021.

289 "When I tried MDMA, it was incredible": "Sebastian," interview by the author, January 2022.

290 "there were just walls and barriers that I'd keep hitting": Michael Pollack, interview by the author, May 2022.

290 gave him methamphetamine instead of MDMA: Michael Pollack, "What Happens When Psychedelic Treatment for PTSD Turns into a Bad Trip," *Slate*, February 2, 2022, https://slate.com/technology/2022/02/psychedelic-treatment -ptsd-dangers-mdma-psilocybin-meth-container.html.

292 for two decades Charley and Shelley have been figureheads: Charley and Shelley Wininger, interview by the author, July 2021.

294 He felt like he was squandering his time and talents: Charles Wininger, *Listening to Ecstasy: The Transformative Power of MDMA* (Rochester, VT: Park Street Press, 2020), 35.

294 "this cute and curvy lady": Wininger, *Listening to Ecstasy*, 38.

294 One of those things, she told Charley, was Ecstasy: Wininger, 42.

294 ran naked through the warm summer rain: Wininger, 45.

295 "stop, drop, and roll": Wininger, xv.

295 vitality, wonder, and play are not things reserved only for the young: Wininger, 172.

296 "extraordinary times call for extraordinary pleasures": Wininger, xvii.

296 "MDMA helps me feel": Wininger, 102, 125.

296 It was a beautiful May day: Charles Wininger, "Can MDMA Heal Grief?" *Lucid News*, March 3, 2022, https://www.lucid.news/can-mdma-help-heal-grief/.

# INDEX

Page numbers with an asterisk (\*), dagger mark (†), or section sign (§) refer to footnotes.

# A NOTE ON THE AUTHOR

RACHEL NUWER is an award-winning science journalist who regularly contributes to the *New York Times*, *National Geographic*, *Scientific American*, and many other publications. Her reporting for the *New York Times* broke the news globally about the MDMA Phase 3 clinical trial and was highlighted by Michael Pollan, Ezra Klein, and Tim Ferriss, among other thought leaders. Nuwer holds master's degrees in applied ecology and in science journalism. Her first book, *Poached: Inside the Dark World of Wildlife Trafficking*, took her to a dozen countries to investigate the multibillion-dollar illegal wildlife trade. She lives in Brooklyn.